Shooting Up

Shooting Up

A Short History of Drugs and War

ŁUKASZ KAMIEŃSKI

OXFORD
UNIVERSITY PRESS

OXFORD
UNIVERSITY PRESS

Oxford University Press is a department of the University of Oxford. It furthers
the University's objective of excellence in research, scholarship, and education
by publishing worldwide. Oxford is a registered trade mark of Oxford University
Press in the UK and certain other countries.

Published in the United States of America by Oxford University Press
198 Madison Avenue, New York, NY 10016, United States of America.

Library of Congress Cataloging-in-Publication Data
Names: Kamieński, Łukasz.
Title: Shooting up: a short history of drugs and war / Kamieński, Łukasz.
Description: New York, NY : Oxford University Press, [2016] | Includes
bibliographical references and index.
Identifiers: LCCN 2015040597 | ISBN 978–0–19–026347–8 (hardcover)
Subjects: LCSH: Medicine, Military—History—Miscellanea. | Soldiers—Drug
use—History. | Drug utilization—History. | Drug abuse—History. | Military art and science—
Miscellanea. | Military history—Miscellanea.
Classification: LCC RC971 .K34 2016 | DDC 616.9/8023—dc23
LC record available at http://lccn.loc.gov/2015040597

3 5 7 9 8 6 4 2
Printed by Sheridan, USA

The book was originally published in 2012 in Polish by Jagiellonian University Press.
This is an edited version translated by Łukasz Kamieński (pp. xv–157, 243–262), Michelle Atallah
(pp. 58–227), and Maciej Czuchra (pp. 227–314).

Of all of civilization's occupational categories, that of
soldier may be the most conducive to regular drug use.
—D. T. Courtwright, *Forces of Habit: Drugs
and the Making of the Modern World*, 2001

The happy warriors. They all sounded as if they were a
little drunk. And they were, though it was on the excitement of the event rather than on alcohol.
—P. Caputo, *A Rumor of War*, 1996

CONTENTS

DETAILED CONTENTS

LIST OF TABLES

PREFACE

Who will ever relate the whole history of narcotica?—It is almost
the history of "culture" of our so-called higher culture.
—Friedrich Nietzsche, *The Gay Science*

Carl von Clausewitz, the greatest and most influential Western thinker on war, reminds us that chance is "the very last thing that war lacks. No other human activity is so continuously or universally bound up with chance."[1] I would argue that academic research is another human activity that is often closely bound up with chance; this study is a product of it. The idea for the book was born unexpectedly as a "side effect" of my other research on the emerging and future applications of biotechnologies designed for military enhancement (namely psychopharmacology, neuroscience, and genetic engineering). Working on the topic of the Pentagon's search for a "magic bullet" drug that could revolutionize soldiers' performance and mood, I was quick to discover that no thorough examination of the history of drugs in combat had yet been written. The same is true even of alcohol, the oldest and most popular military intoxicant. Thus I hope my book will provide some context of the present-day and potential future applications of psychopharmacology in warfare. For as the great eighteenth-century Neapolitan philosopher Giambattista Vico teaches us, only by studying history can we better understand the practices, events, and ideas that shape our own times. What Vico propounded was that we need to go back to the origins of contemporary phenomena or processes should we wish to grasp them.

What is this book about? When one thinks of the two words "drugs" and "war," one almost automatically links them into the "war on drugs," that is, the coordinated efforts to limit the production, smuggling, trade, and consumption of illegal substances both at home and abroad. This volume, however, is not a study about the war on drugs but an attempt to understand the roles that drugs have played in warfare. It is about warriors and soldiers, governments, armed forces, and militant groups of various types making the most of intoxicants. It is a social, cultural, and political history of psychoactive substances on the battlefield.

It is often said that human history is a history of war. This is certainly an overstatement, yet it is true that one of the features of our history is the enormity of the wars humans have fought. I would contend that one of its other vital characteristics is intoxication. Plentiful mind-altering substances have been used in various ways by nearly all peoples through the centuries. Producing a comprehensive history of drugs in warfare is probably infeasible, for such a work probably cannot be written due to the historical and geographical scope of the phenomenon. Mine, of course, is but one of the possible stories, a narrative written with the awareness that there are many other paths that could have been followed.

What I am interested in are potent and rather "controversial" substances, most of which, with the exception of alcohol, are today subject to tight state and international control regimes. I therefore do not focus on traditional and omnipresent psychoactive substances such as nicotine/tobacco and caffeine. Their use by servicemen is still allowed and does not trigger debates as does, for example, amphetamines.

What do pharmacology and war have in common? The etymology of "pharmacology" is usually traced back to the Greek *phármakon*, which means "medicament." But it is important to bear in mind that in ancient Greece the word *pharmākos* referred to a human scapegoat (usually a slave, criminal, or someone disabled or considered ugly) used in state rituals—in public rites of cleansing and in ceremonies aimed at ensuring the well-being and good fortune of a community. The *pharmākos* was manhandled, bitten, driven out, and sometimes stoned to death. So, as the Hungarian-American psychiatrist Thomas Szasz argued, the root of modern "pharmacology" is not "drug" or "medicine" but "scapegoat." When the practice of human sacrifice was abandoned in Greece around the sixth century BC, the word *pharmākos* was transformed into *pharmakeus* and *phármakon*, which came to mean, among other things, a medicine, poison, and panacea.[2] But what of warriors and soldiers? They both sacrifice themselves for their community and are concurrently sacrificed by their society to provide it with, above all, security (i.e., defense and survival) and often also with prosperity and felicity (i.e., expansion, development, and welfare). Of course, they are not scapegoats, but they are ready for sacrifice, even the supreme one—to die in defense of their society and its values. Countless soldiers have given their lives in combat, and war should be seen for what it is: an ultimate "collective ritual." Even so, throughout the centuries individual warriors and entire armies have been enhanced pharmacologically in diverse and remarkable ways. And *phármakon* has been used not only to raise their spirits but also to increase the willingness to self-sacrifice for others. Indeed, as the German physiologist Georg Friedrich Nicolai remarked in his book *The Biology of War* (1918), what makes war exceptional and intoxicating is soldiers' "boundless capacity for self-sacrifice."[3] Their readiness to die for the well-being of their fellow men or for an idea is incompatible with the natural and biological instinct of self-preservation. The Greek hoplites were the first representatives of Western civilization "to overcome the natural human dread" because, writes John Keegan, "fighting face-to-face with death-dealing weapons defies nature."[4] Equally paradoxical and violating of the very "life instinct" is the human pursuit of intoxication motivated not by medical need but by a desire for pleasure and reward. Drugs tend to be poisonous and overdosing on them may be fatal. David Courtwright puts it particularly well:

> Psychoactive plant alkaloids evolved as a defense mechanism against herbivores. Insects and animals who eat them become dizzy and disoriented, or experience hallucinations.... In evolutionary terms, *accidental* intoxication may be valuable: it warns an organism not to go near the plant again. *Seeking* intoxication, let alone profiting from it, is paradoxical. It seemingly defies the logic of natural selection.[5]

So, both intoxication and participation in combat can be seen, to an extent, as inimical to the survival of an individual.

My focus has been, in the first place, on the history of drugs "prescribed" to soldiers by their authorities, not only for medicinal purposes but also most crucially to boost them before and throughout battle and to help them to relax afterward. Uppers, such as alcohol (in small amounts), cocaine, and amphetamines, have been used to improve the fighting efficiency of troops and produce better warriors. By accelerating the tempo of metabolic processes, stimulants increase physical strength—they build stamina, provide energy, eliminate the need to sleep, combat fatigue, and reinforce the fighting spirit. They also enhance courage, improve determination, and fuel aggression. They can, in essence, not only maintain but also, by multiplying human abilities and power, expand the combat performance of the individual soldier. By contrast downers, such as alcohol (in large amounts), opium, opiates, marijuana, and barbiturates, have been used to lessen combat stress and prevent or mitigate war trauma, which ultimately could render soldiers ineffective. Pharmacology, then, has been employed as a means of fighting the most dangerous enemy of combatants, which is to say their shattered nerves.

But despite the fact that the main subject of my research has initially been the official and legitimate administration of psychoactive substances, I could not overlook their unofficial, usually illicit, use by combatants. For centuries, warriors have "self-prescribed" various mind-altering agents, be it uppers, downers, or hallucinogens. Soldiers have usually taken them recreationally to alleviate acute combat stress and mitigate the fear of battle, but also to relieve boredom as well as enhance their performance and thereby increase their chances of survival. As long as self-intoxication did not reduce fighting efficiency and dampen the spirits of the troops, commanders have often turned a blind eye.

In an attempt to present a broader picture of militaries' use of drugs, I will also sketch the efforts made to turn them into tools of war. Intoxicants have, in fact, been employed to undermine the combat readiness and morale of the enemy forces, and to temporarily paralyze its civilian population. The pursuit of nonlethal psychochemical weapons, which greatly intensified during the Cold War, has a long history rooted in the experiments with "magic plants" carried out by shamans. Simultaneously, with the quest for psychoactive weapons, research has been conducted on the pharmacological countermeasures that would allow an effective defense against psychedelic attack. At times intoxicants were also used as a means of subversion since turning portions of the enemy's society into addicts might cause its social tissue to fray.

To sum up, this book is an effort to study three aspects of the "highs" of war:

1. drugs "prescribed" to military personnel and issued by the authorities,
2. drugs "self-prescribed" by combatants, and
3. drugs used as a tool of war—both as feasible psychochemical weapons and as an instrument of subversion.

These three areas do not, however, exhaust the topic as states and armed non-state groups have benefited from drug production and trade to finance their activities, including war-making. Because sometimes this aspect sheds additional light on the main three forms of the military use of intoxicants, and may even condition them, I shall highlight it too, yet mostly as a background issue.

Concepts and Definitions: Drugs and Addiction

When we think about drugs, we instantly have in mind such substances as amphetamine, heroin, cocaine, or marijuana. Drugs are natural or synthetic mind-altering substances that affect the central nervous system. Depending on the particular form of the altered state of consciousness that they bring about, three types of psychoactive substances can be identified:

1. stimulants, which enhance the activity of the nervous system and produce psychical and/or physical arousal (i.e., amphetamines and cocaine);
2. depressants or hypnotics, which retard the activity of the nervous system and have relaxing, tranquilizing, somniferous, or euphoric effects (i.e., alcohol, barbiturates, opium, and opiates); and
3. hallucinogens, which disturb the activity of the nervous system and substantially alter the perception of reality (i.e., atropine, cannabis, mescaline, scopolamine, LSD, and MDMA, commonly known as ecstasy).

Interestingly, there are some substances that, depending on the dose, can have either a stimulating or depressing effect. For example, depressants such as alcohol and opium in small dosages can serve as a mild stimulant.

Drugs have strong habit-forming properties, and their abuse can cause intrinsically harmful physical, psychical, and social effects; therefore, in most countries today, they are illegal and strictly controlled substances with very limited medical applications. The word "addiction" derives from *addictus*— a citizen of ancient Rome who, being unable to repay his debts, was deprived of freedom by the courts and delivered into slavery under his creditor.[6] Intoxicants do indeed have a similar effect; they enslave with their addictive properties.

The concept of a drug is sociopolitical to a degree because it is continually being historically, socially, and politically constructed, deconstructed, reconstructed, and reinterpreted. The deliberate and systematic state policy of prohibiting and penalizing psychoactive substances dates back to the first decades of the twentieth century and in particular to the introduction of early national antidrug regulations (in 1914 in the United States and in 1916 in the United Kingdom) and to the adoption of international agreements (such as the League of Nations International Opium Convention of 1912). Depending on a political, social, and cultural context a substance, which may for ages has been legal and socially legitimized, can suddenly become controlled and illegal except for limited therapeutic applications. The process of the regulation and penalization of some substances has raised a storm of controversies, making the notion of "drugs" highly disputable. Consider, for example, the fact that alcohol is still legal despite its powerful mind-altering properties and fairly strong habit-forming potential. In 1958 Maurice Seevers published his addiction liability ratings for different substances. He assigned points for the ability of each one to produce tolerance, physical and emotional dependence, physical deterioration, and antisocial behavior. The highest score of twenty-one points was for alcohol; barbiturates got eighteen points, heroin seventeen, cocaine fourteen, and marijuana only eight.[7] Why were opium and morphine legal in the United States until 1914 and marijuana until 1937? What makes a

particular substance defined as controlled or illegal is by and large the result of
a political decision and pharmacological knowledge as well as social forces and
mental changes. The essence of this conditioning and sociopolitical discretion
in categorizing and banning intoxicants was particularly well captured by
Thomas Szasz.[8] As one of the most prominent figures in the "antipsychiatry"
movement (which saw many psychiatric treatments as ultimately more harmful than helpful and regarded psychiatry in general as a means of oppression),
he strongly criticized the idea of "mental illness," which he saw as an instrument of the social repression of nonconformists. But Szasz is also well-known
for his full cry against the notions of "addiction" and "narcotism." He enjoyed
provoking his readers, as in this fine passage:

> Formerly, opium was a panacea; now it is the cause and symptom
> of countless maladies, medical and social, the world over. Formerly,
> masturbation was the cause and symptom of mental illness; now it is
> the cure for social inhibition and the practice ground for training in
> heterosexual athleticism . . . the danger of masturbation disappeared
> when we ceased to believe in it: we then ceased to attribute danger to
> the practice and to its practitioners; and ceased to call it "self-abuse."[9]

Like mental illness, addiction is socially and politically constructed, so the
criminalization and penalization of drug use, argued Szasz, aims to target
those nonconformists who fell victim to "ritual persecution."[10] The twin
notions of "addiction" and "drugs" should always be considered and examined
in the interpretative context of the social judgments and values in a particular
period in history. The anthropological approach is, therefore, right in emphasizing the sociocultural frameworks within which an individual or a group
takes a drug and experiences its effects. For we must acknowledge that culture
has affected habits of intoxication, but also that intoxicants have concurrently
inspired a variety of distinct social practices. Hence psychoactive substances
take on an appropriate meaning only in a specific social, cultural, and historical context. Jonathan Shay, writing on the *Iliad* and Homeric warriors drowning their sorrows in wine, used the nice phrase "cultural pharmacology,"
which I find particularly compelling and apt.[11] Indeed, the social application
of pharmacology needs to be understood only through the prism of culture.
The meaning assigned to intoxicants is liquid, being culturally and historically
changeable. The same substance can in one context be called an "illegal drug"
while in another it may serve as a medicine or divine plant. Jacques Derrida
neatly captured the ambiguity inherent in defining and categorizing intoxicants; we must conclude, he writes, "that the concept of drugs is not a scientific
concept, but is rather instituted on the basis of moral or political evaluations: it

carries in itself both norm and prohibition, allowing no possibility of description or certification—it is a decree, a buzzword."[12] It is a decree in a sense of banning certain psychoactive compounds that were previously considered legal and their use was perceived to be normal, often popular, and sometimes even fashionable. In other words, before some substances have been classified as "drugs" and put under state control, they were culturally accepted and commonly used. They constituted an essential and often intrinsic part of a social landscape and were by no means regarded as evil or dangerous. It is important to recognize that it was the culturally sanctioned use of intoxicants that did not allow their abuse to develop into a social problem. The grand passion of governments and societies for controlling various walks of human life has had a very negative effect on the individual's capacity for self-restraint and processes of self-regulation, the most effective and powerful mechanism for repressing the natural human drive for pleasure. It was, after all, the Dutch philosopher Baruch Spinoza who warned that all efforts to restrain personal behavior by force or legal regulation is more likely to arouse vices and dissoluteness than to reform them.[13]

From the very beginning of human history, intoxication has been inherent to cultural life, especially religious, magical, and ritualistic practices. Hence it is for good reason that ecstasy plays a vitally important role in Nietzsche's interpretation of art, myth, religion, politics, and the very concept of the Dionysian. Dionysius was the orgiastic god of wine, pleasure, festivity, ecstatic frenzy, and intoxication. In *The Birth of Tragedy* Nietzsche claims that "the essence of the *Dionysiac* is best conveyed by the analogy of *intoxication*." "The Dionysiac stirrings," Nietzsche goes on to write, that "cause subjectivity to vanish to the point of complete self-forgetting," are awakened "under the influence of narcotic drink, of which all human beings and peoples who are close to the origin of things speak in their hymns."[14] In his famous book *Phantastica* (1931), an impressive review of the use of miscellaneous mind-altering plants, Louis Lewin came to the conclusion that it was the discovery and understanding of the properties of psychoactive substances and the practical application of this knowledge that marked the origins of culture in its primordial stage. He argued that

if it can be taken as a symptom of civilization when men's desires, hitherto exclusively confined to the bare necessities of life, pass beyond these limits, and the individual, no longer satisfied with the crude sustenance afforded by or wrested from nature, finds and delights in stimulants which mainly affect the central nervous system, then a suitable background for such physical cravings must form part of the human constitution.[15]

Aldous Huxley, in similar vein, claimed that

> the urge to escape, the longing to transcend themselves if only for a
> few minutes, is and always has been one of the principal appetites of
> the soul. Art and religion, carnivals and saturnalia, dancing and lis-
> tening to oratory—all these have served, in H. G. Wells's phrase, as
> Doors in the Wall.[16]

Huxley himself experimented with altered states of consciousness induced by
drugs, mostly hallucinogens. Describing his personal experiences with mescaline and psilocybin, he coined the famous phrase "the doors of perception."[17]
Andrew Weil echoed both Lewin and Huxley when in his book *The Natural
Mind* (1972) he contended that the search for "altered and higher states of
consciousness" is a basic human desire that has accompanied the history of
mankind from its very dawn.[18] There is plenty of evidence for this. Take children's love of vertigo-inducing play on roundabouts; or religious people who
in the course of meditation often fall into a trance, losing touch with reality; or
ecstasy, the journey to supernatural worlds, as an essential part of shamanism.
Weil has challenged the commonly held assumptions that the chemical altera-
tion of consciousness is an unwelcome, dangerous, and evil practice. The overwhelming desire to cut loose from harsh, dark, and grim reality is something
humans are fundamentally eager to do. This is one of the things that makes us
human. And intoxication has been one of the important ways of achieving this
goal. In the words of the French artist Jean Cocteau, "Everything one does in
life, even love, occurs in an express train racing toward death. To smoke opium
is to get out of the train while it is still moving. It is to concern oneself with
something other than life or death."[19] In this Cocteau came particularly close
to the truth.

    Intoxication, in its various forms, has thus been one of the distinctive fea-
tures of human beings and an important part of human history. In an article
on Nietzsche, Alphonso Lingis writes of the existential dimension of intoxication, insisting, "[a] life without dreams and without intoxication is a life sick,
rancorous, and without value. One lives for dreams and for festive intoxication."[20] In his quest for the experience of dazedness, numbness, hallucination,
and stimulation *homo ludens* (man the player) experimented with a variety of
plants and substances and in due course transformed himself into *homo narcoticus*. For centuries, psychoactive substances accompanied religious ceremonies and rituals of spiritual enlightenment. Consumed in groups they were
crucial socialization agents that fostered the creation of social bonds and reinforced cohesion. They enabled embedding individuals in social structures (for
example during diverse rites of passage), helped in times of severe hardship

and strain, and allowed people either to relax or boost themselves. In fact, there has been only one society that did not obtain drugs: the Inuit, the indigenous people inhabiting the Arctic regions. This was because of the environment they lived in, which offered no opportunity to grow any psychoactive plant.[21] In the words of Stuart Walton, which I find sum everything up, it is utterly "impractical to separate the efflorescence of Western culture from the intoxication practices in which it is partly rooted, either in classical antiquity or in the raves of today."[22]

As for the military, there are at least two main reasons why I am careful in denouncing the use of psychoactive substances by combatants. First, historically speaking, there was nothing inappropriate about the consumption of intoxicants, most of which could have been easily and legally obtained until the 1930s and 1950s. The substances which today are prohibited and made targets in the global war on drugs, in the past were in common if not everyday use. The "remedies" once dispensed liberally by many armed forces and seen as an effective cure for countless diseases and afflictions, today fall into the category of harmful, habit-forming, and controlled drugs. Formerly the use of mind-altering agents was closely bound to certain culturally defined goals—be they religious, mystical, initiation, or medical—framed within a strong social sanction that prevented their abuse. There were a few factors that contributed to the rise of the modern problem of substance addiction, but the most important were the spread of "narcotic hedonism" (i.e., recreational use intended to promote the pleasure, happiness, or euphoria), the development of policies of regulation and prohibition, and the production and design of more and more powerful synthetic psychoactive compounds. Taking all the above mentioned into consideration, we should not explain, judge, nor condemn the historical practices of drug use by the military through the lens of present-day Western standards. We must not cast the prejudices and generalizations prevalent in today's societies back into the life and customs of previous generations. In essence, the consumption of psychoactive substances by the military has reflected a general social practice of the use of intoxicants, with one exception: it has been based on an utterly practical rationale. It has not only been pragmatic rather than hedonistic but also has usually, though not always, been kept under tight control. Second, because war is an exceptionally dramatic process, many activities, forms of conduct, and customs that would be considered unacceptable, if not immoral, in the world of civilians are fairly normal in military life. The reality of combat and the reality of everyday civilian life are strikingly different. These are two radically distinct worlds. Many of the rules, norms, contentions, and constraints that preserve and keep every society in order and balance do not apply in war. Instead, different rules govern. Not only is war the most extreme, but also the most existential human experience.

Homo furens (a fighting man) finds himself in a life-and-death situation. The experience of combat has a deep personal meaning to which noncombatants can never get close, let alone truly understand. Fighting affects a soldier's body and even more deeply his psyche. It is therefore important to recognize that it has been in the extreme and gruesome conditions of the battlefield that soldiers have been prescribed and have self-prescribed intoxicants of various kinds. Thus often was *homo narcoticus* yet another face of *homo furens*.

I will not conceal my point of view: I am not an advocate of "pharmacological Calvinism" in the military realm. Critics may thus say that I justify the use of psychoactive substances in war, both as a group activity (in armed forces) and as individual behavior (among soldiers). But wouldn't it actually be astonishing if the military had *not* reached for pharmacological support?

The Argument

I contend that grasping the scale of the use of intoxicants by states, armies, nonstate armed groups, and combatants is crucial to the study of military history. For it may change the way we analyze, interpret, and understand war. It is highly problematic to explain the decisions taken under the influence of intoxicants purely in terms of a rational choice approach because drugs are psychoactive chemicals. In this respect we should, if anything, rather talk of "pharmacologically boosted" or "smashed" rationality. Psychiatrists agree that even if the effects of a given mind-expanding substance are well known, we cannot fully predict human reactions. Everything depends on the dose, a drug's degree of purity, the circumstances of its intake, the route of administration, and a person's psycho-emotional condition at the time, as well as specific personal psychophysiological characteristics, such as individual brain anatomy. Ninety-five percent of people will have a textbook response to a drug, but 5 percent might experience an unanticipated bodily reaction.

Both the military use of intoxicants and their application as tools of war have always been surrounded by taboos, hence inevitably studies in military history rarely mention the roles of psychoactive compounds in armed conflicts. It is largely an untold story. Therefore, it is also important to retrace and tell this story to see where we find ourselves in the early twenty-first century. To an extent warfare has always been "pharmacological." Once we realize that chemical doping has for centuries sustained soldiers in the field, we will be able to better understand both the existential and instrumental dimensions of war. Also, we might gain a new perspective on the applications of psychopharmacology in contemporary and future wars. The process of the "pharmacologization of war," which is on the rise in the West and particularly in the United

States, is not as novel as it might seem at first sight. Is it, then, yet another step in the general evolution of war? Even if it is merely a logical continuation of the centuries-long dynamic convergence of drugs and war, its present-day intensification and acceleration may well bring an "ironic grimace" to the changing face of war. Will it trigger a major transformation in its character too? Before attempting to provide the answers we ought to investigate the past first. This book can be then read as a historical background to the study of the present-day warfare.

The Approach

My approach in studying the military history of drugs can be summed up in four points.

First, my perspective derives from an "interpretivist" epistemology. Humanistic interpretation implies that in the debate between "understanding" and "explaining" what is favored is understanding. Of course, facts never speak for themselves because they require interpretation. Yet one must be careful here, for both individual and group behavior can be judged, but according to the moral norms that prevailed at the time in which the event or phenomenon under scrutiny occurred. Such a standing is crucial for the social history of intoxication, especially in war, because, as we know, the social meaning and understanding of drugs and their legal status have profoundly changed over time. Formerly legal, widely available, and commonly consumed even by children (e.g., opium), today they are forbidden, stigmatized, considered harmful, and deemed antisocial. Formerly taken for clearly defined social and cultural purposes (ritual, mystic, religious, etc.), today they are mostly used recreationally. Formerly the consumption of opium, morphine, heroin, cocaine, and amphetamines was pervasive; today they are criminalized except in limited therapeutic use. Put differently, what is needed for the study of "drugs in warfare" is the wider historical, social, cultural, and political context.

Second, I am, to a degree, influenced by the ideas of social constructivism, which build on Vico's view of knowledge. Social constructivism offers a valuable blueprint for interdisciplinary research in historical humanities. A constructivist worldview assumes that the aim of research is to understand social facts, which are never given or constant but instead are socially, culturally, and historically constructed. Individuals and groups might assign multiple meanings to social phenomena. These meanings are not imprinted but "negotiated" through historical and cultural norms, human interactions, and techno-scientific development. Drugs and addiction are such socially, culturally, and

historically constructed "social facts," as are the various myths and stereotypes that surround them. Therefore, studying soldiers' memoirs, recollections, and interpretations is absolutely crucial for discovering the meanings
they assigned to intoxication. Instead of exploring the macro-level of analysis
(that of diplomacy and strategy), we need to descend down to the meso-level
(operations and tactics) and, most importantly, to the micro-level of the individual soldier and his unit. In many instances a research method derived from
the humanistic sociology developed by a Polish sociologist Florian Znaniecki
proves highly useful. His methodological principle of the "humanistic coeffi-
cient" attached the most importance to the perception of the analyzed experience by the participants of the research project.[23] Znaniecki, above all, insisted
that because all social facts are created by social actors, they can only be understood and explained from their own perspective. So, if I am allowed to employ
this approach, I would sometimes take an individual's point of view and present reflections and recollections of the individual serviceman.

Third, although Clausewitz's notion of war as a political activity is commonly taken for granted, I study warfare also as an essentially social and
cultural phenomenon, as do John Keegan, Chris Hables Gray, Christopher
Coker, John Jandora, Patrick Porter, and others.[24] Armed forces are not only
public institutions of the state but also cultural constructs that reflect specific
social settings and culture, with their distinctive values, norms, customs, and
practices at any given time. This view was expressed already by Aristotle in
his epitaph to Lycurgus's system: "The essential object of any social system
must be to organize the military institution like all the others."[25] If war is the
Clausewitzian continuation of politics, then the military is the continuation of
society and its culture. Doubtless Clausewitz would agree.

Fourth, my perspective has been profoundly shaped by a remark by Field-
Marshal Lord Wavell. In his letter to Sir Basil Liddell Hart he wrote:

> If I had time and anything like your ability to study war, I think
> I should concentrate almost entirely on the "actualities of war"—the
> effects of tiredness, hunger, fear, lack of sleep, weather . . . The princi-
> ples of strategy and tactics, and the logistics of war are really absurdly
> simple: it is the actualities that make war so complicated and so dif-
> ficult, and are usually so neglected by historians.[26]

Interestingly enough, the effects of drugs on war may neutralize Wavell's
"effects of tiredness, hunger, fear, lack of sleep, weather." They not only alter
consciousness but, by befuddling the participants, make those hard and troublesome actualities a little less real and thereby more tolerable.

Research Questions

During my journey through the history of the synergy between drugs and war I was guided by a number of questions, in particular:

1. How historically and geographically universal has been the authorized intoxication of combatants?
2. What have been the broader social, cultural, political, and medical contexts of drug consumption by armed services?
3. What specific aims have militaries wanted to achieve by "drugging" their troops?
4. How effective have particular substances been in the war effort?
5. To what extent have the "prescribed" and "self-prescribed" use of drugs shaped soldiering?
6. What have been the side-effects of the military use of intoxicants?
7. What are the ethical issues surrounding drugs in combat?
8. To what extent should the knowledge of the massive consumption of drugs by a given military cause us to reinterpret our understanding of a particular war or campaign?

The Structure of This Book

From ancient times onward, the history of drugs and the history of war have not developed independently. These have been not parallel but rather intertwined stories, as drugs and warfare have coevolved. We shall see how, on many occasions, they have converged in crucial and decisive ways. Because I am telling the history of this synergistic relationship, the structure of the book is chronological. My case studies, I hope, illustrate the most important and vivid instances in which the two processes have come together.

The book is divided into three parts. The first covers history from the pre-modern period to the end of the Second World War, the second explores the Cold War era, while the third reviews contemporary times. The prologue not only sets the framework underpinning this study by exploring the causes and origins of the use of drugs in war but also attempts to provide a brief history of soldiers' favorite intoxicant, namely alcohol.

Part one begins with antiquity and examines the consumption of opium by the ancient Greek warriors; the legend of the hashish-eating Assassins; the use made of a psychoactive alkaloid contained in the *Amanita muscaria* mushrooms by both the Siberian tribes and Scandinavian berserkers; and the traditional use of coca leaves in the Andean regions of South America. The following chapters explore the soldiers of Napoleon Bonaparte seduced by hashish during the famous French campaign in the Orient; the Opium Wars and the employment of opium by Indian and Chinese warriors; the excessive use of opium and morphine in the American Civil War; the practices of intoxication developed by the "savage" and fearless warriors with whom the Western armies engaged during the colonial wars; the experiments conducted by the Europeans with coca leaves; the role of cocaine in the First World War; and finally, the wholesale use of methamphetamine and amphetamine in the Second World War.

Part two turns to the Cold War period and consists of four chapters. In the first three I sketch the major armed conflicts of the Cold War era, namely the Korean War, the Vietnam War, and the Afghan War. In the last chapter I discuss the experiments with psychoactive agents conducted on humans by the American armed forces with the aim of producing nonlethal chemical weapons and the truth serum.

Part three, which is divided into three chapters, turns to contemporary practices, trends, and phenomena. On the one hand, I explore the use of drugs by irregular armed groups: insurgents, terrorists, drug cartels, narco-gangs, and child soldiers in particular. On the other hand, I look at both the authorized and illicit use of psychoactive substances by the American military.

Finally, in the epilogue I invite the reader to look at war as a great metaphor for a potent, habit-forming drug.

I have to admit that my long journey through the meanders of the twin history of war and drugs, of drugs and war—frequently to rarely visited nooks and crannies—has been a fascinating and inspiring intellectual adventure. Still, this epistemologically intriguing expedition into the unknown proved a real challenge full of unforeseen hurdles. In her book, *Writing on Drugs*, Sadie Plant particularly well captured the nature of the problems I had to tackle while working on this book:

> To write on drugs is to plunge into a world where nothing is as simple or as stable as it seems. Everything about it shimmers and mutates as you try to hold its gaze. Facts and figures dance around each other; lines of enquiry scatter like expensive dust. The reasons for the laws and the motives for the wars, the nature of the pleasures and the trouble drugs can cause, the tangled webs of chemicals, the plants, the brains, machines: ambiguity surrounds them all. Drugs shape the laws and write the very rules they break, they scramble all the codes and raise the stakes of desire and necessity, euphoria and pain, normality, perversion, truth and artifice again.[27]

ACKNOWLEDGMENTS

This is an edited version of my book originally published in Polish in 2014. My particular thanks are due to Professors Andrzej Mania, Bogdan Szlachta, and Adam Walaszek from my home institution Jagiellonian University in Krakow for providing funds and support toward translation and proofreading of the manuscript. The book was translated by Michelle Atallah, Maciej Czuchra, and myself. I greatly benefited from the editorial help of Professor Garry Robson from the Jagiellonian University. I would particularly like to acknowledge the scholarly support of my mentor, Professor Christopher Coker at LSE, who strongly forced the idea of making my research on drugs and warfare available in English. A special thank you to Mikko Ylikangas for providing me with detailed information on the use of psychoactive substances in Finland based on his seminal book, unfortunately available only in Finnish, on drugs in Finland from 1800–1950. Mikko read the chapter on the Finns and the Second World War and I benefited greatly from his comments and help. My thanks also go to Norman Ohler, the author of *Der totale Rausch* (2015), the book on the use of drugs by the Nazis, who shared with me the results of his research. I would also like to thank Professor Jonathan Moreno at the University of Pennsylvania, whose works on human experimentation significantly inspired some of my fragments on the Cold War era, for reading the manuscript, providing valuable feedback, and being exceptionally supportive. In closing, I thank the Oxford University Press editors and three anonymous reviewers for their constructive comments and criticism which helped me improve the manuscript, as well as Michael Dwyer at Hurst Publishers for his faith in this project.

Prologue

Pharmacologically Enhanced Militaries

The virtue of the soldiers is worth more than a multitude.
—Niccolo Machiavelli, *The Art of War*

Margaret Mead, Barbara Ehrenreich, David Grossman, and many other authors have argued that killing is not in human nature and that war is not a biological necessity.[1] For centuries, then, societies and states have tried to bring out in their warriors the predator's instinct, the essential trait for the proper conduct of war. This has been achieved through harsh, even brutal, training designed to encourage and trigger aggression, as well as through a range of methods of psychological conditioning aimed at "programming" violence against a dehumanized enemy and "deprogramming" reflection, emotions, and guilt. Militaries have also experimented with various psychoactive plants containing powerful alkaloids, which can boost, hypnotize, or numb soldiers physically and emotionally. This "pharmacological construction" of the great warrior was not of course natural; but, as we are encouraged to believe, neither is the systematic and intentional killing of other members of the same species. As Barbara Ehrenreich reminds us,

> Almost any drug or intoxicant has served, in one setting or another, to facilitate the transformation of man into warrior. Yanomam Indians of the Amazon ingest a hallucinogen before battle; the ancient Scythians smoked hemp, while a neighboring tribe drank something called "hauma," which is believed to have induced a frenzy of aggression. So if there is a destructive instinct that impels men to war, it is a weak one, and often requires a great deal of help.[2]

The aforementioned Yanomamos, the indigenous people who lived in the Orinoco basin on the border between the today's Venezuela and Brazil, fought ritual chest-pounding duels with neighbors at intervillage feasts. The duels were "always conducted between members of different villages and arose over accusations of cowardice or in response to excessive demands for trade goods, food, or women."[3] The duelers, writes Keegan, "took hallucinogenic drugs to foster a fighting mood."[4] The Otomac Indians were another tribal people from the Orinoco basin whose warriors regularly got intoxicated before battle. In his book, *El Orinoco Ilustrado y defendido* (*The Orinoco Illustrated and Defended*, 1731), the Spanish Jesuit priest Joseph Gumilla tells his readers that the Otomacs would "get fighting mad with yupa, wound themselves, and, full of blood and fury, go out to fight like raging tigers."[5] Yupa was a powdered snuff extract from the seeds of the *Piptadenia peregrina*, a tree containing hallucinogenic alkaloids. Among the Otomacs, yupa-induced intoxication played an important ritualistic, shamanic, and therapeutic role, and also one in combat.

Perhaps the practice of getting high by fighting men is as old as war itself. Warriors have always dreamt of gaining superhuman abilities that would bring them estimable victory, particularly when meeting their enemy in a decisive clash. This desire, though varying in shape and intensity, has been integral to the existential dimension of war from premodern times onward. The need to test oneself, one's courage and manhood, in the heat of battle has been common to most dedicated warriors. And the anxiety over one's wish to survive the supreme test of battle, the true test of life, takes on three basic forms.

First, soldiers are afraid of the fear of battle. In the Polish film *Demons of War by Goya* (1998), which tells the story of a Polish contingent in the NATO's Stabilization Force (SFOR) operation in Bosnia, a serviceman explains to his companion: "My father will kill me, if he learns that I was frightened." And his fellow replies to him: "We are all very scared, but no one talks about it." Soldiers are far more often terrified that fear may paralyze them, or at least impair their performance, than they are of the actual fighting. For what is profoundly important is what constitutes the ideal of a fearless warrior: to be tough and preserve one's honor. John Ellis, writing on the Second World War, remarked that "the fear of showing fear was often more powerful than the fear of death itself, and, in a deeper sense, echoes Montaigne's assertion that: 'The thing in the world I am most afraid of is fear.'"[6] Indeed, for there is always a fundamental uncertainty about whether the individual soldier will succeed or fail, whether he will survive the final test of combat. A mistake or mishap may cost lives, or at best his own well-being and that of his fellow men. In military culture, fear has generally been seen as a sign of weakness, a stereotypically feminine trait, a discreditable emotion for a real man; in a word, as something disgraceful to a true warrior. Nonetheless, the fear of failure, death, wounding, suffering, and captivity—in short, an anxiety about grave danger—is a very typical human feeling, a strong emotion that has been biologically and evolutionarily engraved in our nature. It has nothing to do with cowardice. Overall, as Samuel Hynes puts it, soldiers "are simply frightened men."[7] The stress of battle can be so severe that it is an entirely different kind of feeling than the stress of everyday civilian life. Sometimes the emotions associated with combat are so overwhelming and the nerves so shattered that a tragedy occurs, such as the one described by Ernst Jünger in *Sturm* (1923), a short story based on his First World War experience, in which he mentions that "someone shot himself out of fear."[8] Those who have never gone through combat would not understand or experience the cocktail of emotions felt under deadly threat, emotions that can either boost or cripple. Cold calculation and conditioned performance (programmed through military training) can coexist with anxiety, panic, and a trembling of the body or, by contrast, with the stoicism that helps intensify and channel the entire energy of the body. Fighting might be accompanied by either fright or battle frenzy. There is, in short, hardly any other human experience that is associated with an equally wide range of emotions. John Glenn Gray puts it remarkably well: "War compresses the greatest opposites into the smallest space and the shortest time."[9]

As Richard Lazarus claims, people can take on two general types of coping strategy when stressed. They can choose a direct response (problem focused), which aims at modifying, reducing, or eliminating the source of the stress by trying to change the nature of the stressful environment. Alternatively, they can seek to change their reactions to a stressor (emotion focused) to alleviate emotions in order to improve their well-being. In the case of the latter, humans often resort to alcohol and drugs as intoxicants create the impression that problems are less serious than they are in reality.[10] Soldiers must work out their own ways of easing the fear of fear, for they should later be able, to quote a character in Ernst Jünger's novel *Storm of Steel*, to recall what they did: "As we advanced, we were in the grip of a berserk rage. The overwhelming desire to kill lent wings to my stride. Rage squeezed bitter tears from my eyes."[11] Armed forces, as particular social institutions, have developed diverse and culturally rooted means of mustering courage, fostering a fighting mood, and alleviating stress and fear. The use of intoxicants, both stimulants and depressants, has been one such method, and remarkably widespread at that. These were initially magic plants, later pharmacological derivatives, and ultimately synthetic drugs.

Second, a true warrior wants to perform to the best of his ability—wishes to escape from normality and go against the grain. He craves, in a word, the transcendence of his natural limitations and weakness. Stated reductively, this desire can be summarized in the following ambitions: to maintain and improve physical strength and endurance, enhance cognitive abilities, improve mood, and transcend the limits of the human body. Or, to put it differently, to become a superwarrior, who performs almost like a mythological Greek hero and truly experiences his humanity. Still, meeting the physical hardship of fighting and the "inconveniences" of the battlefield is not easy; but here again stimulants offer an effective way out by boosting combat performance. This was not something that was either not thought of or even unthinkable, since through the centuries humans had fed their animals, particularly the draft ones, with psychoactive plants to make them work harder and more efficiently. For example, the Tibetans provided their horses and mules with large vessels of strong tea to improve their ability to work at high altitudes. Fighting cocks were given cannabis mixed with onions to make them more belligerent. And in India, as part of the process of domestication, elephants received opium balls as "rewards for logging tasks executed properly, much as a performing dolphin is rewarded with a fish."[12] Given this, why should warriors not be enhanced and enhance themselves with intoxicants? Stimulants, after all, offer a valuable ergogenic aid by improving physical endurance beyond the normal human capacity. Uppers not only invigorate the body but also strengthen self-confidence, foster bravery and, as Franz Rosenthal commented, albeit on hashish, increase "an inclination toward violent action and taking revenge on one's enemies, and a heightened effort to outdo others in generosity and nobility of character."[13]

Third, soldiers are stressed and anxious not only before battle. Strong and persistent tension during combat and afterward can have severe consequences. The first-hand traumatic experience of killing; seeing wounded, mutilated, and dead bodies; the loss of a close companion; chronic debilitating conditions; enduring stress, and so forth can cause combat trauma, which may develop into posttraumatic stress disorder (PTSD). It was only in 1980, in the aftermath of the Vietnam War and under pressure from mental health professionals and veterans' groups, that the severe nervous breakdown that can develop after experiencing a traumatic event was termed "PTSD" and described in detail by the American Psychiatric Association. Nevertheless, it is certainly as old as war itself. Traumatized behavior during wartime was recorded in ancient times: in ancient Chinese literature, and by Homer, Herodotus, Sophocles, Thucydides, and Xenophon among others. Previously, it was known under various names like "nostalgia," "irritable heart" or "Da Costa's syndrome" (during the American Civil War), "shell shock," "hysteria" or "neurasthenia" (during the First World War), "war neurosis," "battle fatigue," or simply "exhaustion" (during the Second World War and the Korean War).[14] The emergence of modern military psychiatry dates back to the Russo-Japanese War (1904–1905), when the Russians became the first military to establish an independent psychiatric service and to diagnose the mental casualties of war, correctly identifying that psychological and emotional disorders could result from the acute stress of combat. Every war, then, has its toll measured both in the number of soldiers killed and injured, and by the number of those who survive but suffer from invisible wounds. Psychological and emotional scars, which can be much more severe than physical wounds, have a long-term and acute impact on veterans' lives. What Jünger wrote about the soldier's body he could as well have written about his psyche: "under the heavy burden of lengthy war it is unable to bear up its fragile parts any longer."[15] Inevitably, a man breaks down. Many of the adverse effects of battle-related physical disabilities can be mitigated, for example through the use of prostheses. But, most regrettable of all, living casualties of war never quite recover from the ordeal and no "mental prosthesis" has yet been invented to treat the condition. Thus preventing nervous breakdowns has been quite high on commanders' priority lists. Traditional methods for avoiding combat stress reaction have been screening the candidates and selecting the most resistant to mental collapse, realistic and tough training, and the reduction of the duration of soldiers' exposure to fighting (unit rotation remains the most important measure for secondary prevention of combat PTSD).[16] Another means of coping with the emotional burden of war has been the use of drugs, depressants in particular.

My study on the convergent history of psychoactive substances and war begins with alcohol, the most common and, overall, the least controversial intoxicant, which throughout the centuries has regularly sustained soldiers in the field.

Alcohol

The army is a composite of the nation, so that the alcohol problem
there is a matter of the greatest social and governmental importance.
—Dr. Ivan V. Sazhin quoted in Patricia Herlihy, *Alcoholic
Empire: Vodka and Politics in Late Imperial Russia*

Through the ages alcohol has been an integral part of life in many societies. In numerous civilizations, with the major exception of Islam, it has been the intoxicant of choice, consumed in various walks of human activity—from spiritual and religious ceremonies to family gatherings, from everyday diet to medicinal use. It has also been the most popular drug employed by the military. Traditionally, armed forces used it for two general purposes. The first was to suppress uncomfortable and unwanted emotions and mitigate fear-avoidance behavior. The second was to enhance combat performance by reinforcing desirable qualities, abilities, and attitudes. For centuries alcohol has been so common before, during, and after battle that it has entered an almost symbiotic relationship with soldiering. In the course of history, a powerful cultural, social, and political legitimization of drinking has developed in armies, making alcohol truly inscribed into the landscape of warfare.

A moderate consumption of alcohol has long been believed to be highly desirable for raising the fighting spirit of the troops, improving morale, erasing or at least repressing traumatic memories, and helping to cope with the hardships of war. It has also been widely used to anesthetize the wounded, put to sleep the overwrought, warm up the cold, cool down the heated, and nurture the malnourished. Alcohol strengthens the willingness to take risks by increasing self-confidence, undermining prudence, and impairing judgment; therefore, moderately inebriated soldiers might be expected to do things that sober men would hardly risk doing. Feeling all-powerful and invincible, they could, for example, march "over barbed wire waving a bayonet at murderous machine guns."[17]

Group drinking strengthens bonds and builds trust between companions, which is essential for the smooth operation of a unit and the survival of its members. In short, by intensifying intimacy between soldiers alcohol fosters the establishment and maintenance of brotherhood among them. Thus it helps preserve the integrity of small combat units, such as a platoon, and contributes to primary group cohesion. So, if issued under control, alcohol can enhance combat performance; but uncontrolled excessive drinking affects fighting skills and undermines the morale of the troops, and sometimes even ruins an army.

To sum up, alcohol has played four major roles in war. The first one has been medical—for ages it has been employed to anesthetize the wounded, prevent infections (used in the dressing of wounds and as an antiseptic in surgery), and cure (alcohol was long believed to have potent and nearly universal healing properties). The second has been as a stimulant—a moderate dose of alcohol helps alleviate the stress of battle, raise courage, and bring self-confidence in combat. The third has been mental-therapeutic—to relax, induce sleep, numb emotionally, and offer reward for the hardships of battle. After all, in 1846 John Ayrton Paris remarked, "Alcohol, which is properly arranged under the class of exhilarants or excitants, might, without any violation of principle, stand at the head of narcotics."[18] Finally, the fourth role has been physiological. Alcohol strengthens the body by supplying it with considerable extra energy (one liter of wine containing 12 percent alcohol provides between 500 and 700 calories, one liter of pure vodka has 2,800 calories, while the same amount of rum supplies up to 4,000 calories). In 1763 Erasmus Darwin, the English naturalist, physician, inventor, poet, and grandfather of Charles Darwin, proclaimed: "Drink success to philosophy and trade!"[19] Let me develop further his point by adding, "and the conduct of war."

Historically, nearly every society (other than the Islamic society) and its armed forces had their drink of choice, their own source of "liquid courage." So, the ancient Greeks drank wine at feasts, libations, and Dionysian Mysteries but also on the battlefield. Homer portrays his heroes treating themselves with wine during the Trojan War, especially to soften sorrows when mourning their dead comrades. Wine was indeed so popular and omnipresent that Victor Davis Hanson, a prominent scholar of the Greek way of war, raises the question of whether the Greek warriors marched into battle drunk. And he provides his answer: "almost." "It may be naive to assume," writes Hanson,

> that the Greek hoplite, who drank daily both at home and while on the march, would not realize that an extra cup or two of wine at his customary last supper might stanch his fear, dull his sensitivity to physical injury and mental anguish, and make the awful task of facing an enemy phalanx that much easier.[20]

The hoplites drank excessively before battle, and it is most likely that they were often, when the fighting began, drunk. But there was nothing odd or improper in such conduct because in antiquity drunkenness was not seen as reprehensible behavior. On the contrary, it was believed to be a religious-like act that connected man with the gods and liberated his "hidden divinity." Alcohol unleashed man's supernatural powers, which are the most desired traits of a warrior: greater strength and endurance. For, as Iain Gately observes, "Wine was the drink of fighting men, the indispensable lubricant of their culture of death and honor, of sacking cities, of carrying off armor, cattle, and women."[21]

Wine was also a habitual drink of the Roman legionaries, who carried large stocks of it during their numerous expeditions. Because the local sources of water in foreign lands were often contaminated, there was a serious threat of fatal disease, which remained the single greatest risk to a soldier's life in ancient times.[22] Wine, with its germicidal properties, helped protect the health of the legionaries and frequently saved their lives. In short, it was much safer to drink wine than the dubious water.[23] Alcohol played yet another role in the Roman way of war. Aware of the German tribes' great appetite for beer, the Romans often used it as a weapon to beat the barbarians, so that "the tactic of inebriating opponents before slaughtering them seems to have been a standard Roman military stratagem."[24] Tacitus saw the Teutonic passion for intoxication as a major weakness that could, and should, be exploited. Thus he advised: "If you will but humor their excess in drinking, and supply them with as much as they covet, it will be no less easy to vanquish them by vices than by arms."[25] This clever and effective ruse by the Romans of making the barbarians drunk before launching an attack on them was strikingly similar to the waging of unorthodox warfare as strongly advised by Sun Tzu in the sixth century BC. In his *Art of War* this great ancient Chinese philosopher of war declared: "To subdue the enemy without fighting is the acme of skill."[26] Speaking of the times of Sun Tzu, Chinese soldiers got in the fighting mood also by drinking wine, while "their ardor was aroused by gyrating sword dancers."[27] The Aztec warriors, too, drank before battle a wine-like beverage known as *pulque*, made of the fermented syrup of American Aloe (*maguey*). In addition, they boosted themselves with *teooctli* (the divine drink), which was strong *pulque* amplified with herbs and spices for greater intoxicating effect.

Medieval chronicles report that before the battle of Hastings in 1066, the knights of King Harold II were so exhausted by a long march that they spent most of the night preceding the fight drinking heavily. So, when the battle did come, they must still have had alcohol in their blood. The French knights also drank themselves into a stupor prior to the battle of Agincourt in 1415 during the Hundred Years' War (1337–1453).[28] They calmed themselves down in preparation for combat, but in the end were crushed by the English forces. It is probable that heavy drinking the night before impaired their combat performance.

Moving in time to the Napoleonic wars, two French infantry divisions under the command of generals Louis Vincent Saint-Hilaire and Dominique Vandamme, who were charged with the task of seizing the Pratzen Heights during the battle of Austerlitz (1805), were "given triple rations of brandy, nearly half a pint per man."[29] The effect was mostly desirable, because, as a French officer observed, the troops "burst with eagerness and enthusiasm."[30] And before the battle of Waterloo in 1815, the troops of the anti-Napoleonic coalition attempted to make soldiers enthusiastic for combat by dispensing decent rations of rum to the troops.[31] The precise role of alcohol in their victory as yet remains unknown.

An Empire Built on Rum

What does Ian Williams have in mind by remarking: "There is no doubt that rum was indeed a weapon of war"?[32] Well, for a long time it was a drink commonly issued to English sailors and soldiers. In the eighteenth century it replaced the traditional alcoholic beverages distributed to seamen and infantrymen, namely the more common beer and the less common wine and brandy. Rum proved to be much more attractive than these old drinks because it was not only very cheap in the Caribbean but also had a higher alcoholic strength; thereby significantly less room was required for storage and transportation when compared with beer or wine. In short, rum was a more cost-effective option, because it helped save both space (precious aboard ships) and money. Until the beginning of the eighteenth century, the regular ration in the Royal Navy was one pint of wine or a half pint of brandy. After the introduction of rum, sailors were issued a half pint a day. Yet in 1740 Admiral Edward Vernon considered the suggestions forwarded by captains and doctors, who insisted that swallowing the whole ration of liquor at a single draught had a bad effect on sailors' health and behavior. Thus he ordered that rum be diluted to half strength with water (half a pint of rum and a quart of a pint of water).[33] At first sailors disliked the new drink and called it "grog" after Admiral Vernon's nickname "Old Grog," which he got from his coat of grogram cloth. But they soon got used to it. In 1825 the ration of rum was reduced to a quarter of a pint, and in 1850 it was further cut down to one-eighth. Beginning in 1928, under the provisions of the special instruction of the Admiralty, sailors could request a money equivalent of their alcohol allowance.[34]

It was estimated that in the second half of the nineteenth century, the British Army of 36,000 men required some 550,000 gallons of rum annually, including extra alcohol allowances issued before battle (distributed for better combat) or in its aftermath (for celebrating victory).[35] After all, every occasion for heavy drinking was welcomed, no matter whether it was a royal birthday or the anniversary of a major event. Thus rum played an important role in the management of the army's manpower for, as Major General James Wolfe, known for his training reforms in the British Army, declared in 1758, it was "the cheapest pay for work that can be given."[36] The year 1875 was a remarkable one, in which the British armed forces consumed the exceptionally large amount of 5,386 million gallons of rum, but later the level of authorized drinking began to drop.[37]

Rum was issued to soldiers because it was believed to make them better fighters, and the battlefield experience did indeed seem to prove it. This favorable and highly desirable impact of alcohol on the fighting spirit of the troops was commonly known as "Dutch courage." The phrase derives from the English soldiers who fought in the Netherlands in the English-Dutch wars of the seventeenth century, and who got their courage up by one or two sips of a Dutch gin called "genever." Originally, the English troopers used the expression when referring to Dutch soldiers, who drank both heavily and frequently.[38]

In the 1760s the ration of rum in the British forces deployed in the American colonies was half a pint per soldier per day, which came to twenty-three gallons per man per year.[39] When the American War of Independence broke out in 1776, it was self-evident to both the English and the colonists that soldiers could not be expected to fight without being provided with regular supplies of rum. Another explanation for the widespread use of alcohol was the climate; a German officer remarked in a letter sent in 1780 from New York: "This is a bad country, this America, where you always have to drink, either to get warm, or to get cool."[40] And it was a commonplace belief that alcohol had valuable healing properties, particularly in that it secured the body against both overheating and hypothermia. General George Washington, the commander in chief of the Continental Army, was firmly convinced that troops must be regularly supplied with alcoholic beverages. Because he saw alcohol as an indispensable military provision, when in 1777 the supplies of rum for his units were delayed, Washington sent an urgent letter to the Continental Congress, in which he argued that "the benefits arising from the moderate use of strong liquor have been experienced in all Armies and are not to be disputed."[41] He also advised that, in order to secure a regular and undisrupted supply of alcohol for the military, public distilleries should be established in various states. By the time the war ended in 1783, as many as 2,579 distilleries had been registered in the newly independent country.[42] The hostilities, therefore, significantly contributed to the development of the distilled spirits industry in America.

Being such a critical military commodity, rum also became a tempting strategic target. Cutting the enemy off from its rum supplies could destroy the troops' morale and thereby facilitate victory. Unsurprisingly then, the British forces sought with great determination to destroy American stocks of the commodity, hoping to break the fighting spirit of the rebel colonists. Attempting to achieve this goal, the British 64th Regiment of Foot resolutely "destroyed no less than 400 hogsheads of rum in Washington's stores on the Hudson."[43] The importance of rum as a strategic asset is also well illustrated by the story of American general Israel Putnam, a hard and unyielding commander, who was only once reported to be distressed in the battlefield—when "a shot had passed through his canteen and spilt all his rum."[44] After Britain introduced a blockade on rum importation to America, the colonists turned to the production of whiskey, the beverage that later, especially in the course of the American Civil War (1861–1865), proved a crucial war asset.[45] Early in the Civil War, both the Union and Confederates systematically supplied their armies with whiskey.[46] And although the troops did not generally get drunk before battles, the Confederate commanders noticed a harmful effect of drunkenness on overall combat efficiency and began prohibiting the use of alcohol. In 1861, for example, Confederate general Braxton Bragg introduced a ban on sales of alcohol within five miles of Pensacola, where his troops were stationed. The general argued that "distilled evil" not only brought demoralization but was also causing death and disease. Thus he proclaimed: "We have lost more valuable lives at the hands of the whiskey sellers than by the balls of our enemies."[47] Following Bragg's advice bans on alcohol were initiated in other Confederate camps, but it was impossible to rigorously enforce them as soldiers smuggled alcohol, for example, in the barrels of muskets or in watermelons (large fruits could absorb as much as half a gallon of injected whiskey).

In the mid-nineteenth century the British Army also noticed the alarming problem of alcohol abuse.[48] Instead of providing Dutch courage, alcohol increasingly caused health problems and a diminution of esprit de corps. Scott Hughes Myerly notes, "For most soldiers, alcohol was the only escape; it was customary in many regiments to pay the men once a month, and most would then drink until their money was gone."[49] As early as in the eighteenth century, alcoholism had become a nightmare for both the army and the navy, although it was not yet officially recognized as a social problem. In the nineteenth century drunkenness in the ranks took on epidemic proportions.[50] Armed forces were largely recruited from among the working class (often in the taverns), and the newly enlisted men brought with them the culture of heavy drinking.[51] Moreover, the custom of daily rations of alcohol encouraged drinking, yet the officers were convinced that without the standard government allowance their men would laze and refuse to follow orders. Alcohol, the liquid means of army management, went out of control, so that its abuse required new forms of control and administration.

To conclude, in the colonial and imperial age, the use of alcohol in war was prevalent. Victor Gordon Kiernan puts this particularly well in his study of European imperialism: "Alcohol was almost as indispensable as food. It supplied some nutrition, mollified hardships, and sharpened appetite for battle: there must have been a dash of Dutch courage in all Western armies in action. . . . Without this solace the empire could not have been won."[52] After all, the British writer H. Warner Allen did not exaggerate when in 1931 he wrote:

> Rum is the Englishman's spirit, the true spirit of adventure. Whiskey belongs to Scotland and Ireland, Brandy to France, Gin to Holland, but Rum is essentially English, despite its tropical origin. The very word calls up heroic memories of the iron seamen who on the lawful and unlawful occasions built up the British Empire overseas, and if ever Rum were to disappear from navy rations, a great tradition would be tragically broken.[53]

Many nations, then, had their alcohol of choice, which was closely bound to tradition but also inscribed into their military culture.

The Vodka Ethos

The Russian military was a large consumer of spirits. The customs and practices of the tsarist army should, however, be considered in the more general context of Russian culture, with one of its distinctive patterns being the remarkably liberal consumption of alcohol. Drunkenness in Russia has been so excessive that it came to be regarded as a habit, a norm, and an integral part of the national character. Unsurprisingly then, alcohol remained an inescapable element of the tsarist officers' daily lives. It is, in fact, hard to find an officer's memoir that does not mention either individual or group intemperance.[54] Uniform heavy drinking did not, however, affect officers' careers adversely. Quite the contrary—the requirement that they drink themselves into a stupor was a central part of the initiation rituals for new officers. Overall, alcohol abuse was rampart. John Bushnell describes how in the nineteenth century "officers in Siberia were notorious drunks because there was nothing else to do. Officers in Poland drank inordinately because units were based, for strategic purposes, far from major cities."[55]

Drinking vodka was embedded in the ethos of the imperial Russian officer corps to such an extent that it might be seen to have been an officer's duty. Those who did not drink or drank in an unreasonably moderate fashion were considered eccentrics and unfit for the job. Junior officers "who drank but moderately were likely to be reproved by their commanders."[56] Temperance was seen as an act of political deviance, while heavy drinking was by no means regarded as incompatible with the proper performance of military duties. Paradoxically, as some historians, such as John Keep, observe, in the eighteenth and nineteenth centuries private soldiers "had a better reputation for sobriety than their officers or most civilians" because they usually drank kvas (a fermented nonalcoholic beverage made from bread) or native beer rather than the much more expensive vodka.[57] This pattern of uniform drinking was, however, soon to change, as there was no better way of boosting soldiers' fighting spirit than through government rations of vodka. Early in the eighteenth century, Peter the Great, known to drink between thirty to forty glasses of wine a day, allowed that Russian sailors be given vodka rations three times a week.[58] By 1761 the custom of providing daily portions of alcohol for the navy, called charka (one-hundredth of a bucket, or 0.125 liters), had already been set up. In 1797 Emperor Paul I "institutionalized" charka by introducing the right to a daily provision of alcohol into naval regulations.[59] Daily rations of vodka had also become commonplace in the infantry, although initially it was issued only in combat or under extremely harsh battlefield conditions. For example, in 1812 during the fighting against Napoleon's forces, Russian soldiers were given three charkas (almost 0.4 liters) of vodka every day.[60] Sometimes, prior to a major battle or in the aftermath of victory, generous commanders substantially increased the rations. The custom of rewarding the troops with alcohol was well described by Leo Tolstoy in War and Peace: in November 1805, after the Russian army seized the city of Wischau (today the Czech Vyškov) and captured a whole French squadron, "The sovereign's gratitude was conveyed to the avant-garde, honors were promised and a double ration of vodka was issued to the men. The bivouac campfires crackled and the soldiers' songs resounded even more merrily than on the previous night."[61]

Most privates who before joining the army had not abused alcohol became, after the prolonged administration of *charkas*, alcoholics. The majority of recruits began drinking early, usually immediately after learning of being called by a conscript committee; thus the Russian expression arose: "drunk as a recruit."[62] Because Russian soldiers received very modest pay, they were legally allowed to earn extra money and frequently hired themselves out as laborers or artisans. In fact, they would take any job to get some money. Critics claimed that they worked only for drink money because the official administration of vodka had turned them into drunkards.[63] Indeed, the privates regularly drank to intoxication on leave, and the nineteenth-century Russian army can well be described as a great "school of drinking." After sipping *charka* there often came a desire for the next one, which soldiers had to buy themselves. During the Crimean War (1853–1856) the drunkenness among the troops turned into a grave disadvantage. Leo Tolstoy, who fought in the Crimea as a young officer, recalled leading a "dissipated military life."[64] So did the entire officer corps.

At times alcohol led to tragicomic events, like the one during the Russo-Japanese war (1904–1905) which, by the way, Russia funded largely with revenues from the sale of alcohol, since from 1895 the state held the monopoly on the production and distribution of spirits.[65] Late in the war, the commander of the Russian garrison at the fortress of Port Arthur surrendered after he was sent, instead of the expected and badly needed supplies of ammunition, 10,000 chests of vodka.[66] Liquid courage apart, the bottles could not save the garrison. This was a telling event, as many foreign war correspondents found the scale of drunkenness among the Russian ranks absolutely astonishing. A German reporter correctly observed: "'Who defeated the Russians?' ask foreigners, and they answer, 'The Japanese did not conquer, but alcohol triumphed, alcohol, alcohol.'"[67] And a Russian journalist of the *Vilna Military Leaflet* reported that "the Japanese at Mukden found several thousand dead-drunk soldiers, whom they bayoneted like pigs."[68] Indeed, as a Russian officer recalled:

> Drinking and more drinking—what victories could there be? All, or almost all of our forces suffered from alcoholism. That is why we lost battles. And can it be that this poison has become less pervasive after the war? The Treasury can go on enriching itself on revenues from the monopoly, but what's the sense of that if the military will not be able to prevent the Treasury from being seized by foreign forces?[69]

To make the story even worse, the commander of the Russian fleet, Grand Duke Aleksei Aleksandrovich, the younger brother of Tsar Alexander III, was in drunken stupor at most of the critical moments of the war. Some historians even see his alcoholism and poor decision-making as responsible for the Russians' ultimate defeat.[70] The devastating impact of alcohol on Russian fighting effectiveness was, however, nothing new. As early as 1758, during the Seven Years' War (1756–1763), the Russians did not manage to crush the Prussian forces at the battle of Küstrin, most probably because their left wing unit had gotten heavily drunk on vodka, which the overjoyed soldiers had accidentally discovered. Ultimately, some 20,000 Russians were captured and the battle ended indecisively.[71] The question of the extent to which vodka can be held responsible for this outcome remains unanswered. Yet the examples of the catastrophic impact of vodka on the Russian conduct of war are plentiful.

Total War in the Fog of Prohibition, Rum, and Wine

In 1906, in order to reduce drinking among officers and to combat the plague of alcoholism in the ranks, the Russian Ministry of War issued regulations prohibiting the sale of alcoholic beverages in the regimental canteens. Most crucially of all, and much to the dismay of soldiers, in 1908 the government rations of vodka were terminated.[72] There were two main reasons for the abolition of *charka*. The first was the diminution of fighting power, poor combat efficiency, and breakdown of military discipline of the Russian army in the aftermath of the humiliating defeat by Japan in 1905. The second was the increasing weakening of the authority not only of the individual officer-alcoholics but also of the tsarist officer corps in general.[73] In 1914, after the outbreak of the First World War, the government imposed restrictions on the trade in spirits, wine, and beer by revoking the manufacturers' licenses and permits issued before the war.[74] In addition, the maximum permitted strength of alcohol was reduced from 40 to 37 percent, and its sale was prohibited in public places of entertainment. The previous year the navy had abandoned the custom of dispensing vodka to sailors as part of their rations, except in emergency situations such as very long periods at sea, bad weather, or for specific medical indications.[75] This antialcohol crusade resulted, basically, in the rise of the homemade production of spirits, as the Russians massively resorted to running hooch. By the same token, the Russian state deprived itself of considerable revenues from the sale of alcohol, which could have significantly added to a stretched budget (in 1913 it accounted for as much as 26 percent of state incomes).[76]

The London *Times* acknowledged this unprecedented tsarist prohibition-like policy and on September 21, 1914, offered a somewhat overly optimistic commentary:

> The great victory over drunkenness in Russia has received far too little attention in this country [Britain]. Since China proscribed opium, the world has seen nothing like it. We have been well reminded that in sternly prohibiting the sale of spirituous liquor Russia has already vanquished a greater foe than the Germans.[77]

It is, however, difficult to properly assess the Russian temperance measures. For, unfortunately, the restrictions placed on the military supplies of vodka had a highly demoralizing effect on the troops, as they were deprived of what since the times of Peter the Great had been a customary soldierly allowance. At the same time it was demanded of them that they invest great effort in combat, and they were expected to make a supreme yet sober sacrifice. But this was too much to be demanded from "Ivan" (the nickname for a Russian soldier), so whenever the fighting stopped temporarily on the Eastern Front, soldiers eagerly traded with their German counterparts bread, sugar, and other items for vodka.[78] Unsurprisingly, when the Bolshevik Revolution, which overthrew the tsar, broke out in November 1917, the troops indulged in the most excessive orgies of drunkenness. Thus was the boomerang effect of the tsarist anti-alcohol campaign—a total breakdown of military discipline and utter chaos in the ranks.

Although under the 1908 tsarist edict, soldiers could have been discharged for alcoholism and drunkenness, it was only the Bolsheviks who launched a firm, though yet again fruitless, antialcohol crusade. Soldiers of the Red Army, established in 1918 and recruited mostly from the peasantry, were not only trained in discipline but were also taught the basic principles of personal hygiene, being encouraged to bathe and brush their teeth regularly. On the other hand, recruits were strongly dissuaded from drinking vodka. New regulations adopted by the Bolsheviks ruled out alcohol in the barracks, and Krasnoarmeets (Red Army men) could even be sentenced to death for drinking while on duty. They were also discouraged from drinking in their free time.[79] The communists considered alcoholism to be one of the distinctive features of the old oppressive order, as the instrument of the debasement and impoverishment of the working class. It was for this very reason that it had to be wiped out because, as chairman of the Military Revolutionary Council S. I. Gusev explained, "when the Communist gets drunk, the Menshevik can celebrate."[80] Certainly, alcoholism was a nightmare, and the Bolsheviks reasonably feared that uncontrolled drinking could make soldiers unfit for combat and

thereby unable to prevail over the Whites. The following episode well illustrates that these concerns were taken very seriously. When the fighting moved
to Ukraine, Leon Trotsky, the head of the Red Army, was extremely anxious as
the region was "well-stocked with alcohol in all its forms," and the Bolsheviks
might have taken a heavy fall in 1919 as a result.[81] Trotsky, therefore, issued an
order, and soldiers caught drunk were shot immediately in many Red Army
units on the southern front during the Ukraine campaign.

Russia was not the only state which restricted the manufacture, sale, and
consumption of alcohol during the First World War, because, as was believed,
it stood in the way of the total mobilization of societies and the ultimate utilization of their productive energies. By threatening to hinder efficient war
production, drunkenness could have posed a grave danger of losing the war
on the home front. Coal dealer Vergil Gunch, a character in the novel *Babbitt*
by Sinclair Lewis, which is a biting satire on American culture, society, and
lifestyle, says cynically while sipping a drink: "You don't want to forget prohibition is a mighty good thing for the working-classes. Keeps 'em from wasting
their money and lowering their productiveness."[82] The manufacture of alcoholic beverages was viewed as a waste of crucial resources that could otherwise
be used and sent to the war front. Moreover, was not it highly improper if not
downright immoral to drink for pleasure at a time when soldiers were risking
their lives and dying on the battlefields of the World War? Hence drunkenness
came to be presented as utterly unpatriotic and unethical behavior, particularly in the United States, where the nationwide campaign for temperance was
perceived as a crucial component of America's global moral crusade in defense
of freedom and democracy.

The prohibition on the consumption of alcohol extended to cover also
American soldiers, as they were to stand out from their European counterparts, who were regularly given alcohol. Drinking was said to be evil because,
for example, it rendered combatants incapable of shooting accurately. Already
in 1901 the Canteen Act (or more precisely the Anti-Canteen Act) prohibited
"the sale of, or dealing in, beer, wine or any intoxicating liquors by any person in
any post exchange or canteen or army transport or upon any premises used for
military purposes by the United States."[83] After the United States entered the
First World War in April 1917, Congress extended these regulations to cover
the sale of intoxicating beverages beyond military camps where American
troops were stationed. As a result, total prohibition covered an area of up to
five miles around each army post, which made the sale of alcohol to servicemen in uniform clearly illegal. As an "exceptional nation," the United States
adopted an exceptional stance on the military consumption of alcohol, even
in small amounts. Contrary to the European military drinking culture, the
Americans deemed alcohol as having a degenerative effect on combatants. The

overall goal then was, as the secretary of the Navy Josephus Daniels insisted, to give America "the soberest, cleanest, and healthiest fighting men the world has ever known."[84] The *U.S. Army Manual of Military Training* issued in 1917 instructed servicemen as follows:

> Do not drink whiskey or beer, especially in the field. It will weaken you and favor heat exhaustion, sunstroke, frostbite, and other serious troubles. Alcohol muddles the mind and clouds thoughts, and so causes a feeling of carelessness and silliness that may ruin some military plan, or give the whole thing away to the enemy and with it the lives of yourself and your comrades. The soldier who drinks alcohol will be among the first to fall out exhausted.[85]

However, given the ubiquity of alcohol on the Western Front, it was quite impossible to keep military personnel completely dry. Therefore, the commander of the American Expeditionary Forces, General John Pershing, allowed his men deployed in France light wine and beer.

Unsurprisingly, with the United States joining the war, the "priests of temperance" from the Anti-Saloon League put forward the most powerful argument, claiming that "sobriety is the bomb that will blow kaiserism to kingdom come."[86] Thus was the war grist to the mill for the entire temperance movement. The Eighteenth Amendment to the American Constitution, which entered into force in January 1920, banned the production, importing, sale, and consumption of alcohol beverages throughout the United States for nearly thirteen years. Still, this astonishing experiment with forced sobriety, which brought exorbitant profits for the Mafia and caused significant losses to the federal and state budgets, could have by no means contributed to the Allied victory.

Meanwhile in Great Britain Prime Minister David Lloyd George proclaimed: "[W]e are fighting Germans, Austrians, and Drink; and, so far as I can see, the greatest of these three deadly foes is Drink."[87] Following Lloyd George's declaration King George V joined the abstinence campaign and announced the "King's Pledge," which, "as an example to the nation," banned all alcohol from the royal households until the war came to an end. Under the 1914 Defence of the Realm Act, civil servants were empowered to impose limits on the sale of alcohol, and they went on to perform their duties very eagerly. Interestingly, the wartime restrictions on pub opening times survived until the late twentieth century. The production of beer, which during wartime was three-quarters weaker than usual, declined by one-third, from thirty million barrels in 1914 to nineteen million in 1917.[88] Lloyd George kept an all-out propaganda offensive on the boil by declaring, for example, that drinking deteriorated society's productive powers and was doing England "more damage in the War than all the German submarines put together."[89]

The temperance campaigns undertaken not only in Britain but also in France and Germany are yet further evidence of the total character of the war. The divide between home front and war front was transgressed, and the conflict encompassed all spheres of social life. At the same time, however, contrary to the goals of the crusades for sobriety at home, governments (except the American and Russian) continued to regularly supply their forces in the field with daily rations of alcohol, be it rum, wine, brandy, or beer. Many combatants managed to survive the sheer brutal reality of industrial warfare and keep their shattered nerves under control due to the rations of alcohol provided by the army. When compared to the wars of the past, much greater stocks of alcoholic beverages were required given the totality of the First World War, and at times the rations distributed to the troops were really substantial. In addition, of course, the combatants supplied themselves with supplementary bottles of every shape, color, size, and alcoholic content.

In the British Army the distribution of the daily allowance (a standard one-sixteenth pint of rum) belonged to the commander of a division. Although he was formally required to consult the military doctor, almost all commanders were ready and willing to unconditionally grant rations to their men.[90] The rum rations were small but quite regular, and officially the army considered it in purely medical terms: as a remedy for fatigue, stress, and hardship. Rum was delivered in ceramic jars marked with the initials S.R.D., which officially stood for Special Rations Department, but which soldiers read as Services Rum Diluted, Seldom Reaches Destination, Sadly Rarely Distributed, or Soon Runs Dry. This only shows how vital rum was for military life on the front line. Even minor shortcomings and delays in the daily supplies almost automatically caused a slight diminution of morale and fighting spirit or, at best, disappointment and discontent. As British soldier Gerald Burgoyne confessed, even "a drop of rum in our tea works wonders."[91] Most men, of course, wished to receive much bigger rations of liquid courage, especially before leaving for combat, and complained about the poor provisions. A comment by Thomas Penrose Marks, who fought in the infantry lines, is representative: "The second ration [administered before battle] is supposed to give us Dutch courage. It might fulfill its purpose if it were handed out in more liberal doses . . . It does not even make us merry. But every one of us welcomes it."[92]

Rum, being inherent to the military life of the "Tommy," the proverbial British soldier, became intoxicatingly synonymous with combat. In his splendid book *The Great War and Modern Memory*, Paul Fussell describes life on the front line. Most mornings in the trenches began about 4:30 a.m. Soldiers were then given tea, bread, bacon, and

[i]f the men were lucky enough to be in a division whose commanding general permitted the issue of the dark and strong government rum, it was doled out from a jar with the traditional iron spoon, each man receiving about two tablespoonsful. Some put it into their tea, but most swallowed it straight. It was a precious thing, and serving it out was almost like a religious ceremonial.[93]

Before battle, in order to foster a fighting mood, soldiers were given a larger, usually a double, dose of government rum. Siegfried Sassoon, the poet and British infantry officer, recalled his first days on the front line: "The raiders had been given only a small quantity, but it was enough to hearten them as they sploshed up the communication trench."[94] Another soldier powerfully and eloquently evoked rum's vital part in the British war effort, writing that during an attack "pervading the air was the smell of rum and blood."[95] In 1922 a medical officer, who was heard by the parliamentary committee investigating the problem of "shell shock" (PTSD in today's psychiatric terminology), testified emphatically: "Had it not been for the rum ration I do not think we should have won the war."[96] Speaking of combat stress, even before the outbreak of the war, in articles published in the renowned *British Medical Journal*, doctors recommended alcohol as the only proven, traditional, and effective cure for most of the soldiers' mental disorders.[97] The British praxis of moderately enhancing the troops with rum gave rise to the fables of soldiers who fought bravely but at times recklessly. But this is precisely how myths are created.

What rum was for Englishmen, wine (colloquially known as *pinard*) was for Frenchmen. But before it became a standard provision of the French army at the beginning of the twentieth century, soldiers had received a small daily ration of distilled alcohol (one-sixteenth of a liter).[98] This change in the French military's alcohol of choice was pushed through mainly by grapevine growers and wine producers, who suffered badly from overproduction, low prices, and a steady decline in earnings. The government contracts for wine secured the producers lucrative income benefits. At the outbreak of the First World War, every French soldier was entitled to a quarter of a liter of wine a day. As the war progressed, the rations increased to three-quarters, and in 1918 some units issued as much as one liter per man per day, which was the amount approved by the French Academy of Medicine as a maximum safe dose, that is, having no harmful effects on human health.[99] In the course of the war, the lobbying by the wine manufacturers, who had been successfully developing a national cult of wine, intensified even further. In the fall of 1914, the Midi producers donated to the army substantial stocks of *pinard*, on which occasion a special song was composed. Its refrain urged soldiers to drink eagerly the wine of victory to

enable the entire nation to celebrate "a lovely drunkenness of glory."[100] One of
the song's verses pledged:

In drinking this generous wine
They will forget all of their misery.
In its warmth, they will feel
Strength, energy, courage.
For wine revives the heart
And inspires arms to take up their task.[101]

The essence of this vital liquid element of the French national identity was captured by Dr. Edouard Bazerolle, who claimed that wine "is one of the ingredi-
ents from which our race and national temperament was formed." Should the
French give up wine, he argued, "the French race would lose its true character
and become a bland people without any personality."[102]

In 1936 the Nicolas wine company published a stylish illustrated booklet
entitled *Mon docteur le vin* (*My Doctor, Wine*), presenting the views of prominent physicians on the health benefits of moderate wine drinking. In the
preface the publisher used the poem *Hommage au vin* (*A Tribute to Wine*),
composed by the First World War hero Marshall Philippe Pétain, in which he
declared that "of all the supplies sent to the army during the war, wine was
surely the most highly anticipated and appreciated by the soldier."[103] The ado-
ration and mythologization of wine sometimes gave rise to fantastic and ridiculous claims, such as the opinion expressed by a military doctor who served on
a recruiting board: "We were able to note that among the young men called for
army duty, those from wine growing regions were the most muscular, alert, and
lithe, as well as the strongest, biggest, and leanest."[104] Overall, wine drinking
was popularly seen as a patriotic duty. In his path-breaking book *Mythologies*
(1957), Roland Barthes remarked that, for the French, wine is "a totem-drink,
corresponding to the milk of the Dutch cow or the tea ceremoniously taken by
the British Royal Family." In his view, for all Frenchmen "to believe in wine is
a coercive collective act" because the beverage had grown into "the foundation
of a collective morality" and been established as a great national myth.[105]

It was believed that in the First World War, wine, a highly sophisticated
drink, had significantly contributed to the defeat of the beer-drinking Germans.
Popular mythologies and patriotic rhetoric fed crudely stereotypical opinions
with a strong nationalist tinge. For example, it was claimed that while rum
helped bring victory to the British and wine did the same for the French, it was
beer that was somehow responsible for the miserable defeat of the German army.
The French openly despised beer as a primitive beverage. Playing on the antag-
onism between wine drinkers and beer drinkers was, however, nothing new.

Consider a verse from *Livre de vie et de mort* (*The Book of Life and Death*), a French poem composed in the thirteenth century: "[T]he poor resort to ale . . . and the richer folk resort to wine."[106] And writing about the Middle Ages, Léo Moulin went on to explain that the "noblemen drink wine, the common people drink beer."[107] Nevertheless, beer was for the Germans what wine was for the French, namely the essential substance of their national identity. Beer drinking was a vital catalyst of social binding but also one of the manifestations of the national community, especially after the unification of Germany in 1871. An almost patriotic habit of beer drinking was largely grounded in the specific Prussian understanding of Germanness. The famous view expressed by King Frederick the Great was very much in line with the tradition of Prussian militarism. In his *Coffee and Beer Manifesto* issued in 1777, he strongly advocated beer drinking: "His Majesty was brought up on beer and so were his ancestors and his officers. Many battles have been fought and won by soldiers nourished on beer, and the king does not believe that coffee-drinking soldiers can be depended on to endure hardship or to beat his enemies."[108] In the aftermath of the First World War, the French could have claimed that the Germans would have been better off had their troops drank more coffee than beer.

The Second World War

"Wine, the pride of France," argued the French politician Èdouard Barthe, "is a symbol of strength; it is associated with warlike virtues," for it makes soldiers more courageous.[109] Because, as was commonly believed and publicly proclaimed, *pinard* saved France during the First World War, in the preparation for the next inevitable clash of the great powers, the French army stored not only weapons, ammunition, food, and fuel, but also vast amounts of wine. So after the Germans launched their attack in May 1940, every day 3,500 trucks supplied the French troops in the field with two million liters of wine.[110] A typical ration was three-quarters of a liter per man per day.[111] This time, however, the salutary and invigorating effects of the splendid drink did not save France against the German blitzkrieg. Marshall Philippe Pétain, the leader of the collaborating government of Vichy and a great eulogist of wine's role in the First World War effort, discovered, as he believed, the reason for this defeat. Paradoxically, he insisted, what undermined the morale of the troops was the prevailing drunkenness. France lost because at the decisive moments of the critical struggle its troops were severely inebriated. Instead of assisting the French army in waging a defensive war, *pinard* severely weakened it. Wine, argued Pétain, destroyed the very spirit to fight. After all, if in 1918 wine was believed to be a source of victory, why could it not be blamed for the disastrous defeat in 1941? The Vichy government, then, launched the first large-scale anti-alcohol campaign in France's history. Immoderate drinking was now deemed extremely unpatriotic.

Just as rum accompanied the British troops in the Great War, it also supported them in the Second World War. The infantryman John Horsfall honestly acknowledged: "We simply kept going on rum. Eventually it became unthinkable to go into action without it."[112] Yet while moderate drinking could sharpen appetite for battle, excessive drinking undermined fighting power and military discipline. Heavy abuse of alcohol was recorded as a problem jeopardizing discipline in the American armed forces. In 1944–1945 as many as 44,420 servicemen were diagnosed with alcohol dependence.[113] But it was the Wehrmacht that suffered from addiction of epidemic proportions.[114] Drunkenness in the German ranks often led to quarrels, fights, insubordination, violence against superior officers, sexual offenses, or death from drinking lethal methyl alcohol (normally used as a fuel, solvent, and antifreeze). The statistics gathered by the Wehrmacht medical corps revealed 705 military deaths induced by alcohol between September 1939 and April 1944. This was an official figure which obviously excluded suicides, traffic accidents, and friendly fire casualties caused by drunken soldiers. The actual rate must have been much higher.[115] Following the defeat of France in July 1940, the growing scale of the alcohol problem impelled Adolf Hitler (who was almost a total abstainer) to issue an order that all Wehrmacht soldiers found guilty of crimes committed under the influence of alcohol were to be severely punished, including the death penalty. But in reality the appeal of alcohol-induced escape from the horrors of war significantly reduced the fear of harsh punishment. The temptation to get drunk was more powerful than the need to fulfill the führer's demand. Moreover, most field commanders were much more lenient than the commander in chief for, as a general in the medical corps, Walter Kittel, put it openly, "only a fanatic would refuse to give a soldier something that can help him relax and enjoy life after he has faced the horrors of battle, or would reprimand him for enjoying a friendly drink or two with his comrades."[116]

In his autobiographical account of a German soldier on the Eastern Front, *The Forgotten Soldier* (1971), Guy Sajer recalls, "Those who were neither asleep, on guard, playing cards, nor writing letters were absorbing the alcohol which was freely distributed along with our ammunition." Sajer quotes a wounded German infantryman, who tells us:

> There's as much vodka, schnapps and Terek liquor on the front as there are Paks [antitank guns]. It's the easiest way to make heroes. Vodka purges the brain and expands the strength. I've been doing nothing but drinking for two days now. It's the best way to forget that I've got seven pieces of metal in my gut, if you can believe the doctor.[117]

As long as alcohol consumption was kept within bounds without causing general drunkenness amongst the troops, officers turned a blind eye to drinking and from time to time even issued some extra allowances to their units as a reward for good performance.

And what of the Red Army? The explanation for the unimaginable determination, devotion, and sacrifice of the Soviet soldier in the Second World War was not merely discipline (further strengthened by the presence of the NKVD officers and the threat of harsh punishment for insubordination, which often meant immediate execution) and ideological indoctrination but also the numbing effect of alcohol. Because the Bolshevik temperance campaign was doomed to complete failure, beginning in August 1941 soldiers on the front line were again administered vodka rations, the standard allowance being one hundred grams a day.[118] Of course, Krasnoarmeets supplemented these small rations of the "water of life" with almost everything that contained ethanol (be it a solvent, brake fluid, or antifreeze). Thus the Red Army produced its own distinct drinking culture, which actually—contrary to all ideological premises—represented a direct continuation of the tsarist military tradition. A report on the officer corps compiled in 1940 by the Central Committee of the Communist Party confirmed that drunkenness remained the bane of the armed services.[119] One soldier put it bluntly: "[E]ven if you are not an alcoholic when you go into the Army, you are when you come out."[120] The Red Army, in a word, provided its men with an advanced training in heavy drinking. In the areas liberated from the German occupation the Krasnoarmeets were drinking steadily both on and off duty. Adhering to the old rule of *bellum se ipsum alet* (war feeds war), they looted all alcohol and components useful for the production of hooch. A Soviet colonel admitted in 1945: "When our soldiers find alcohol, they take leave of their senses. You can't expect anything from them until they have finished the last drop." He went so far as to argue that "if we hadn't had drunkenness like this we would have beaten the Germans two years ago."[121] He was, of course, exaggerating, but there was some truth in his words. Drinking was so excessive that it gave rise to plentiful anecdotes and jokes. Take one postwar example: the Soviets built a computer with artificial intelligence and asked it what would be the perfect diet for a private soldier, assuming that a meal is cheap, calorific, and improving of morale. The computer gave this answer: "A kilogram of potatoes and a liter of vodka."

Moving to the Pacific theater of war, we also uncover the role of alcohol in combat. Prior to their take off, the Japanese *tokkōtai* (kamikaze) pilots participated in a number of rituals and ceremonies. They were bid an emotional farewell at the airstrip with music, songs, and hugs from their commanders and local inhabitants. The culmination of the goodbye ceremony was toasting the emperor with small shots of sake. During the special farewell parties directly preceding the mission, the tokkōtai pilots tried to enjoy the last hours of their lives. The day before falling in battle, like "cherry blossoms," most got duly drunk. Hayashi Ichizo, who died on April 12, 1945, wrote in his letter to a friend:

> The farewell party was fun. I, the brave warrior, will definitely destroy our enemy, even if it takes seven lives. Hopefully, you won't forget about me after I go. Since I am intoxicated, I don't know what I write. I am sure you understand. Forgive me if I said anything nasty to you. As long as you are alive, it is OK. I am lonely.[122]

Alcohol enabled most of the kamikaze pilots to endure the wait until their one-way mission. From the moment of becoming members of the special attack force, or even from the time of enlistment, they were painfully aware of their fate as they stood in line for death. How to live while feeling constantly torn by the conflict between the patriotic duty they had grown up with and the sheer will to live, so essential to youthfulness and often coupled with a strong opposition to vulgar militaristic propaganda? On April 27, 1944, about a year before his death, Takushima Norimitsu noted in his diary:

> It is difficult to hope for the glory of returning from the battlefield. Believing that a shortcut to eternity is to perish as a dew drop on the battlefield, and not having any guarantee of being alive the next day, it is only too human to take some drink, become intoxicated, and sing songs with passion. No one could laugh at such behavior.[123]

Thus alcohol helped the tokkōtai pilots live as the final day approached. Most photographs showing their last moments, especially of drinking sake just before taking off, were confiscated by the authorities and stamped "not permitted."[124] Why were the officials afraid of the public image of the plainly inebriated kamikaze pilots who sacrificed their lives for the emperor and the nation? Theirs, after all, was a "high" sacrifice.

Alcohol and Soldiering since 1945

The Second World War was the last conflict in which armed forces extensively supplied the troops with daily rations of liquid courage. The practice has been gradually, yet not entirely, abandoned after 1945. Although today's institutional military culture does not in general allow for alcohol use, this does not, of course, imply that drinking problems have been nonexistent or that at times commanders have not tended to look indulgently on their drinking subordinates, who should otherwise be prosecuted.

In the course of the Vietnam War (1965–1973), the gravest threat causing a breakdown of discipline among American troops was not the highly publicized drug addiction but a rather concealed issue of drunkenness. The overall extent of alcohol abuse was much more pervasive and rampant than drug abuse.[125] Commanders regularly turned a blind eye to soldiers' excessive drinking, in part because an inner war within the American forces in Vietnam was waged not against alcohol but against marijuana and heroin, which were considered public enemy number one. Research commissioned by the Department of Defense revealed that 88 percent of soldiers admitted drinking on duty, often in "prodigious amounts." As much as 73 percent of junior enlisted men and 30 percent of officers were either "problem drinkers" or "heavy or binge" drinkers.[126] The military recognized that alcohol abuse was, as the Army chief of staff General William Westmoreland admitted, a "serious problem." And serious it was, for the commanders were overtolerant toward drinking, as had been the case in the Second World War. In Vietnam, soldiers received a modest government ration of alcohol—two cans of beer per man per day. In December 1970, in addition to this small allowance, to boost the morale of the troops, drinking in barracks was approved. So from now on, servicemen could buy cheap alcohol in the base stores, the so-called PXs (Post Exchanges).

Officers themselves frequently encouraged alcohol abuse by offering their men free beer or whiskey in return for greater combat efficiency, thereby stirring an appetite for drinking. In other words, alcohol was issued as a reward for proven proficiency in enemy kills. This largely explains why soldiers cut off the ears and penises of their dead enemy, because showing the trophies on their return to base camp entitled them to more reward-alcohol. Private David Tuck testified that "the person who had the most ears was considered the number one 'Vietcong' killer. When we'd get back to base camp, they would get all the free beer and whiskey they could drink."[127] In short, drinking, often excessive drinking, was prevalent in the combat zone in Vietnam. Indeed, as Marc Levy recalls,

> While there were rumors about soldiers fucking up because of drugs, the only cases I knew of were with alcohol; guys drunk or hung-over who couldn't do their jobs or [who] made mistakes like stepping on a land mine, which cost lives. Drinking was simply part of the culture in Vietnam and it was everywhere. A beer was cheaper to get than a soda.[128]

Soldiers used alcohol for self-medication, as a means of numbing themselves emotionally and physically. Here is how one Vietnam veteran described his way of dealing with traumatic experiences: "I did it with the alcohol. And I did it when I was in the 'Nam. For that two days I stayed fucking shitfaced, just to numb it. Just so I wouldn't have to think about it."[129] Most American servicemen in Southeast Asia experienced the therapeutic power of alcohol as it enabled escape from the painful intrusive thoughts and images that only worsen combat trauma. Gonzalo Baltazar, a private serving in the 2nd Squadron, 17th Cavalry, 101st Airborne Division, was not exaggerating when he honestly said, "Everybody in Vietnam drank like fish, and every chance you got you drank yourself silly. Us infantry guys, we were a bunch of alcoholics."[130] Thus many returned to the United States as alcohol addicts. In fact, 53 percent of veterans interviewed by Lee Robins in 1973 had a serious alcohol problem.[131]

Overall, drinking for courage has remained one of the most popular means of self-medication by soldiers for relieving the stress of combat. Take, for example, the case of Lieutenant David Tinker of the British Army, who fought in the Falklands War in 1982 and admitted that "the best thing to do is to have a few wets before an attack." He went on to recall: "I'd had a drink before the [Argentinean] Exocet attack and the pulse rate stayed very normal."[132]

When drinking ceases to be under control and assumes epidemic proportions, alcohol use develops into a severe institutional problem. In the early post-Soviet times the propensity for alcohol dependence and misuse in the Russian military was an important factor not only in eroding morale, destroying esprit de corps, and weakening fighting effectiveness, but also literally deteriorating the material base of the army's combat capabilities. This became plainly evident during the Chechen wars (1994–1996, 1999–2006). Despite the fact that the Russian army provided servicemen with huge amounts of free vodka, it was not sufficient to satisfy the enormous appetite of the troops. Thus soldiers regularly traded weapons, ammunition, and military equipment for alcohol with the enemy fighters. Chechen leader Imran Ahhayev recalled that the Russians sold them an armored vehicle in exchange for two chests of vodka and the promise not to fire at their site for a week to permit "leisurely consumption."[133] In this way Russian soldiers supplied the Chechens with light and heavier weapons; the very same arms they were subsequently fired at with.[134] Frequently, it was the case that Russian commanders returned the bodies of killed Chechen fighters to their families but only in exchange for a bottle of vodka.[135]

Chechen fighter Akhyad D. is quoted by Valery Tishkov as saying, "We never drank vodka in action, but Russians were always drunk to ward off fear."[136] This chronic intoxication loosened moral constraints and facilitated acts of brutal violence. Furthermore, sometimes drunkenness at all levels of command caused terrible military mistakes. Let me take a particularly telling example. During an attack on New Year's Eve night in 1995, Pavel Grachev, the former defense minister who personally commanded the Russian troops in Chechnya, was pompously celebrating with his staff officers in Mozdok not only the new year but also his own birthday. Heavily drunk, Grachev made a fateful decision. He sent a column of tanks into Grozny that resulted in many Russian casualties, and, after a week of fighting, the city was reduced to ashes. Grachev was (in)famous for his heavy drinking, as he rarely showed up sober at press conferences. To sum up, the best description of the overall condition of the Russian forces in Chechnya might be a comment by one of the journalists: "They are nearly all drunk out there, 'no limits' appears to be the order of the day."[137]

And what of the American military today? The number of army personnel covered under the programs for alcohol abuse doubled between 2003—that is, the beginning of Operation Iraqi Freedom (OIF)—and 2010. The rate of soldiers with a drinking problem increased from 6.1 percent per 1,000 men in 2003 to 11.4 percent in 2009.[138] Nearly 9,200 soldiers sought treatment for alcohol abuse in 2009, a 56 percent increase since the war in Iraq began. This rapid growth can be in part explained by the fierce intensity of combat stress caused by the confrontation with an enemy who fights asymmetrically. At present, alcoholism remains a far greater problem than drug abuse: 85 percent of military personnel covered by the army substance-abuse treatment program are reported to have an alcohol problem.[139] As many as 43 percent of active-duty American military personnel admit to binge drinking, compared to 27 percent of national household residents.[140] In general, soldiers on missions in Afghanistan and Iraq drank both excessively and frequently. Brian, a three-tour Fort Hood area soldier, bluntly confirms this view: "I realized I wasn't ever going to have a job that was going to enable me to drink like in the military."[141] Of course, one must be careful here in overestimating the problem, because, as we already know, alcohol abuse has a long tradition in the American military. Heavy drinking has been, in essence, an intrinsic part of its culture. Let me quote Larry Scott, an army veteran, who jokes, "Back when I was in the Army, back in the 1970s and 1980s, we assumed drinking was mandatory." He further observes, "Drinking was as big a problem then as it is now. It just wasn't as highlighted."[142] This should not surprise, for, after all, the military is "an institution largely comprised of young Americans at those ages where drinking is seen as a rite of passage, and where peer pressure found in social networks is a prime determinant of alcohol use."[143] As recent reports confirm, male American military personnel indeed drink more than civilians.[144] And patterns of heavy drinking usually continue after servicemen leave the military.[145] To conclude, military service in the United States and alcohol use remain positively related, especially for men.

Conclusion

To sum up this brief discussion of the synergistic relationship between drinking and combat: alcohol has been the oldest and most popular intoxicant of war. Both administered by armed forces and self-prescribed by soldiers, it has propelled troops into battle and helped them bear the burden of fighting. By bringing temporary and virtual escape from violent battlefield reality, alcohol has been an almost universal liquid way of masking the horrible face of war. The Polish literary man Tadeusz Boy-Żeleński said that "the human animal likes to get drunk to shed the burden of humanity."[146] His saying gains additional meaning in the context of combat and military life. Throughout the centuries, a peculiar social understanding and acceptance have developed for combatants using alcohol to support themselves in the field. Above all, the government custom of rationing rum, vodka, whisky, wine, beer, and other beverages somehow legalized the additional self-administration of alcohol by soldiers and licensed their moderate drinking. Richard Holmes is perfectly right to remark that the military use of alcohol has been "infinitely more widespread than bland official histories might suggest."[147] As we will see in the course of the book, this has been even truer with regard to nonalcoholic drugs.

PART ONE

FROM PREMODERN TIMES TO THE END OF THE SECOND WORLD WAR

Premodern Times

Opium, Hashish, Mushrooms, and Coca

Human cultures have always experimented with extracts from plants and animals with which they co-existed. Some of these extracts were poisonous, others produced hallucinations, and many had medicinal properties.

—John Mann, *Murder, Magic, and Medicine*

The history of mind-altering substances is as old as humanity. In the times when people had not yet mastered agriculture or animal husbandry, they lived on what they managed to hunt, fish, or gather. By trial and error they discovered the strange, often hallucinogenic properties of many plants and also some animals. Ancient peoples such as the Greeks, Assyrians, Persians, Siberian tribes, Vikings, American Indians, and others made quite extensive use of a variety of disparate intoxicants. Hence psychoactive plants became commonly used, largely for ceremonial and religious purposes. As they evolved into an important, even essential, part of culture, they promptly found their way also onto the battlefield.

Homer and a Miracle Drink of Oblivion

For the Greek civilization, opium was a commonplace.
—Martin Booth, *Opium: A History*

Opium, the juice extracted from cut seedpods of the opium poppy plant (*Papaver somniferum*), was already known and used by the Assyrians and the Sumerians (in ideograms dated 4000 BC, the poppy is called the "plant of joy").[1] In ancient Greece, to which opium came from Egypt, it was both well known and common—used for fumigation at temples and oracles, sacrificed to gods, and taken to induce hallucinations during mysteries and rites. The Greeks also benefited from the healing properties of opium juice, and its medicinal use was widely reported by Hippocrates, Heraclitus, Theophrastus, and others. Most crucially of all for this study, the Greeks discovered the physically enhancing properties of opium that, mixed with wine and honey, was given to invigorate athletes during hard training in preparation for the Olympic Games.[2]

The first reference to the opium poppy in Greek literature occurred in Homer's epics, and it focused on its depressant properties. There is a passage in the *Odyssey* that describes how grief and sorrow for companions who died in the Trojan War were drowned in the "drink of oblivion" called "nepenthes." What is particularly telling about this story is that the attempts to relieve the pain of war—the symptoms of war trauma and combat stress—date back as early as the times of Homer. For the psychological costs of war are, we are told by psychiatrists and anthropologists, similar today as they were over 2,000 years ago, since these emotions and feelings are inherent to humankind. Helen offers nepenthes, a "liquid relief of trauma," to the son of Odysseus, Telemachus, who over the course of his long journey in search of his father comes to the court of her husband King Menelaus. The poem reads:

> Then other things were devised by Helen the daughter of great Zeus:
> straightway into the wine they were drinking she cast an elixir
> banishing sorrow and anger and ridding the mind of all evils.
> He who swallowed the potion when it had been mixed in the wine bowl
> would not shed any tears from his cheeks for the day that he drank it,
> even although his mother and father had both of them perished,
> even although his brother or much loved son in his presence
> were to be killed with a sword, while he with his eyes was observing.
> Such were the subtle and excellent drugs that the daughter of Zeus had.[3]

Contrary to what had previously been thought, nepenthes, the drink that quiets all pains and quarrels, was not hashish but opium. The Greeks dissolved it in alcohol, obtaining a mixture that was later known as "laudanum" (the name derived from the Latin *laudare* meaning "praise"), a splendid opium tincture invented around 1525 by Paracelsus, the famous "father of modern pharmacology." In the 1760s laudanum was popularized by Thomas Sydenham, the English doctor reckoned to be the founder of modern clinical medicine. He based his alcoholic opium tincture on sherry; strong wine; port, or other liquor, made of spices such as cinnamon, saffron, and cloves.[4] Paracelsus, who referred to opium as "the stone of immortality," declared: "I possess a secret remedy which I call laudanum and which is superior to all other heroic remedies."[5] To return to antiquity, the Greeks used the solution of opium in alcohol not only in the aftermath of battle—to calm down their nerves, quiet their sorrows, cope with grief, and relieve hateful memories—they might also have taken it in advance, to inspire greater courage in warriors going into battle, which is highly probable given the use made of opium by athletes.[6]

In his remarkable book *Odysseus in America* (2002), Jonathan Shay offers an analysis of veterans of the Vietnam War generation through the lens of one of Homer's great poems. Shay's is a moving interpretation. He reads the *Odyssey* as a grand, epic allegory of a warrior's long and tormented homecoming and finds a detailed description and examination of the plentiful hazards, challenges, and problems that warriors returning home have to face. One such challenge is war trauma. It manifests in the profoundly disturbing memories of the battlefield experience and horrific images stored in the veteran's visual memory, which torture the psyche when they appear involuntarily. What often makes homecoming particularly difficult is the return to the family, as relatives generally do not and cannot understand that the person they welcome back is not the same one who left for war. Veterans frequently turn to drugs as a means of self-medication—for coping with severe emotional problems and repressing harmful memories. This, in turn, provokes new difficulties, particularly that of addiction. Homer portrays this remarkably well in Book 9 of the *Odyssey*. The fruit of the lotus tree, which induces a pleasant state of relief, numbness, and drowsiness, is the only food eaten by the inhabitants of the Island of Lotus-eaters, to which Odysseus and his decimated fellows arrive at some point of their journey back home. Thus we read:

> For these comrades of ours, those Lotus-eaters devised no
> loss or destruction but gave them flowers of lotus to feed on.
> Any of them who ate of the honey-sweet fruit of the lotus
> wished no more to return us a message or take his departure;
> rather, they wanted to stay right there with the lotus-eating
> people to feed on lotus and always forget their returning.[7]

The addictive potential of the lotus turns out to be so great that Odysseus must exert force to prevent his men from staying on the island. He binds them and drags them to the ships; only then can they leave for the onward journey. The lotus symbolizes a narcotic that brings relief, albeit simultaneously a powerful habit-forming substance that may trap veterans on their road back to civilian life. The fellows whom Odysseus sends to check the land of the lotus become so attracted by the plant of forgetfulness and alleviation that they no longer wish to return home. Thus intoxicants, in a word, can significantly slow down the journey to Ithaca, which taken literally stands for home. When read metaphorically, the story can be seen as a convenient allegory of the civilian world or society at large. The problem with drugs is that, having a powerful appeal as a means of coping with the symptoms of trauma, as the miracle elixir of oblivion, they soon emerge as a formidable obstacle to adjusting to civilian life. Jonathan Shay superbly sums up the essence of the lotus (i.e., the addiction) story: "You get into lotus abuse and you lose your homecoming. Forget your pain—forget your homecoming!"[8] The narcotic lotus not only offers a false forgetfulness, but it also precludes Odysseus and his crew from a true comeback or, at best, considerably delays their return.

The Assassins and the Archetype of the Non-Western Intoxicated Warrior and Terrorist

> The Assassins no longer appear as a gang of drugged dupes led by scheming impostors, as a conspiracy of nihilistic terrorists, or as a syndicate of professional murderers. They are no less interesting for that.
>
> —Bernard Lewis, *The Assassins: A Radical Sect in Islam*

The popular stories go that the premodern Muslim terrorists of the Nizari Ismaili group regularly got high on hashish. It was for this very reason that they were initially referred to as *hashishi, hashishiyya,* or *hashishiyyin* (from the Arabic word *al-hasziszijjin,* meaning "hashish eaters"). The oldest known written source describing the group as *hashishiyya* dates probably to 1123.[9] It was Christian crusaders returning from Syria to Europe who called them the "Assassins," and this word entered many languages. The English term "assassination" means a religious or politically motivated murder committed in an abrupt or secretive attack.[10] And this was precisely how the Nizaris killed their victims. The legend has it that the Assassins took intoxicants for spiritual stimulation and to sharpen their minds. Drugged with hashish, utterly devoted to the sect, particularly its leader, and blindly committed to their faith, they were ready to give their lives for the cause of radical Islam. They were calculating, competent, ruthless, disciplined, unbribable, and fanatical.[11] But was this really due to intoxication?

The Nizari Ismaili was established in the 1080s as a radical sect of Shia Muslims, a minority within a minority. After the group captured the Alamut castle in Persia in 1090, the fortress became its main base. At first, the Assassins fought against the Sunni but later also against the Christian crusaders in the area of today's Syria and Iran. The sect survived until its decisive defeats in the second half of the thirteenth century at the hands of both the Mongols and the Mamluks. For over two centuries the ferociously anti-Sunni and extremely anti-Christian Nizaris had terrorized the Middle East. Their principal purpose was to disrupt and destroy the Sunni order, and they sought to achieve this through their basic method of action: assassination. Their tactics were based on treacherous killings, usually carried out with a dagger by the fedayeen (*fidai*), that is, those "committed to the cause" who occupied the lowest level in the seven-grade scale of initiation. Today, they would perhaps be called hitmen, but for centuries they have been perceived as the archetypal religious terrorists.

In the Western imagination, these young fighters were habitual hashish users. The drug was long believed to put them into a narcotic trance, thus helping to overcome fear before their murderous actions. In the twentieth century, however, this formerly prevalent view has been called into question. It was probably the Nizaris' fanatical bravery, writes David Morgan, and the fact that they rarely attempted to escape after committing a killing that gave rise to the popular belief that the group operated under the influence of drugs.[12] Perhaps these stories were made up and promulgated by their antagonists to discredit the Assassins. It is likely that the Westerners mistakenly grasped the meaning of *hashishiyya*. And it was this false understanding that came into being in Europe. The twelfth century brought numerous Muslim treatises on the adverse effects of hashish, which was widely claimed to cause severe harmful physical and mental changes in the body. More importantly, however, it was believed to destroy religious faith and undermine morality. Hashish was, in a word, corrupting. So addicts were assigned a low social status and were often treated as heretics and criminals. The description of the Nizaris as *hashishiyya*, insists Farhad Daftry, was not literal but rather metaphorical and symbolic, for what it emphasized was not their secret use of hashish. Instead, it indicated their low social position, amorality, profanity, and the nature of the real threat they posed to Islam.[13] The very term "hashish-eaters" was used to pompously reveal that the group did not adhere to the principles of Islam, acted extravagantly, and had very extreme views. In a word it located itself outside Islam proper. For, as Franz Rosenthal reflected in his study on hashish and medieval Muslim society, the herb "may have been not as dirty as wine by nature, but the general opinion was that it made the addict physically dirty."[14] Hence hashish-eater was a deeply offensive name. In fact, none of the surviving Islamic sources charged the group with the habitual use of psychoactive substances.[15]

There are two basic arguments that debunk the popular image of the Assassins as drugged terrorists. The first is that the typical effects of hashish, such as insensibility, relaxation, and decreased aggression, do not necessarily facilitate the accomplishment of the demanding and precise task of assassination. Because the fedayeen's tactics required them to patiently hole up for long hours awaiting a good opportunity to attack, they would need a stimulant rather than a sedative. And hashish is a downer that impairs rather than enhances concentration. If the Nizaris were primed with hashish before going on their missions, they would not have been the perfect killers that they were.[16] The second argument is that the group was extremely ascetic, just like its leader Hassan-i Sabbah. The most telling testimony to his austerity and purity of morals is the execution of one of his sons, who had to die after being accused of drinking wine as alcohol was strictly forbidden in Islam. Although when compared to drinking, hashish was seen as a lesser evil, no narcotic consumption was allowed at Assassin castles in Persia. Hence the free, not to say deliberate, use of drugs by the group seems highly improbable.

Rather than hashish, the Nizaris' truly powerful intoxicant was their deep religious faith, coupled with crazed fanaticism. What propelled them to action were a sacred duty and the need to bring the divine message to the infidel. Thus violence grew into a sacramental duty, fulfilled in obedience to the ultimate teleological imperative. What strongly motivated the fedayeen to give their own lives was the promise of a heavenly prize after death. They were led to believe they would go straight to paradise, where Allah would reward them with dozens of beautiful virgins.

There was probably little truth in the commonplace belief, which persisted in the West down through the centuries, that after the great master (the legendary Old Man of the Mountain) selected the fedayeen for the next mission, they were drugged and removed to a beautiful secret "heavenly garden." In the West it was Marco Polo who, on recounting his visit to Persia in 1273, reinforced the legend that the Assassins used narcotics. There is a key passage in his *Description of the World* (1299):

> Sometimes the Old Man, when he wished to kill any lord who made war or was his enemy, made them put some of these youths into that Paradise . . . For he had opium to drink given them by which they fell asleep and as if half dead immediately as soon as they had drunk it, and they slept quite three days and three nights. Then he had them taken in this sleep and put into that garden of his . . . And when the youths were waked up and they find themselves in there and see themselves in so fine a place . . . and the damsels were round each one always, and all the day were singing and playing and making all the caresses and dalliance which they could imagine, giving them food and most delicate wines, so that intoxicated with so many pleasures and with the little streams of milk and wine which they saw, they believe that they are most truly in Paradise.[17]

Having spent some time in the wonderful garden they were drugged again, put asleep, and moved to the great master's palace. After waking up from their narcotic-induced sleep, they recounted the paradise that they had visited and "how they had great desire to return there" permanently. When the Old Man wanted to kill someone, according to the legend, he sent those fedayeen who already knew that if they died, they would immediately go to paradise, an earthly foretaste of that which they had already experienced. Thus, writes Marco Polo, "none feared death . . . and they exposed themselves like madmen to every manifest danger, wishing to die together with the king's enemy and despising the present life," crazily desperate to return to paradise for good.[18] Polo himself, who for twenty-two years traveled through Asia, continued the rich tradition of myth-making narratives on the Assassins. Among his predecessors were such influential figures as Benjamin of Tudela (1167), Burchard of Strasbourg (1175), Arnold of Lübeck (before 1210), and James of Vitry (c. 1216–1228).[19] All of them drew an image of the Nizaris that became built into European culture as a powerful myth. Marco Polo significantly added to this myth, telling yet another version of it, and contributed meaningfully to the growth of the Assassins legend. The story of the Old Man of the Mountains and his frenzied followers thus became deeply rooted in the Western imagination. It reproduced itself over the following centuries and survived essentially untouched into the nineteenth century. When in May 1809 the prominent French linguist and orientalist Silvestre de Sacy spoke at the Institut de France, he confirmed that the term "assassin" derived from the Arab word for "hashish."[20] Reinforced by the authority figure, the myth continued to flourish, inspiring among others Charles Baudelaire, who in his *Poem of Hashish* (1860) wrote:

> I will not repeat his story of how the Old Man of the Mountain, having first intoxicated them with hashish (whence Hashishins or Assassins), locked up, in a garden full of delights, those of his youngest disciples to whom he wished to give an idea of paradise, as a glimpse, so to speak, of the reward they would earn for their passive and unreflective obedience.[21]

Even if, as Bernard Lewis insists, and I agree with him, the Assassins did not boost themselves with hashish before attacking their victims, even if they did not use narcotics (be it opium or hashish) to send the fedayeen to sleep and manipulate their consciousness, there still remains a powerful legend. Most crucially of all, this legend grew into a peculiar archetype of the fanatical, vicious, fearless, and intoxicated non-Western warrior, terrorist, and partisan. In a premodern manner it brings together politics, religion, violence, and drugs. What is essential about an archetype, as Mircea Eliade reminds us, is the historical recurrence of specific patterns of human behavior and thought, for it embodies their social, cultural, and political "reproduction."[22] In essence, it is all about the intergenerational imitation of customs, practices, and behavioral patterns. Carl Gustav Jung, who developed the notion of the psychological archetype, explained that the concept can never be reduced to a single formula. This is simply because an archetype is a sort of vessel that cannot be completely emptied or filled. There is always some room left for a new reading, for a new meaning. An archetype is a possibility, a potentiality that materializes by taking on a different, distinct shape in a particular age. It remains in a state of constant flux, always ready to emerge as an enriched reflection of the original pattern. For Jung, not only was an archetype inherent to consciousness, but it was also intrinsically dynamic in the sense of its incessantly changing form. It is continually reinterpreted and translated into the language and symbols congruent with the specific historical stage of culture. Thus the archetype of drugged, savage non-Western warriors revealed itself, for example, in the indigenous peoples fighting with the imperial armies through the period of Western expansion in the nineteenth century. And today it reveals itself in the religious-motivated postmodern terrorists, insurgents, and members of other violent nonstate armed groups.

The Mushroom-Eaters

In a letter from a native of Zurich in 1799, in which year a Russian army under Korsakov was stationed there, the amazing statement was made that the Russians gathered and ate fly amanitas on the Zürichberg [a wooden hill overlooking Lake Zürich]. Of course, the Russians must have learned to do this in their own country.
—C. Hartwich, 1911 quoted in Valentina Pavlovna Wasson and R. Gordon Wasson, *Mushrooms, Russia and History*

The indigenous inhabitants of the North Asian steppe, particularly the Siberian tribes of Chukchi, Yakuts, Yukaghirs, Kamchadals, Koryaks, and Khanty, belonged to the peoples whom Valentina Pavlovna Wasson and Gordon Wasson, prominent experts on the role of mushrooms in various cultures and societies around the world, called the "mycophilic peoples" or the mushroom lovers, in direct contrast to the "mycophobic peoples."[23] They used muscimol, the psychoactive constituent contained in the *Amanita muscaria* mushroom. It was the German Dominican philosopher Albert the Great (Albertus Magnus) who, in the thirteenth century, discovered the poisonous property of the fungus, which attracts flies to kill them with its toxins, and gave it its popular name of "fly agaric." "He fed some flies with milk," writes Maguelonne Toussaint-Samat, "in which he had infused pieces of the fungus;

not one of them survived."[24] In Siberia the fungus was not eaten raw but either swallowed as a dried ball, eaten as a mushroom soup, or consumed soaked in a fermented brew of the Siberian northern bilberry. The raw mushroom has mild psychoactive properties, but when dried it develops potent neurotoxic effects, because in the process of decarboxylation, one of its compounds, ibotenic acid, is converted into muscimol, the alkaloid which is a sedative-hypnotic agonist of the GABA receptors. The toadstool was therefore eaten dried, because in this form it assumes the ultimate potency to anesthetize, improve stamina, and sharpen the brain. In essence, muscimol has both a powerful boosting and a strong hallucinogenic effect. A proper dose of *Amanita muscaria* provides such potent motor stimulation that initially the intoxicated person cannot control an overwhelming need to move. The first hallucinations are experienced about fifteen minutes after the ingestion of the mushroom. However, when the effects of muscimol fade away, some acute symptoms of hangover occur: numbness, sleeplessness, exhaustion, and headaches.[25]

According to a Chukchee myth, there is a cosmic link between *Amanita muscaria* and thunder. In their monumental study *Mushrooms, Russia and History*, the Wassons write that "lightning is a One-Sided Man who drags his sister along by her foot. As she bumps along the floor of heaven, the noise of her bumping makes the thunder. Her urine is the rain and she is possessed by the spirits of the fly amanita."[26] The picture of fly agaric growing in the place hit by lightning is popular in numerous Eurasian myths, tales, and legends. Over fifty distinct species of this hallucinogenic fungus occur in Europe, Asia, Africa, and North America. In almost the whole of Eurasia—from Scandinavia to Kamchatka—*Amanita muscaria* was used for ceremonial and cultural purposes (mostly in shamanistic rituals), for recreation and stimulation, and, at times, also at orgies. More important, the mushroom was also regularly taken by warriors, bestowing upon them the power of a thunderbolt.

Because in the Siberian intertribal trade the dried fly agaric was very expensive (a single specimen could be worth as much as a few reindeer), only the wealthy could afford it. Yet the poor discovered relatively early a truly outstanding feature of the fungus: the urine of its eater retains surprisingly strong psychoactive properties since muscimol is not affected by the kidney-filtration process. Equally important is the fact that urine is cleared of the toxic alkaloids contained in the mushroom. Thus, remarkably, drinking the urine of an eater of *Amanita muscaria* not only produced an almost equally strong psychoactive effect but was also much safer. To quote Richard Rudgley: "This property was known to many Siberians, who avidly drank their own or others' urine to achieve a state of intoxication, much to the disgust of many Russians and other observers of this curious custom."[27] The Swedish officer Philip Johan von Strahlenberg, who explored Siberia geographically and anthropologically during his long years as a prisoner of war after being captured at the battle of Poltava in 1709, was the first European to describe this astonishing practice, which aroused almost as much disgust as interest among foreigners. In 1730 he reported:

> When they make a feast, they pour water upon some of the mushrooms, and boil them. Then they drink the liquor, which intoxicates them. The poorer sort . . . post themselves round the huts of the rich, and watch for the opportunity of the guests coming down to make water; and then hold a wooden bowl to receive the urine, which they drink off greedily, as having still some virtue of the mushroom in it, and by this way they also get drunk.[28]

The urine of one person who had eaten *Amanita muscaria* could produce a mind-altering effect in up to six other men.[29] Moreover, when the psychoactive effects of mushroom eating faded away, to prolong the state of inebriation people often drank their own intoxicating urine.

This practice of collecting and drinking urine was very popular among the Siberian warriors, especially on the eve of battle. Muscimol significantly enhanced their fighting performance for, according to oral tradition, it raised stamina without affecting mental acuity.[30] Legends and tales say that those tribes who ate *Amanita muscaria* produced truly fierce and brutal "mushroom warriors." Despite marching long distances with heavy loads, they still showed extreme endurance in battle. Intoxicated and vicious, they fought and won in a battle frenzy.

The most fearless and ferocious fighters are, however, known from the history of the Vikings. This elite caste of Germanic warriors was called the "berserks" after the mythical Berserk. The legend has it that this mighty hero of the old Scandinavian (Norse) mythology, the grandson of the eight-handed Starkadder, went into battle only in bearskin (*ber sark*), without any armor, and fought with reckless boldness and fury.[31] The "berserks," who appear in many sagas and poems and whose existence is attested to in various iconographic sources, wore the skins and fur of wild animals, and—just like the mythical Berserk—were fierce, raging, and madly courageous.

The eighteenth century gave rise to a theory explaining the way in which the fearless Scandinavian warriors worked themselves into a state of nearly uncontrollable, trance-like fury. In 1784 Samuel Lorenzo Ødman, after comparing the descriptions of the *berserksgang* (berserk-raging) with the stories about mushroom intoxication among the Siberian tribes, especially the Koryaks, came to the conclusion that they both behaved similarly. He supposed that berserks must have induced in themselves the state of amok by eating *Amanita muscaria.* "I am inclined to believe," wrote Ødman, "that the Berserks had knowledge about such an intoxicating means, and that they made use of it and kept it secret so that their prestige would not be reduced by the general populace's knowledge of the simplicity of the technique."[32] His thesis seemed further confirmed by sources which indicated that after a wild battle frenzy, berserks insulated themselves from the world and rested for a couple of days in a state of numbness and hangover. They might, indeed, have suffered from mushroom poisoning. In addition Ødman, a theologian at Uppsala University, also found religious links between the Siberian tribes and Scandinavian berserks. His point was that Odin, the main Norse god of war and warriors, was introduced to Scandinavia by peoples who migrated from Asia. According to the mythology, the Norse berserks, that is, the best of warriors, were chosen by Odin, who gave them fury by making them like wild animals.[33]

In the late nineteenth century, the prominent Norwegian physician and botanist Frederik Christian Schübeler agreed with Ødman's thesis that prior to battle berserks drank a ritual drink made of fly agaric. In 1994, however, John Mann came to the conclusion that berserk-raging might have been induced by *Amanita pantherina* rather than by *Amanita muscaria*. While the latter induces hallucinations, the former contains higher levels of muscimol. The greater concentration of psychoactive constituents in *Amanita pantherina*, which is known to produce mania, makes this fungus a better candidate for explaining the berserks' battle fury and their sensation of turning into wild animals.[34] The hallucinations induced by the ingestion of *Amanita* mushrooms are perhaps similar to those caused by the plants of the *Solanaceae* family, which contain such alkaloids as atropine, scopolamine, and hyoscyamine. One feature of the psychosis induced by these plants is, as the noted German toxicologist Erich Hesse put it in 1946, "that the intoxicated person imagines himself to have been changed into some animal, and the hallucinosis is completed by the sensation of the growing of feathers and hair, due probably to the main paraesthesia."[35]

Although some authors continue to claim that it was not intoxicants that transformed warriors into berserks but their exceptional psychopathic personalities and a remarkable ability to produce psychotic states (something along the lines of shamanic ecstasy) further reinforced by religious rituals, the Ødman-Schübeler thesis has gained popular academic recognition in Scandinavia. In this view, it was psychoactive agents that enabled a magical transformation of warriors into berserks.[36] Hence the ideal of a sturdy and brave warrior, who wreaks terror and death, fights in a wild frenzy, and is capable of superhuman effort and deeds, came into being through deliberate intoxication. It was an important, though of course not the only, factor behind the phenomenon of *berserksgang*.

Berserks seemed to be invulnerable to the blows of their enemies, almost insensible of wounds. The local people were desperately afraid of their attacks and raised their prayers: "God save us from the Fury of the Northmen." In the Western tradition, berserks have been closely associated with the terrifying image of the pagan warrior-beast. Schübeler described them in the following words:

> In the old Norwegian historical writings it is mentioned, in many places, that in olden times there was a specific kind of giants who were called *Berserks*, that is, men who at certain times were seized by a wild fury, which, at the moment, doubled their strength and made them insensible to bodily pain, but which also deadened their humanity and reason, and made them like wild animals ... Men who were thus seized performed things which otherwise seemed impossible for human power. This condition is said to have begun with shivering, chattering of the teeth, and chill in the body, and then the face swelled and changed its color. With this was connected a great hotheadedness, which at last went over into a great rage, under which they howled as wild animals, bit the edge of their shields, and cut down everything they met, without discriminating between friend or foe. When this condition ceased, a great dulling of the mind and feebleness followed, which could last for one or several days.[37]

The English word "berserk," meaning "wild," "crazed," "violently frenzied," but also "battle frenzy," derives from the name of the premedieval and medieval Scandinavian "furious warriors." For when a warrior goes berserk, his humanity regresses to animal divinity or divine animalism. Often infuriated by the death of his fellow comrades-in-arms, a frenzied warrior loses control and with no inhibition whatsoever burns with a desire for revenge. Not paralyzed by fear but feeling empowered by a divine might, he wreaks astonishing slaughter by causing brutal death and destruction. In the frenzy of battle he often violates the norms and principles essential to the warrior ethos, sometimes also betraying his own honor. Running amok or berserk is quite common in the heat of combat; it is, in fact, universal among men at war since it may happen to any soldier in the field. Achilles, a "wild god," embodies the prototype, if not the archetype, of such a pattern of battlefield behavior. While seeking to avenge the death of Patroclus, his close friend and, as some argue, also his lover, he goes berserk. In the darkness of his fury Achilles turns to outrage and defiles Hector's body. He first allows others to mutilate the corpse and then hitches it to his chariot and drags it around the walls of Troy in view of Hector's family.

In his animal-like conduct the great Achilles deviates from the Greek warrior ethos, which assumed that the enemy should be hated but must be respected. Homer seeks to portray here Achilles as an antihero, an antiexemplary figure. But we must also acknowledge that the ancient Greek idea of a hero was immensely complex and deeply mixed. A hero was both needed by the people (by fighting courageously he secured their survival and well-being), and dangerous to them (his impetuous character and fierce behavior often brought death to bystanders). Achilles is one such example—he went against his own army in the Trojan War because his withdrawal resulted in many Greek deaths. Or take the case of Odysseus, who, in the course of his incredibly long journey home to Ithaca, made many unwise and fateful decisions, causing the death of most of his companions. Jonathan Shay seized upon this point to argue that "Achilles harmed the Greek army during the war; Odysseus harmed his people after the war."[38] Yet they were both great Greek heroes. A hero embodies the best and worst in humanity.

Descriptions of battle frenzy quite frequently occur in the literature on war. Consider the memoirs of the Vietnam War veterans, one of whom wrote: "December 22, 1967, is the day that the civilized me became an animal . . . I was a fucking animal."[39] A berserk person not only loses control over himself and his violent behavior but, most crucially of all, also loses his human face. Lawrence Tritle reminds us that running amok, indiscriminate killing, and mutilation of the body of the enemy has been known across time and culture. Certainly, "it is not something that only primitives practice. It is in fact a very human thing."[40] What usually triggers the berserking of fighting men under fire is the death of a comrade-in-arms, friend, or a relative. Today's example of berserking is pictured in Nick Broomfield's film, based on real events, *Battle for Haditha* (2008). In November 2005 a U.S. Marine corporal well liked by his colleagues was killed by a roadside bomb in the city of Haditha in Iraq. His crazed and furious companions took savage revenge by indiscriminately attacking civilians who lived on a nearby hill, killing twenty-four people, including nine women, five children, and a crippled old man in a wheelchair. It is easy to qualify their act as a war crime. For those observers who have never heard of war amok, battle frenzy, or going berserk, this was but a savage murder. Yet, notwithstanding criminal liability, it was a striking example of men going berserk under fire—a mental condition that involves immensely complex psychophysical and neurobiochemical reactions. Jonathan Shay offers an ambiguous, yet even still more telling, comment on berserk-raging:

No one has ever drawn a syringe of blood or cerebrospinal fluid from a berserk warrior nor mapped the electrical activities of his nervous system. No one knows how much of the large literature on the physiology of extreme stress can be applied to berserking, on which there is no established physiological literature. It is plain that the berserker's brain and body function are as distant from everyday function as his mental state is from everyday thought and feeling.[41]

For berserking is like getting intoxicated—it strengthens physical endurance and stamina by using up the body's reserves of energy, reduces the feeling of pain, lessens stress, and eases fear. Most crucially of all, it removes both physical and moral restraints, which, in turn, often lead to unpredictable behavior. The point is that berserks are intoxicated endogenously by the cocktail of biochemical substances produced in their bodies, mainly in their brains. Even so, prior to running amok they have often hopped themselves up exogenously, so that their battle madness is drug-induced in a double sense.

Let me return to the "mushroom warriors." The extraordinary courage, and often bravado, of both Siberian and Scandinavian fighters might have also resulted from one of the hallucinogenic effects of fly agaric: micropsy. This produces a distorted perception of the surroundings as significantly diminished, which, in turn, brings greater self-confidence and a feeling of omnipotence over a tiny and feeble foe—micropsy shrinks the world to a less threatening size. But muscimol can also produce the opposite effect, called macropsy, which is the perception of objects as considerably larger than normal. Many researchers link the origins of unnaturally tiny creatures that inhabit the worlds of fairy tales, folktales, and legends precisely with this perception-altering property of hallucinogenic mushrooms. *Amanita muscaria* is also one of the favorite themes of the illustrators of fairy stories. So are dwarfs, whose headwear usually looks like a mushroom head. Thus have literary stories clearly been inspired by the hallucinogenic effects of fly agaric. Consider Lewis Carroll, who carefully studied the works on fungi by the English botanist and mycologist Mordecai Cubitt Cooke. John Mann points out that Carroll's description of the psychoactive effects of hallucinogenic fungi "is so accurate that it is tempting to speculate that he may have experienced the effects himself."[42] It was probably micropsy that influenced him to write *Alice's Adventures in Wonderland* (1865) and *Through the Looking-Glass* (1871). A kind of leitmotif of these books is that the girl grows and shrinks after eating a piece of mushroom and other things, like cakes. Take, for example, this passage describing the aftermath of taking a bite of a mushroom: Alice

> nibbled a little of the right-hand bit to try the effect. The next moment she felt a violent blow underneath her chin: it had struck her foot! She was a good deal frightened by this very sudden change, but she felt

that there was no time to be lost, as she was shrinking rapidly: so she set to work at once to eat some of the other bit.[43]

The motifs inspired by the influence of fungi upon man are also evident in *Gulliver's Travels* (1726) by Jonathan Swift, whose characters include the tiny Lilliputians and the giant Brobdingnanians. It looks as though Swift was also fairly familiar with or had even experienced micropsy and macropsy as induced by *Amanitas*. Yet one might wonder what the worlds of fairy tales have to do with the mushroom warriors. Well, the berserks who fought hooked on *Amanita muscaria* or *Amanita pantherina* must have experienced the world in exactly the same way as does Gulliver in the country of the Lilliputians—they must have felt an overwhelming predominance over a weak and miniscule enemy. In a word, they turned into giants, excelling their adversary in every single respect.

The use of "magic mushrooms" by fighting men has also been recorded in modern history. Consider these few examples. The Tatars produced a special drink made of hemp and *Amanita muscaria*, which they drank before combat to induce trance-like fury and raise the spirits.[44] During the war between Sweden and Norway in 1814, some Swedish soldiers of the Varmland regiment were reported to be fighting hopped-up, most likely on *Amanita muscaria*, "seized by a raging madness, foaming at the mouth."[45] And in 1945 a group of Soviet infantrymen, perhaps Siberian, was intoxicated with the mushroom and performed equally fearlessly at the battle of Székesfehérvár in Hungary. They were said to be fighting in a wild frenzy like "rabid dogs" and then falling into a deep sleep.[46] Even if we never ultimately find enough evidence to confirm the authenticity of these stories, the very existence of such oral traditions affirms how firmly rooted in culture the archetype of the intoxicated, mad warrior has been.

Controversies aside, there is plenty of evidence to support the claim that it was psychoactive mushrooms, originally used mainly in religious ceremonies, that helped create the famous great warriors of Siberia and Scandinavia. To sum up, fly agaric became a meaningful part of the sociocultural history of psychedelics, as it played an interesting role not only in rituals and fiestas but also in warfare. The coca plant served similar functions for the people in South America. Very much like *Amanita muscaria*, it originally played a sacred and magical role, but its use was more widespread while its intoxicating effect was far weaker (the plant served as a mild stimulant). Westerners discovered coca leaves during the conquest of South America, brought them to Europe, and later made them widely popular in the purified and intensified form of cocaine. This development from coca to cocaine, however, took the Europeans three and a half centuries.

The Incas and Their Invigorating Coca

When the whites came, our ancestors consulted the Sun God. He
told them to trust in the coca leaf. The coca will feed you and cure
you, he said, and give you the strength to survive. . . . I ask God to
give us always plenty of coca.
—A Peruvian Indian in the film *Coca Mama: The War on Drugs*, 2001

In 1499, on his first encounter with the Indians on the coast of what is today
Venezuela, Amerigo Vespucci was absolutely astonished to see the locals pas-
sionately chewing a weed. In a diary of his second voyage he wrote that the
Indians reminded him of cattle constantly chewing their cuds. He reported:

> They were very brutish in appearance and gesture, and they had their
> mouths full of the leaves of green herb, which they continually chewed
> like beasts, so they could hardly speak; and each had round his neck
> two dry gourds, one full of that herb which they had in their mouths,
> and the other of white flour that appeared to be powdered lime.[47]

We should not be surprised that for Vespucci, the eminent Florentine, the customs and behavior of the natives were barbarous and strange. While he and
his companions could not understand this weird habit of the locals, Francisco
Pizarro shed more light on the issue. During his conquest of Peru in 1533,
he discovered that the "green herb" chewed by the Inca warriors was coca
leaves and, most crucially of all, that the plant enabled them to fight off fatigue,
increase endurance, and build up resistance to pain. Today we know that they
had been doing so for several thousand years.

In 1566 Juan Matieza de Peralta made the persuasive remark, "Without coca
there would be no Peru."[48] He was right, for without coca the pre-Columbian
Inca civilization may not have survived at the altitudes in which it had developed and flourished. The legend says that the coca plant was the gift of gods;
it was therefore assigned a magic meaning and used mainly by warlocks
and soothsayers. In the Incan culture, coca served many other crucial functions too, namely religious and ritualistic (from the thirteenth century it was
regarded as a divine plant, indispensable in spiritual ceremonies and sacrificial
rituals), therapeutic (commonly used as a means of preventing disease), and
energizing (a traditional physical enhancer during exhausting activities). The
stimulating, invigorating, antidepressant, and anesthetizing properties of the
leaves could be reduced to this formula: coca gives power and alleviates hunger, thirst, and the feeling of cold. Coca leaves contain not only many valuable
vitamins (particularly vitamin B), proteins, and minerals (mainly iron and cal-
cium), but also some fourteen alkaloids, including one-half to one percent of

cocaine. And it is cocaine that, by affecting the central nervous system, accelerates the use of inner energy stored in the body and at the same time reduces hunger, thirst, and fatigue.

The half-Andean Jesuit Blas Valera, son of a Spanish conquistador and a native Peruvian mother, writing in 1609 on the beneficial medical properties of coca, observed that it

> preserves the body from many infirmities, and our doctors use it pounded for applications to sores and broken bones, to remove cold from the body or to prevent it from entering . . . It is so beneficial and has such singular virtue in the cure of outward sores, it will surely have even more virtue and efficacy in the entrails of those who eat it![49]

Valera was not exaggerating, because coca allows for better performance, especially at high altitudes where the air is rarefied (about 3,600 meters above sea level), by speeding up the heart rate it improves respiratory function. On long missions the Inca messengers (*chasqui*) chewed coca leaves regularly, which immensely improved their endurance and stamina. Coca empowered them to cover as much as 240 kilometers a day. The *chasqui*, who also supplied the royal family with high-value goods, were exceptionally fast sprinters, so that, for example, fish caught in the Pacific "could be eaten in Cuzco the following day—300 miles from the coast and all uphill."[50] The sixteenth-century chronicles written by Pedro Cieza de León, José de Acosta, and Juan Montien contain records which confirm that the custom of chewing coca (known as *chacchar*) was a routine way of combating fatigue during high-altitude travels in the Andes. For example, in 1590 Father José de Acosta, a Spaniard Jesuit missionary, recorded that coca imbued the Indians with "force and courage."[51] All of these reported enhancing effects of coca were essentially the same as the ones that have always been highly prized and desired by the military. Unsurprisingly then, the Peruvian and Bolivian armies made substantial use of the leaves, especially during long and exhausting marches at high altitudes. The exceptional examples of the military application of coca include a Bolivian soldier who in 1837 managed, in just twenty days, to travel an incredible distance of 2,200 kilometers and, more remarkable still, arrived with no major signs of fatigue.[52]

Recent research and archaeological evidence suggest that chewing coca in South America began in at least 6000 BC.[53] In the Inca Empire the privilege of *chacchar* was at first exclusively limited to the Inca, peerage, and priests. Over time, however, it became slightly more widespread. During the conquest, the Catholic Church struggled to introduce a total ban on the use of coca, which initially also became a policy of the Spanish conquistadors. The Europeans realized that the only effective way of detaching the Indians from their "savage" Incan rituals was to deprive them of the right to use coca leaves. In 1569 the bishops' conference in Lima damned the plant, denouncing the habit of chewing it as evil. It was believed that by eliminating the ancient custom the colonizers would manage to destroy ancient Inca spirituality. Deprived of their identity the natives could, ultimately, be subdued. But when the conquistadors discovered that coca could help increase the productivity of their colonial slave workers and simultaneously cut down by 20 to 25 percent the necessary food rations, they quickly abandoned the policy of eradicating the coca habit. What followed was the ruthlessly pragmatic use of the boosting effects of coca and the centuries-old custom of *chacchar* by the Spanish colonists. Regular rations of the leaves helped improve the efficiency of the Incan workers at the mines located at 4,000 meters above sea level. The Creole plantation and mine owners gave their workers as many as three breaks a day to chew coca leaves.[54] By turning coca into a crude instrument for maximizing the productivity of the encomienda system (which allotted a certain amount of indigenous slave labor to the Spanish settlers), and thereby for multiplying profits, the colonists stripped coca of rite, religion, magic, and the social values that had previously accompanied its use.

Max Weber might have argued that coca was demagified by the inexorable march of Western instrumental rationality and its globalizing spillover. This was an inevitable effect of modernity. Of the original five major functions played by coca in the Inca culture, paramount importance was assigned to its role as a mild stimulant. There is a striking passage in Golden Mortimer's classic text *Peru: History of Coca* (1901) that sums up well this forced transformation of the coca habit in the Andes: "Labour was found to be utterly impossible without the use of Coca, so that the Indians were supplied with the leaves by their masters, just as so much fuel might be fed to an engine in order to produce a given amount of work."[55] Furthermore, in the process of its instrumentalization coca became a valuable currency. The Andean planters commonly paid their workers with the leaves, and this practice survived in some regions of the Andes to the twentieth century.[56] This, in turn, caused even further impoverishment of the Indians because they were not paid in cash and therefore could not buy food. Instead of coins, they were given coca leaves that alleviated hunger but did not satisfy it. The next step in the dual process of instrumentalization and demagification of coca was therefore its commercialization.

The Spanish conquest of the Inca Empire prompted the widespread use of coca, which changed under Spanish rule from being reserved for the use of privileged individuals of the elite into a stimulant for the masses. *Chacchar* ceased to be a festive ritual and turned into an everyday necessity. A strikingly similar historical change in the social role assigned to drug taking occurred in nineteenth-century China regarding opium. At first its smoking was limited to the ruling elites, but over time it became more common, if not almost universal. The British greatly contributed to this mass consumption of opium, which eventually led to the spread of large-scale abuse and addiction. What was at stake, however, were the interests of the British Empire (I will explore this story further in the third chapter).

The Americans too, with the utmost pragmatism, made instrumental use of the alkaloids contained in the coca leaves to maximize the productivity of quasi-slave workers. In an article published in 1912 in *Century* magazine the American physician Charles B. Towns reported that "in the Deep Southern States, overseers in the cotton fields were putting cocaine into (free) midday soup fed to fieldhands, the better to improve their output in the afternoon."[57] Thus the black laborers in the American cotton plantations shared a similar experience of coca(ine)-assisted exploitation with the Incan slaves working in the Andean silver mines. In 1902 an American medical journal mentioned one planter who, instead of the traditional allowance of whisky, issued his workforce regular rations of cocaine.[58] In fact, the cocaine habit spread to the South from New Orleans where, as early as the late 1880s, black stevedores began taking the drug to cope with harsh working conditions and the inhospitable climate. These poor and malnourished laborers soon discovered highly beneficial, invigorating effects of the stimulant. While on cocaine some could work as much as "seventy hours at a stretch without sleep or rest, in rain, in cold, and in heat."[59] And when these "cocaine workers" got drafted into the U.S. Army, they took their habit with them. Over time the use of cocaine by soldiers became such a pressing issue that during 1910–1912 military doctors published many articles urging that the army be cleaned of addicts. Nonetheless, the real convergence of coca and war dates back to the eighteenth century. So, let us go back in time.

Coca and the Siege of La Paz

Coca's performance-enhancing effects were widely recognized during the Indian revolt against Spanish rule in South America, particularly at the time of the anti-Spanish rebellion of Túpac Amaru II in the second half of the eighteenth century. Don Hipólita Unanue, the editor of *Mercurio Peruano* magazine, reported that a group of Indian warriors was tasked to get through one of the coldest plateaus in Bolivia to return to their division. During this extremely exhausting march they found themselves deprived of provisions and eventually "only those soldiers were in condition to fight who had from childhood been accustomed to always carry with them a pouch of Coca."[60] From March to the end of June, and again from August to mid-September 1781, a force of

40,000 rebels led by Julián Apasa Nina, known as Tupac Katari, laid siege to the Bolivian city of La Paz. As the encirclement continued, the Indian militants refused to carry on fighting unless they were regularly supplied with sufficient stocks of coca. Katari had no choice but to send special expeditions to bring the leaves from the Andean plantations. This was a brilliant decision as he contrived to prevent the revolt of his men, managing to maintain discipline, and combat performance.

Coca, which helped those involved endure the strenuousness of the long siege, was equally important for the besieging Indian troops and the besieged civilians, mostly the Spanish. Behind the city walls both the garrison soldiers and the populace endured the hardship of defense and stayed alive after the exhaustion of food stocks only through the chewing of leaves, which relieved hunger, thirst, and built up physical endurance. And the conditions in La Paz were truly extreme—up to 10,000 of the 25,000 people trapped behind the walls died, many starved to death. The commander of the city's defense recalled later that the starving people ate horses, mules, and donkeys; then they took to cats and dogs; and once there were no more animals left, they fed themselves with the bark of trees. Cases of cannibalism were also reported. Unsurprisingly, the large stocks of coca gathered in the city turned out to be a critical commodity for those who were lucky to survive. It was the first time that the power of coca was revealed to the world in such a spectacular way.

When the Jesuits' written reports of the dramatic events in La Paz reached Europe, they much intrigued the Westerners and were carefully studied, mostly by medical doctors and military men. What were the conclusions drawn from these accounts? In 1787 a Jesuit, Father Antonio Julián, came up with a fairly humanitarian, as he saw it, answer to the problem of the poor. He suggested that European paupers should be fed with coca leaves to suppress their hunger and thirst, and thereby reduce their frustration, discontent, and anger. In 1793 Don Pedro Nolasco Crespo encouraged the supply of coca to European seamen to sustain them during long and debilitating voyages.[61] And what of soldiers? A few more decades would pass before European militaries first seriously experimented with coca, the story that I continue in chapter 6.

Napoleon in Egypt and
the Adventures of Europeans
with Hashish

Can you imagine a state in which all the citizens get intoxicated with hashish? What citizens! What warriors! What legislators! Even in the Orient, where its use is so widespread, there are governments which have realised the necessity of banning it. Indeed, it is forbidden to man, on pain of degradation and intellectual death, to disturb the primordial conditions of his existence, and to destroy the equilibrium between his faculties and the environments in which they are destined to operate.

—Charles Baudelaire, "The Poem of Hashish"

The Europeans began to study the Jesuit testimonies on the amazingly empowering effects of coca at about the same time as the veterans of the famous but unfortunate Napoleon Bonaparte's Egyptian expedition were returning to France.

When, in June 1798, Napoleon arrived in Egypt, the conquest of which was thought as smoothing the way for an attack against British India, his Army of the Orient (*Armée d'Orient*) of 36,000 men faced the challenge of adapting not only to the local climate but also to Egyptian tradition, culture, and the local lifestyle, including drinking strong coffee and smoking water pipes. The strict ban on the use of alcohol turned out to be one of the most noticeable features of Islamic custom. It soon appeared to be an acute problem because, as we know, the armies of the eighteenth century were heavily "dependent" on daily rations of drink. The situation came to be even more discomforting, given that during the sea voyage to Egypt soldiers were issued as much as 0.7 of a liter of wine a day.[1] Nonetheless, the French troops quickly became familiar with the local equivalent of alcohol, that is, drinks and dishes made of hashish (a product produced from the resin of the flowering tops and leaf fragments of *Cannabis sativa*) and the habit of inhaling the vapors of roasting cannabis seeds. Its widespread availability and low price had made hashish the most popular hallucinatory substance commonly used by Muslims from the Middle Ages on. By strictly forbidding the use of alcohol, Islam had to offer its believers some kind of substitute and the choice fell on the intoxicating resin derived from cannabis.[2] The thirteenth-century jurist Alam-ad-din Ibn Shukr remarked:

> O soul, turn to amusement,
> For by play does a young man live.
> Do not get fed up with daily drunkenness.
> If it cannot be wine, let it be hashish.[3]

The practice of using cannabis for nutritional and medical purposes and, above all, as an intoxicant, originated in Central Asia. From Herodotus we learn that the Scythians discovered that hemp can be smoked and built special tents in which they roasted cannabis seeds with red-hot stones and got drugged on the smoke and odor. Indeed, as Baudelaire observed, "the pleasure they derived from it was so intense that it drew from them cries of joy."[4] Cannabis then moved down to India and Africa. In India, which can actually be called the world's first cannabis-oriented culture, the plant was used orally not only as a cure (to treat diseases like malaria and rheumatism) and relaxant (to ward off boredom) but also as an enhancer (to combat fatigue, especially during the harvest). To mitigate fear and increase energy before battle Hindu warriors drank *bhang*—a milk or water infusion of dried flowers from female cannabis plants, and leaves, seeds, and stems from male and female specimens, often mixed with sugar and black pepper.[5]

But what of Napoleon's army? In the course of the acclimatization and cultural adaptation of French soldiers, hashish promptly replaced alcohol as the military intoxicant of choice.[6] The commanders were, however, quick to observe that its use was undermining fighting power and jeopardizing the morale of the troops. Half a century later, Charles Baudelaire compared alcohol and hashish by pointing to the desirable effects of the former and the harmful impact of the latter. It is worth quoting at length the argument he put forward in his *On Wine and Hashish* (1851), as it illustrates the seriousness of the challenge that the French army faced in Egypt:

> On the one hand we have a drink that stimulates the digestion, fortifies the muscles, and enriches the blood. Even taken in great quantities, it will cause only slight disturbances. On the other hand we have a substance that troubles the digestion, weakens the physical constitution and may produce intoxication that lasts up to twenty-four hours. Wine exalts the will, hashish destroys it. Wine is physically beneficial,

hashish is a suicidal weapon. Wine encourages benevolence and socia-
bility. Hashish isolates. One is industrious, in a manner of speaking, the
other essentially indolent. . . . Finally wine is for those people engaged
in honest labour, those who are worthy of drinking it. Hashish is among
the solitary pleasures, and is favoured by miserable idlers. Wine is useful and produces fruitful results; hashish is useless and dangerous.[7]

Unsurprisingly then, the officers of the *Armée d'Orient* correctly recognized the
"uselessness and dangerousness" of hashish, which was generating laziness and
sluggishness among their men. For, as one writer put it, the drug "turns a lion
into a beetle and makes a proud man humble and a healthy man sick. If he eats, he
cannot get enough."[8] Determined to maintain the esprit de corps of the troops,
they sought to somehow provide them with their traditional, well-known, and
much less dangerous companion and comforter, alcohol. So the army commissioned the construction of a factory for the production of brandy and rum. Soon
stills for making alcohol from dates, one of the most common fruits in Egypt,
were set up. Soldiers became fond of the beverages, and the business quickly
proved profitable.[9] Although the drink satisfied their needs, the troops did not
want to give up hashish as the pleasures induced by cannabis were more intense
and of a different kind than the ones produced by alcohol. Above all, many soldiers had become habituated to hashish, for once tried it is difficult to do without
it. In order to prevent disobedience and the demoralization of his men, which
could have called into question the prospects of the entire campaign, Napoleon
issued a prohibitive order. Signed relatively late, in October 1800, it was intended
to discipline the troops and dissuade soldiers from inducing altered states of consciousness by using local hashish products. There is a passage that comes to mind
in this context in Baudelaire's "Poem of Hashish" that supports these regulatory
measures: "Hashish, like all solitary joys, makes a man useless to other men, and
society superfluous to the individual, impelling him to admire himself cease-
lessly and propelling him day by day towards the gleam of the abyss in which he
may admire his face like Narcissus."[10] Therefore, the threat to fighting power and
military discipline was quite real and grave.

Napoleon's anti-hashish order aimed to prevent the army from being
reduced to a clumsy "cluster of beetles." The following excerpt makes us realize how significant was the problem the army command had to deal with:

Article 1. Throughout Egypt the use of a beverage prepared by certain
Moslems from hemp (hashish), as well as the smoking of the seeds of hemp,
is prohibited. Habitual smokers and drinkers of this plant lose their reason
and suffer from violent delirium in which they are liable to commit excesses
of all kinds.

Article 2. The preparation of hashish as a beverage is prohibited through-out Egypt. The doors of those cafés and restaurants where it is supplied are to be walled up, and their proprietors imprisoned for three months.

Article 3. All bales of hashish arriving at the customs shall be confiscated and publicly burnt.[11]

On examining this order one cannot help but have the impression of reading the guiding principles of today's war on drugs. The prohibition was absolute, as the importation, manufacture, sale, and consumption of hashish were for-bidden under threat of severe punishment. Still, the ban should be seen for what it was: the European invaders penalized practices that had been inherent to local tradition and customs from the early thirteenth century. What once had been part of the way of life in Egyptian society became considered evil and thus outlawed by the newcomers. Despite these repressive anti-hashish measures, however, in the spring–summer of 1801, the soldiers of the appar-ently demoralized French army were leaving Egypt, and they were taking home with them a hashish habit and the drug in plentiful supply to sustain it.

Napoleon's expedition was joined by a group of 151 scientists, members of the Commission of the Sciences and Arts. The task of these scholars, who today would be called "field anthropologists," was to explore and describe the secrets of Egyptian history, art, and technology; in short, to conduct a study on the ancient civilization of Egypt. They too were attracted by hashish and seduced by its intoxicating effect. To discover the secrets of processed cannabis resin, numerous samples were sent for analysis to laboratories in France.[12] A mem-ber of the Commission, the pharmacist Pierre-Charles Rouyer, reported in an article published in 1810 in the *Bulletin de Pharmacie*: "For the Egyptians, hemp is the plant par excellence, not for the uses they make of it in Europe and many other countries, but for its peculiar effects. The hemp cultivated in Egypt is indeed intoxicating and narcotic."[13] Thus Napoleon's campaign in the Orient made the Europeans interested not only in the history, art, and culture of Egypt but also in cannabis.

Curiously enough, British propaganda spread rumors that it was hash-ish that powerfully fueled the Napoleonic armies and enabled them to move quickly over vast distances and maneuver effectively in the hot Egyptian weather. Some British believed, then, that intoxication could bring victories, which was, of course, not true because hashish had exactly the opposite impact on the combat readiness and fighting effectiveness of the *Armée d'Orient*. Anyway, the French efforts to conquer Egypt and later also Algeria (in 1830–1847) were joined at the hip with the introduction and spread of hashish, first in France and then in the rest of Europe. The subsequent recreational use of cannabis followed.

Perhaps the earliest stories about the use of cannabis as a euphoriant came to Europe with knights returning from the Crusades, and it was Marco Polo who, in his *Description of the World*, popularized the knowledge of hashish. Nonetheless, the drug had not really been used in Europe until the end of Napoleon's Egyptian enterprise.[14] We might well ask why, in spite of the large-scale production and widespread use of hemp rope (mostly in shipping), which in Europe dated back to the first–second centuries AD, the Europeans had not themselves discovered the intoxicating properties of cannabis. This is especially striking given that for a long time they had been experimenting with various mind-altering substances. In the nineteenth century the German natural history scientist Ernst von Bibra, who is considered the father of modern ethnobotany, offered a fairly convincing explanation for this question. In the landmark book *Die Narkotischen Genussmittel und der Mensch* (*Plant Intoxicants: A Classic Text on the Use of Mind-Altering Plants*), published in 1855, he described the methods of cultivation, preparation, and consumption of seventeen different psychoactive plants, including cannabis. Bibra explained:

> The Indian hemp plant...has very different chemical properties than the European plant. It contains substances that do not mature in our colder climate, or develop only in small amounts. In short, it is a situation similar to that of the poppy plant, which yields only small amounts of opium here in Europe, or of the rose, from which hardly a drop of rose oil can be extracted, whereas large quantities are extracted from it in the Orient.[15]

Today we know that he was perfectly right, since in a hot and desert climate the cannabis plant produces in large quantities the resins which contain psychoactive alkaloids, particularly the principal one of THC (tetrahydrocannabinol). And this is for a reason, because their main task is the protection of flowers and leaves from the excessive loss of water. In essence, these alkaloids constitute a defensive mechanism that enables the plant to survive in dangerous environmental conditions.

It was the veterans of the French campaign in the Orient who made hashish fashionable and popular among Parisian artistic circles. The exclusive Club des Hashischins, set up in 1844, was a secret society that counted famous bohemian artists among its members, including Honoré de Balzac, Charles Baudelaire, Alexandre Dumas, Eugene Delacroix, Gustave Flaubert, and Théophile Gautier. In a gentlemanly and generally modest way they experimented with altered states of consciousness. A few members of the club made hashish the main theme of their work, above all Baudelaire ("The Poem of Hashish," 1860) and Gautier (*Le Club des hachichins*, 1846). During the monthly meetings at the Hôtel Pimodan the artists ate hashish, a green paste, which they called "jam," made of—just as in the Muslim countries— hash, butter, herbs, and peanuts. Through these hashish sessions they sought inspiration, new artistic sensitivity, and exceptional spiritual experience. They exchanged views on drugs and talked about personal mind-expanding adventures.[16] Thanks to hashish, wrote Baudelaire—whilst still painfully aware of its "devilish" properties—"[t]he spiritual world opens up vast perspective, full of brilliant new possibilities" as "the simplest words, the most trivial ideas assume a bizarre new appearance; you are even surprised to have found them so simple before now."[17]

The case of Napoleon's soldiers, who had a hand in the spread of hashish in France and other European countries, is an interesting and telling historical example of what might today be called "civil-military relations." The main interest in the analysis of the relationship between the civilian and military worlds has usually been the impact of social customs, norms, tradition, and culture on military organization and the ways of war. However, as the history of the French troops returning from Egypt illustrates, the military frequently went ahead of their societies in experimenting with psychoactive substances. More importantly, soldiers often played a substantial role in spreading the practices of recreational intoxication and drug habits. We must, therefore, acknowledge that when it comes to the social history of drugs, the relationship between the civilian and military spheres has been a complex one.

Hashish began to flood France and Europe more intensively following yet another war, the war waged in defense of the honor of the French consul in Algeria, a country which formally was part of the Ottoman Empire. In 1827 a ridiculous diplomatic incident took place, which was not as trivial as it might seem at first glance because it had far-reaching consequences. During an audience with the Dey, the French consul, Pierre Deval, writes Richard Davenport-Hines, "was so rude that the reigning Dey of Algiers flicked him with a fly whisk."[18] Three years later this tragicomic episode resulted, though indirectly, in the French military expedition against Algeria. The motives behind this operation were, of course, more serious than the humiliating treatment of the French consul, which itself served as the casus belli. On the one hand, France presented its military operation as a part of a war against the pirates who used the Algerian seacoast as a base from which to wreak terror on the high seas, thereby severely jeopardizing the colonial powers' interests in North Africa. Historians have, however, dismissed this argument, because as John Donnelly Fage insists, the war on pirates was authorized in 1815 by the Congress of Vienna in response to Great Britain's request for the right to protect its commercial interests on the seas, but in 1830 it could hardly be seen as a justified cause for the invasion of Algiers. The real reason for the French attack was the efforts undertaken by King Charles X, who sought to check the social and political ferment in France and restore his authority through an overseas military expedition that would stir up patriotic sentiment.[19] Yet these hopes proved futile, as Charles X was dethroned in 1830 by the July Revolution. On the other hand, the Dey of Algiers demanded that the French repay their debts incurred between 1793 and 1798. The story was that two Algerian merchants from the Bakri and Bushnaq families supplied the French army, including Napoleon's troops prior to the Egyptian expedition, with grain but were never paid. The merchants were indebted to the Dey and insisted that their insolvency was due to the French not fulfilling the contract. It was during a heated conversation on these issues that the Dey lost control of himself after the French consul, speaking on behalf of his government, categorically refused to pay the debt.[20]

The French expedition that began in 1830 ended in the ultimate conquest and colonization of Algeria, which in 1847 was finally incorporated into the administrative structure of France. A massive migration of about 50,000 French people (known as *colons*), who settled in Algeria from the mid-1820s, greatly intensified direct contact between the overseas territory and France. These close connections enabled more and more Europeans to discover and experience the intoxicating proprieties of hashish. The drug was becoming increasingly popular, eventually crossing social divides and ceasing to be a luxury reserved exclusively for the artistic and intellectual cream of the crop. The use of cannabis quickly came to be so prevalent that Théophile Gautier fulminated that "hashish is replacing champagne." And in 1845 he urged that "we believe we have conquered Algeria, but Algeria has conquered us."[21] Baudelaire, too, saw the threat of hashish developing into an acute social problem. Being an eager experimenter with drugs, he drew on his personal experience and went on to compare opium and hashish, offering the following disturbingly vivid conclusion: "The one is an easy-going seducer, the other a dissolute demon."[22] Yet for the Chinese, opium ultimately came to be more of "a dissolute demon" than "an easy-going seducer," particularly as it turned into a tool of their colonial exploitation.

3

The Opium Wars

Without opium, Chinese history in the nineteenth and twentieth centuries would have been far different.
—Timothy Brook and Bob Tadashi Wakabayashi,
"Introduction: Opium's History in China"

The first major war in which psychoactive substances played a central role was the conflict between Great Britain and China in 1839–1842. As the British fought to retain the right to supply the Chinese with opium, the London *Times* quickly called the conflict the "Opium War." The hostilities resumed again in 1856–1860 (the so-called Arrow War), this time with France joining England. The British won every conflict, further opening the Chinese market not only to opium exported from India but also to international trade in general.

A "Free Trade in Poison"

Opium repeatedly became a casus belli because it was crucially important to the British Empire. What was at stake was its commercial expansion, access to Chinese ports, and the reduction of tariff barriers—in short, concessions for merchants involved in trade with China. Because opium represented the most lucrative business, it became a reason for the wars. In their immediate aftermath, the export of this commodity to China flourished significantly. In 1858, following the second Opium War, Britain imposed on China favorable changes in tariffs, including those for opium, which prompted its ultimate legalization. In this way Britain managed to "secure an important financial pillar of its far-flung political empire."[1]

Whereas in the first half of the eighteenth century the value of Chinese exports to England was almost three times the value of the British exports to China, by the mid-nineteenth century it was already more than nine times.[2] Indian opium was supposed to be the commodity that would help reduce or even eliminate such an unfavorable imbalance. Because China would trade only in silver, the English needed to sell it Indian opium in order to obtain enough bullion to purchase tea and silk.[3] The Opium Wars should, then, be seen for what they were: wars waged in defense of England's dominant position in global trade, or, to put it differently, they were harsh manifestations of "free trade imperialism."[4]

For the Chinese, not only did Britain's actions represent ruthless economic exploitation, there was also something else involved. Britain, it was believed, pursued a deliberate policy aimed at bringing Chinese society under foreign control through its physical and moral debilitation and demolition. What the West attempted to achieve through its opiate-based "moral poisoning" was numbness, impoverishment, demoralization, and the destruction of the centuries-old Confucian values. In the twentieth century the Chinese coined a special term to describe the British opium policy: *duha zhengce*, meaning "empoison," or imperial poisoning. In the West, it was Karl Marx who introduced into the general discourse the notion of drug-founded imperialism by describing the nineteenth-century British policy toward China as a "free trade in poison."[5] It is an irony of history that while the present-day wars on drugs are waged against drug production and trafficking, in the nineteenth century "drug wars" were fought to impose free trade in substances that are illegal today. Opium had come to represent a powerful symbol of both the oppression of the Chinese state and its chronic inability to undertake reforms that would facilitate the development of a capacity to resist Western intrusion and exploitation.

What the Empire of Free Trade insisted on was to secure the operation of the classic law of supply and demand. The East India Company, which for a long time enjoyed the monopoly on trade in India, provided the opium supply, while the constantly growing popularity of opium smoking in China fueled the demand. What, then, was the demand and supply of opium in China? The drug arrived in the country most likely in the first century BC with sailors traveling to Africa or India through Burma, but its large-scale supply began in the Middle Ages and is credited to the Arab merchants.[6] Until the seventeenth century opium had been used for medicinal purposes as a cure for diarrhea and impotence (it was believed to be a powerful aphrodisiac) and as a common ingredient in cakes. The recreational smoking of *madak*—opium mixed with tobacco, which not only had a greater addictive potential but also brought more intense pleasures than pure opium—was brought to China by European sailors.[7] It was probably the Dutch in Java who were the first to smoke tobacco mixed with opium as a remedy for malaria. The habit was later introduced into Formosa (present-day Taiwan), from where it found its way to China.[8] Because smoking opium pipes (or narghiles) became widespread and troublesome, the emperor, who earlier in 1637 had outlawed the smoking of tobacco, also banned opium smoking in 1644.[9] The prohibition, however, had the opposite effect than that intended: the consumption of opium increased so much that by the end of the seventeenth century every fourth Chinese used the drug.[10] Its growing popularity stemmed from the fact that it was cheaper than alcohol and that by reducing hunger and thirst it "enabled the poor to do with less food."[11]

As the rapidly growing demand for opium could not have been met by local poppy cultivation, the Portuguese seized the opportunity and began to export Indian opium to China. The English and Dutch merchants soon followed and from the seventeenth century opium became a high-value commodity in the Far East. In 1729 the Chinese authorities responded to the ominously spreading drug habit by introducing a highly restrictive anti-opium edict that targeted the "dealers and keepers of opium shops" who "were to be strangled."[12] This attempt to control opium trafficking was, however, a complete failure. Whereas in 1729 some 200 chests of opium (of about 63.5 kilograms each) entered China, in 1735 imports doubled and in 1767 amounted to as many as 1,000 chests.[13] This upward trend did not stop, and while in 1800 the number of chests entering China was 1,800, in 1838 it peaked at 34,000.

The East India Company, which until 1833 secured a monopoly on trade in India, recognized China as a potentially highly profitable market for Indian opium. After 1763 the Company, which can be seen as the first "drug cartel," established an extensive trade network based on contracted dealers who, given the official ban on opium importation, smuggled the commodity into China. This commercial system worked exceptionally well, particularly until 1796, when the emperor Kea-king issued another decree that reintroduced a ban on the importing of opium.[14] The mechanism was as follows: under the monopoly the Company produced opium in India and sold the chests at auctions in Calcutta to private buyers who would then ship the commodity to China. The agency houses received and sold chests to the smugglers, who distributed the drugs across China.[15] While in 1773 opium earned the Company 39,000 pounds, in the 1830s it brought it about one million pounds a year, which was roughly one-sixth of its total annual profits from the Indian trade.[16]

Originally, opium smoking was confined largely to the upper classes, but the practice quickly spread to the lower strata of society. At the beginning of the nineteenth century the smoking of pure opium was already fairly common too. Between 1820 and 1835 the number of people taking opium in China increased sixfold.[17] This "poppy" intoxication crossed the barriers of social class and was so rampant that one author has gone so far to speak of the "McDonaldization" of opium consumption.[18] In the 1830s James Holman offered the following description of the pervasiveness of opium smoking: "The use of opium has become so universal among the people of China, that the laws which render it penal ... have not the slightest effect in decreasing the prevalence of so general a habit."[19] He went on to report, "Smoking houses abound in Canton, and in every town and village in the empire: the inhabitants of every class, who can furnish themselves with the means to obtain the pipe, are seldom without this article of general luxury."[20] So, in the late 1830s there were about four million people, or 1 percent of the total Chinese population, addicted to the drug.[21]

Ultimately, faced with the increasingly dangerous and rapidly expanding epidemic of addiction, the Chinese authorities stepped in to take firmer action. Lin Zexu, appointed as the commissioner responsible for halting the illegal import of opium, unequivocally expressed his position: "If we still hesitate to take any determined action to ban it, within ten years there would be no soldiers that can be deployed to defend the country from foreign invasion; nor would there be any money left to maintain our army. Could we remain unfrightened when we think about that?"[22] His was, of course, a rhetorical question. In 1838 Lin took decisive steps by destroying the confiscated British opium and closing the port of Canton to British shipping. These actions jeopardized the economic interests of not only the East India Company but also of the entire English Empire, giving the British no choice but to force China to cease its hostile anti-opium activities. This conflict of interests resulted in the first Opium War. So what of the Chinese army, whose future so much worried Lin Zexu?

The Opium Armies

The Opium Wars are an exceptional example of the complex connections between international politics, war, and drugs; the use of opium by troops is part of this complexity.

Given the pervasive consumption of opium in China it is hardly surprising that many soldiers of the emperor's army who were fighting in the Opium Wars to defend the country against the flood of Indian opium were, paradoxically and tragically, drug addicts. A decade after the first Opium War, the Taiping Rebellion (1851–1864) took power in southern China. Its success was the result not only of the weakening of the country and the military caused by the war but also of the epidemic addiction rates of nearly 90 percent among the ranks of the emperor's army.[23] The Chinese armed forces in the mid-nineteenth century can therefore be well described as the world's largest "opium army." But, of course, they were not the first military to use opium routinely.

The Sikhs, among the greatest Indian warriors, were regularly slightly high on opium for the same reasons as the Ottoman soldiers, earlier in the sixteenth century. In 1546 the French naturalist Pierre Belon, while documenting his travel experiences to Asia Minor and Egypt, reported the abuse of opium by the Turks. Belon's account was slightly exaggerated, but it is still worth invoking:

> There is not a Turk who would not purchase opium with his last coin; he carries the drug on him in war and in peace. They eat opium because they think they will thus become more courageous and have less fear of the dangers of war. At the time of war, such large quantities are purchased it is difficult to find any left.[24]

Henry Waterfield, a general major who served in India from the times of the great anti-British mutiny in 1857–1859, testified that 80 percent of Sikh soldiers were "occasional opium takers," 15 percent used it regularly, and about 0.5 percent were heavy abusers. Another British officer, William Biscoe, reported that in his Sikh regiment nearly 60 percent of men "took it and left it off as occasion required." In fact, in terms of combat performance "it was not considered a defect in a man if he took opium occasionally."[25] When the drug was elusive, it was the army's responsibility to supply soldiers because moderate opium eating had a positive and desired impact on the attitude and fighting performance of the troops. Sometimes the use of the intoxicant in India was so deeply rooted in everyday life and customs that it was a cultural norm. Take the case of the Rajputs, the descendants of the Hindu warrior caste of North India who, probably from the 1720s on, used opium regularly and had a habit of sharing it with their horses and camels before leaving for a mission to patrol the desert.[26]

The Indian commander, Sirsubha Sakharm Martand, testified that

> [m]y long connection with and intimate knowledge of the State army enables me to say unhesitatingly that a moderate dose of opium is an unmixed good to the consumers. Opium eating does not necessarily lead to immorality or crime. It gives staying power under great exertions such as long marches and hunting excursions. As compared with alcohol drinkers, I found opium consumers to be steady, quiet, reliable, and obedient soldiers. In my time I found 40 to 50 percent using opium in the State army.[27]

Also the general in command of the Indian state army in Indore, Balmukund Gayadeen, confirmed:

> Opium is eaten as well as drunk in the army. The percentage of consumers in my opinion is 50. A moderate use of opium is known not to tell against the physique of soldiers. Opium-eaters are sober, quiet,

obedient, enterprising, and attentive to their duties. They can stand hard marches under the influence of the drug . . . If the use of opium is accompanied by the use of milk, sweetmeat, or any substantial food as is usually the case, it is not only harmless but positively beneficial. It staves off hunger, and keeps the user from the effects of exposure to cold or heat. . . . Opium is also useful to animals and makes them capable of undergoing hard work and long journeys.[28]

Unlike the Indian military, which generally saw the moderate use of opium as enhancing fighting spirit and combat performance, opium abuse had a severe impact on the Chinese troops. This was clearly in evidence already in the 1830s during the quelling of the Rebellion of the Yao ethnic group in South China.[29] Xi En, the governor responsible for the suppression of the Yao uprising, repeatedly sent disturbing messages to the emperor reporting that seven in ten Chinese soldiers were opium addicts. He was pessimistic for a reason; how could an army of opium-eaters achieve any victory? The imperial investigative censor, Feng Zhanxun, wrote in a similar fashion that "[m]any Cantonese and Fujianese soldiers smoked opium, there are even more among the officers. They are cowards and they have spoiled our operation. They are really despicable."[30] Opium made the soldiers forget about hunger, withstand the cold, endure the hardships of military life, and numbed them emotionally. Also, it was used for medicinal purposes to relieve a whole range of illnesses and was often taken prophylactically, especially by the troops posted in the empire's southern provinces. Most soldiers, however, took opium because of their addiction. The remarkable difference in the impact of opium on the Indian and Chinese troops—positive and negative, desirable and unwanted, invigorating and debilitating—can be explained partly by the different culture of drug use, that is, the Indians being more temperate than the Chinese. There was also another phenomenon at work, because, as mentioned, depending on such factors as dose, capacity of the body to tolerate and withstand intoxicants, and the expectations and attitudes of the user, opium can have either stimulating or tranquilizing effects.[31] Medical and clinical studies have focused mostly on the drug's sedative properties; therefore its boosting effects, the ones that the Indian warriors took great advantage of, at first glance might be surprising. While the Indian fighting men used opium advisedly and for the pragmatic reason of gaining combat advantage, the majority of Chinese troopers were hooked on the drug and rendered ineffective for duty. What is more, the habit in the army had snowballing consequences: from the 1860s on, Chinese troops had been a major force that triggered the further diffusion of opium smoking among the civilians in the southern provinces.[32] The Imperial Army, in short, turned into a powerful catalyst for the spread of the epidemic of addiction throughout society.

In his book *The Social Life of Opium in China*, Yangwen Zheng firmly argues:

> Opium had demilitarized the fighting machine, as soldiers found the best way to escape boredom and combat responsibilities. Given seven thousand soldiers out of ten thousand were invalids, any battle would have been lost. Here, however, it was not only the battle against the Yao people that was lost but also the first Opium War itself.[33]

It was not wise to send heavy opium-smokers to battle, for they lacked the will for combat. Drug abuse destroyed individual fighting spirit and the morale of the troops. Feng Zhanxun observed that "the poison of opium is that when the people smoke it, they waste themselves and ruin their business, and when the soldiers smoke it, they become tired and break the army's discipline."[34] In the same vein, the English physician C. Toogood Downing, who lived in Canton, noted that "the class of people who consume opium in China are those of the male sex, chiefly between twenty and fifty-five years old, and of all ranks in society . . . It affects soldiers very much, rendering them weak and decrepit."[35] In that respect, it is worth mentioning the ancient Chinese thinker on war, Sun Pin, active in the fourth century BC, who grasped the ultimate truth: "When an army is internally exhausted, even numerous expenditures of energy will not result in solidity. When you see the enemy is difficult to subdue, if the army still acts wantonly between Heaven and Earth, it will be swiftly defeated."[36]

Lieutenant Alexander Murray remarked that he believed that the Chinese soldiers took opium to raise their courage and prepare for battle. To his surprise, and contrary to what he had expected, Murray did not see them being euphoric or numbed but only insanely manic. He recounted:

> About twenty wounded men were taken into our hospital, where their wounds were dressed; but several died from the immense quantity of opium they had taken to get their courage up to the fighting point. Most of the attacking party were mad with excitement, produced probably by this abominable drug.[37]

What Murray also expressed was actually the prevailing view among the English soldiers and officers at the time, namely that a proper enemy has his natural courage grounded in character, values, intrinsic fortitude, and proper training. During the "opium punitive expedition" against China, a well-armed British army encountered an enemy that proved to be composed of "half-humans driven mad by an abominable drug."[38] For the British, an unnaturally boosted enemy was not a worthy opponent. Although military technology gave the European soldiers a decisive advantage, they did not see it in terms of an unnatural enhancement. The point is that technology was considered merely as an extension of their human abilities while opium changed the body from within. The issue was not about artificial tools of war but about the artificially created condition of a soldier. Of course, the British were somewhat hypocritical in their reasoning—it was, in fact, they who had substantially contributed to the opium addiction they later criticized. Their expedition, moreover, was an important element of England's drug-funded imperialism, prompting the expansion of the opium habit in Chinese society and the armed forces.

Undoubtedly, the widespread addiction to opium was neither the sole nor a dominant cause of Chinese military defeats. It was, to be sure, a significant factor, indicating the utter depletion and collapse of the army. Yet something else was involved, too; the condition of the Chinese military organization reflected the general bankruptcy of a corrupt political system and the social and economic breakdown in the eighteenth and nineteenth centuries under the Qing dynasty (1644–1911). The Chinese army faced myriad military problems: it was ill-prepared, badly organized, and its structure was defective and inefficient at all levels. Because soldiers were miserably paid, it was often difficult to fill vacancies with a sufficient number of volunteers. In addition, troops were armed with obsolete weaponry, which in turn helped prevent them from becoming an effective fighting force and could not compensate for organizational malfunctioning, poor command, and low morale. While the Western forces were equipped with rifles and guns, the Chinese army relied on an infantry armed with spears, pikes, bows and arrows, knives, and rattan shields. Thus was its typical armament in the Opium Wars. Rifles did not become standard issue in the Chinese military until the 1880s.[39]

Also, the army, it seems, had departed far from the traditional Chinese values and ethos grounded in Taoism and Confucianism; the troops that fought the British and French forces were generally unfamiliar with the ancient Chinese art of war and military methods depicted in the classics like Sun Tzu and Sun Pin. One can go even further and claim that the nineteenth-century Chinese army actually embodied a negation of most of the military classics' advice, while exhibiting many of the weaknesses and faults against which they warned. Sun Tzu wrote in his *Art of War*:

> Thus a victorious army is as a hundredweight balanced against a grain; a defeated army as a grain balanced against a hundredweight. It is because of disposition that a victorious general is able to make his people fight with the effect of pent-up waters which, suddenly released, plunge into a bottomless abyss.[40]

Regrettably, it would not be possible to portray his nineteenth-century successors in this way. The Chinese army fighting the British was more like "a grain balanced against a hundredweight"; it resembled, if I may employ this comparison, a streamlet and on occasion a puddle. Water is an often-used Taoist image and symbol, a kind of ideal, so to speak. In the *Daodejing* (or the *Book of the Way*), the key classic Taoist text composed around the sixth century BC and considered one of the most profound and important works of Chinese philosophy, Laozi taught: "The highest goodness is like water: Water benefits the myriad things and rests in the places everybody detests."[41] It was Sun Tzu, whose *Art of War* is a typical example of Taoist writing, who claimed that a good army should also be like water—formless, flexible, and compliant; seemingly soft but easily adaptable to a turbulent, ever-changing battlefield environment; and responsive to the enemy's moves. In the nineteenth century, however, the Chinese army was as anything but water. It was fossilized and curiously wreathed in chaos and failure, unable to flexibly adapt to its enemies' tactics. It might rather be likened to smoke—the opium smoke—blowing, numbing, and vanishing.

An army is a representation of the society for which it fights; also, the way of warfare reflects a society's culture at a given period. In Chinese society, where both the elites and the lower ranks often lived in the fumes of opium, its army also marched and fought in an opium haze. A weak state and a debilitated society can only raise a sluggish army. What the Chinese soldiers were missing was *ch'i* (the spirit, refreshing breath, or essential vital energy). *Ch'i* is a broad term understood as motivation, determination, and morale and fighting spirit. *Ch'i* can counteract material deficiencies, as it is the energy that boosts the troops. That was long ago discovered by ancient commanders and philosophers, and was also fully recognized and experienced by Napoleon Bonaparte, who used to say that in war the moral (human agency and the will to fight) is to the physical (weaponry and equipment, training, and military capability) as three to one. Even the best trained and equipped army cannot prevail if it lacks *ch'i*. Let me return to Sun Pin as his words perfectly illustrate the tragic condition of the Chinese Imperial Army at the time of the Opium Wars: "If their *ch'i* is not sharp they will be plodding. When they are plodding they will not reach their objective. When they do not reach their objective, they will lose the advantage."[42] In China, like in India, it was hoped that opium would facilitate soldiers' endurance and lift their fighting spirit. Yet, contrary to this original intent, its abuse only weakened their *ch'i*. In 1836 Yuan Yu-lin warned that if opium addiction were to continue and spread, the social consequences would be damaging. He wrote with little exaggeration that "[f]athers would no longer be able to admonish their wives, masters would no longer be able to restrain their servants, and teachers would no longer be able to train their pupils."[43] He might have gone even further as Lin Zexu and added that soldiers would no longer be able to fight nor defend the empire.

To conclude, opium had a highly demoralizing and harmful impact not only on Chinese society but also, worse still, on its upholders. The opium troops hopelessly struggled to protect the society against the opium dictate of the West. At the time, the British and French generally abstained from opium, although some records mention its intentional use in the French army, and not only for anesthesia. For example, writing in 1843 the famous English physician John Ayrton Paris reported that during the Napoleonic wars French army surgeons "were in the practice of administering opium and Cayenne pepper to the soldiers who were exhausted by fatigue" to improve the performance of their combat-weary troops.[44] Nevertheless, it was only during the American Civil War and in its aftermath that opium, as well as morphine, went into common, though mainly medical, use among the armies of the West.

The American Civil War, Opium, Morphine, and the "Soldiers' Disease"

> But, even if taken under a doctor's orders, the opiates could produce addiction. During the Crimean War, the American Civil War, and the Franco-Prussian War, many of the wounded returned home as habitual users. After the Civil War, for example, the number of American addicts was estimated at 400,000—about one percent of the population; morphine addiction became known as "army disease."
>
> —John Frederick Logan, "The Age of Intoxication"

Opium did not have as long and turbulent a history in North America as it did in Asia. Nevertheless, the surgeons of both the Continental Army and the British Army were making the most of it by the time of the American War of Independence (1775–1783).[1] Nearly eighty years later, in the American Civil War, opium and morphine were routinely employed to treat wounded soldiers and subdue physical and emotional pain. The character of this first total modern war of the industrial age manifested itself in sheer brutality and massive bloodshed. The conflict generated a large number of injured and sick combatants who were badly in need of life-saving medical treatment. The severity of the wounds and mutilations inflicted by modern weapons (such as rifles, machine guns, and artillery) posed a formidable challenge to war medicine. Given that both the medical and nonmedical use of opium had been fairly common in prewar America, the character of the Civil War was conducive to their widespread distribution to the troops, which in turn resulted in the pervasive use and abuse of opium and morphine by soldiers and veterans.

Medicine, Opium, and Morphine

Thomas De Quincey reminds us that in the nineteenth century opium was generally seen as a panacea for almost all human pain and suffering.[2] Its regular

use was regarded as quite normal, and it was commonly applied to treat conditions such as asthma, bronchitis, chlorosis, cholera, depression, dysentery,
gripe, headache, hemorrhoids, insomnia, malaria, menstrual disorders, rheumatism, and syphilis, and also as a preventive against diarrhea and malaria,
and even as an antiemetic.[3] The famous early American physician Nathaniel
Chapman, the author of *Therapeutics* (1817), one of the first systematic treatises on pharmacology, declared opium the most useful remedy in the whole
materia medica. In fact, in the 1830s it ranked as the single-most widely prescribed drug in America, recommended for both adults and children as a cure
for nearly any medical malady, even in the treatment of masturbation, which
at that time was considered a disorder.[4] Even the most hardened skeptic of
the use of drugs, such as the American physician and writer Olivier Wendell
Holmes, prized opium as the one and only medicine "which the Creator himself seems to prescribe."[5] Morphine, which has a nearly tenfold stronger effect
than opium, was an equally common medicine, frequently used in the treatment of any disorder accompanied by pain.

How to explain this great attractiveness of, and almost universal belief
in, the "healing properties" of opium and morphine? To begin with, medical
knowledge, education, and training in the United States were generally of a low
level and inadequate. Most physicians were not only ill-informed but lacked
diagnostic skills; moreover, the available medicines usually proved largely
ineffective. Thus they were not well prepared to treat their patients. Secondly,
physicians were, by and large, indolent. Why trouble with the earnest examination and diagnosing of patients when they could instead be prescribed a
remedy that almost always brought rapid, if only apparent, improvement? An
experienced physician spoke with disarming candor about his professional
colleagues: "When a doctor is called near a patient complaining of pains and
he does not want to bother about making a diagnosis, or he wants to go fishing,
he simply resorts to the ever-ready hypodermic of Morph. Sulp. 1/4 grain."[6] In
this way, the noticeable enhancement of health proved the treatment effective,
so opium and morphine enabled physicians to retain and even raise patients'
confidence in their knowledge and skills. In short, because of their ability to
alleviate the symptoms of numerous ailments, opium and morphine grew
into a near wonder-remedy in the nineteenth-century materia medica. They
emerged as an amazing magic elixir, eagerly and routinely administered by
doctors. And the medical men themselves accounted for the majority of male
addicts in the United States. According to conservative estimates, up to 10 percent of physicians were opium inebriates who were "notoriously tempted to
treat their own headaches, insomnia and anxiety with opium and morphine."[7]

The regular taking of these drugs for only ten to fourteen days can cause
physical dependence. The time required to become a habitual user is, of course,

an individual matter and has to do with, among other factors, the dosage, type, and form of the narcotic (a powder, tablet, liquid, or injection) and the circumstances of its introduction to the system. Patients suffering from chronic conditions, such as dysentery, malaria, rheumatism, syphilis, or even insomnia were particularly vulnerable to addiction.

In the West opium and morphine were also used for nonmedical purposes, most notably to brighten the mood, heal "existential pain," sink into oblivion, and provide artistic inspiration. In 1821 Thomas De Quincey published a landmark, and extremely popular, book called *Confessions of an English Opium-Eater*, in which he described his fantastic opium dreams. He wrote: "Thou only givest these gifts to man; and thou hast the keys of Paradise, oh, just, subtle, and mighty opium!"[8] De Quincey's amazing visions encouraged many to experiment with the drug. Considered as a perfect means of stimulating imagination and enriching spiritual experience, opium was used enthusiastically to escape from the grim reality of everyday life. Take for example, Hector Berlioz, who confessed: "I must take my ten drops of laudanum and forget things until tomorrow."[9] So he took it and composed his romantic symphonies and operas. In 1830, being in a cheerful mood and feeling a sheer opium-induced ecstasy, he wrote the *Fantastic Symphony*, which bore a telling subtitle: *An Episode in the Life of an Artist*. Leonard Bernstein nicely called Berlioz's symphony "the first psychedelic musical trip." It is an autobiographical piece that reveals the experiences and emotions surrounding the artist's unrequited love. An unhappy man, whose love is unappreciated, poisons himself with opium in an unsuccessful attempt to commit suicide. An inadequate dose of the drug suffices only to plunge him into a strange hallucination.

In the nineteenth century, when the addictive potential of opium and morphine was not yet thoroughly understood, the drugs were so popular among American women that it was they who accounted for over 60 percent of all addicts. Frustrated women could not overtly numb their psychical pain with alcohol, because it was indecorous for females to drink and get drunk. Yet with opium and morphine it was different, so they were both taken by those women who wished to put themselves in a more cheerful and euphoric mood. Lydia Gwilt, a character in the novel *Armadale* (1866) by Wilkie Collins, an author who liked to intoxicate himself with opium, declared: "A man, in my place, would find refuge in drink. I'm not a man, and I can't drink."[10] Hence morphinism was predominantly a female domain, for as an anonymous lady remarked: "I am the last woman in the world to make excuses for my acts, but you don't know what morphine means to some of us, many of us, modern women without professions, without beliefs. Morphine makes life possible. It adds to truth a dream."[11]

When the Civil War began medicine was still at the dawn of a new, modern era, so it should not surprise us that soldiers displayed a bitterly critical attitude to the medics who, overall, had a poor reputation and were unpleasantly referred to as "butchers." An Alabama infantryman made a telling remark: "I believe the Doctors kill more than they cure." And an Illinois private observed that "our doctor knows about as much as a ten year old boy."[12] There was considerable truth in this. Only in the aftermath of the conflict, following the discoveries of Louis Pasteur and Robert Koch, did the revolution in bacteriology begin to emerge on the horizon. Of course, it arrived too late for the victims of the war. The historian of medicine Richard Harrison Shryock raised a basic question: "Compared with the great innovations in commerce, transportation, and industry, what certain benefits could medicine offer to the people of the 1860s?"[13] The answer is "relatively little." Even so, over the four years of the conflict military medics treated some ten million patients.[14] In the course of the war medicine developed somewhat, with significant progress occurring especially in the system of caring for the wounded, particularly in the Union. What before the conflict had been an utterly chaotic and ill-organized army medical service was transformed into a decent bureaucratic structure. Also, the huge demand for medicines during the war vastly contributed to the development of the American pharmaceutical industry. While in 1860 there were eighty-four chemical manufacturers, including pharmaceutical companies, by 1870 their number had increased to 300. Over the same decade, the product value of drugs rose from 3.4 million to 16.2 million dollars, with the most common therapeutic agents being quinine, opium, and morphine.[15] The former two were also the most popular drugs of choice during the Civil War and were widely distributed and used excessively in the extreme battlefield environment. David Courtwright cites a report produced in 1865 by the secretary of war which indicates that the Union soldiers alone were issued ten million opium pills, nearly eighty tons of powdered and liquid opium, and 850 kilograms of morphine.[16] Drugs were used routinely for wound dressing, in surgery (mostly amputations) and during recovery treatment. And the medical personnel had a lot of work on their hands, as the gunshot wounds inflicted by modern firearms were extensive, deep, and serious.

The Soldier's Wounded Body

Rifles had been known from the mid-fifteenth century, but it was only in 1847 that the problem of the time-consuming and complex process of loading the barrels with helical grooves was solved by the French Captain Claude-Étienne

Minié. He changed the bullet's shape, sharpened its ending, and added a small iron plug and a lead skirting, which expanded under the gas pressure, and pushed it against the barrel wall, thereby increasing the muzzle velocity. These improvements, that is, smaller bullets that had greater kinetic energy, not only enabled faster loading and firing but also increased accuracy. In short, Minié managed to considerably improve the lethality of firearms. James H. Burton, working in an arms factory in Virginia, slightly further improved the Minié ball and spread its use in the United States, so that it became the most common bullet used in the Civil War.

The wounds inflicted by Minié balls were, however, much more severe than were those caused by conventional round bullets.[17] The Minié balls did not simply enter and exit the body, but most often got stuck in it, causing more extensive tissue damage. On the whole, wounds of extremities most often meant traumatic damage to bones, blood vessels, and nerves. Frequently the only medical treatment was amputation. According to the *Medical and Surgical History of the War of the Rebellion*, the detailed six-volume compilation of the Union's medical sources published in 1870–1888, nearly 30,000 of the 175,000 gunshot wounds of extremities recorded in the Union forces resulted in amputation and, overall, 75 percent of soldiers who suffered an amputation survived.[18] The statistics for the Confederate forces were most probably similar, although it is difficult to provide exact data as the archives of the Confederate Army surgeon general were almost entirely destroyed in the great fire in Richmond, Virginia, in 1865.[19] As amputations were very painful surgeries, subjects were given strong doses of whisky, opium, and morphine. Inevitably many patients, and not only the amputees, developed an addiction after being regularly administered the drugs during the postoperative treatment. Take, for example, the case of a Confederate veteran who, after being shot in head, was put on morphine and from that time on remained hooked on the opiate, and at the age of eighty-two still required special medical supervision.[20]

Alfred Jay Bollet, a historian of medicine, noted that for each man killed on the battlefield there were four to five soldiers wounded in action.[21] These are estimates, of course, but even the most conservative figures point to the immense scale of pain and suffering from the injuries wrought by the war. Unfortunately, being wounded often meant a slow death in a poorly organized field hospital, where the most basic standards of hygiene were not met. Before having their wounds dressed, soldiers were usually given alcohol, which was believed to prevent traumatic shock, and oral opium pills, while their wounds were dusted or rubbed with powdered opium or morphine. Later, at the end of the war, the intravenous injection of morphine slowly emerged as a popular means of delivery. This was a more practical and potent technique, which brought an immediate and strong painkilling effect.[22]

Despite the well-known stories of the limited use of anesthesia in surgery, particularly in the Confederate Army, most historians agree that it was, in fact, generally available in both Union and Confederate hospitals. And even though the South had more limited access to anesthetic drugs because of the blockade, it managed to secure more or less regular supplies, quite often obtaining them as the spoils of war. Consider, for example, Stonewall Jackson and his army, who, during the campaign in the Shenandoah Valley in the spring of 1862, took possession of some 15,000 portions of chloroform, an amount that considerably eased the work of the Confederate surgeons. In essence, chloroform (in use from 1847) was more favored in the field hospitals than ether (in use from 1842), which was a much more explosive anesthetic and thereby more dangerous at locations close to the frontline.[23]

Anesthetics were used for the first time in combat settings by Edward H. Barton during the Mexican–American War (1846–1848).[24] Yet the history of their widespread application in battlefield care began with the Crimean War, during which they were often, sometimes even routinely, applied by Russian and French surgeons. In the British Army, by contrast, physicians were at first deeply skeptical and even hostile toward anesthetics. Chloroform was initially seen by British military surgeons as a sinful substance, for a man is born in pain and must endure the suffering. A memorandum issued by Sir John Hall, the principal medical officer of the British Army, well illustrates this resistance to the anesthetic. Warning against its use he insisted, "However barbarous it may appear, the smart of the knife is a powerful stimulant; and it is much better to hear a man bawl lustily than see him sink silently into the grave."[25] Hall's position could be understood as a defense of the warrior ethos and the traditional pattern of masculinity—a warrior must remain tough and courageous until the very end. Anesthesia was thought to discredit a real man and soldier. Hall could have argued that it stripped him of valor and other noble warrior qualities. Eventually, however, even in the British Army tradition had to give way to modern anesthetics. As the Crimean War was the first conflict marked by the relatively widespread administration of anesthesia during surgery, by the outbreak of the American Civil War it had already become commonplace in military medical care.

Minié balls brought not only death and severe injuries, but they also transmitted dirt and germs that caused nasty infections, mainly gangrene. Unfortunately, wound infections were at the time something endemic and extremely dangerous as 46 percent of patients who developed gangrene died.[26] Because the mechanism of disease causation was not yet known, the available antibacterial measures, such as iodine, were not used properly. Instead of applying antiseptics immediately to disinfect wounds, doctors lingered, thereby unwittingly allowing infections to develop. In short, bactericides were not used preventively, as we now know they should be, but were administered only when the symptoms were already noticeable, too late to achieve any positive healing effect.

Deadly Diseases

Those who managed to survive battle and retain their lives despite serious injuries were still exposed to a high risk of infection. Viruses and bacteria do not abide by human frontlines and, statistically speaking, the most severe threat to soldiers was not an armed enemy but germs. Indeed, more men died from sickness (419,000) than in combat (204,000).[27] This rate was 110,000 battle and 250,000 disease casualties in the Union forces and 95,000 and 165,000 respectively in the Confederate Army.[28] So, on average, for each man killed in battle there were two soldiers claimed by diseases. For example, in a brigade of the 4th Vermont Infantry Regiment under George P. Fosters, 280 soldiers died from disease and 162 from battlefield injuries. Or take the case of Henry Lawton's unit of 1,126 men from the 30th Indiana Infantry Regiment—275 were fatally defeated by bacteria and viruses, and 137 were killed in combat.[29] This list could be extended unit by unit.

The alarming rate of infectious diseases stemmed not only from the absence of effective remedies and prophylactics but also from poor sanitary conditions. American doctors did not know how to sterilize surgical instruments. Worse still, because of the frequent lack of water, surgeons quite often did not wash their hands or tools for days, thereby transmitting deadly germs from patient to patient. A telling example is the battle of Perryville, Kentucky, in October 1862; in the aftermath, water was so scarce that some surgeons were unable to wash their hands for two long days.[30] Given this utter disregard of the most elementary rules of hygiene, germs spread like wildfire, causing deadly epidemics. Thus microbes waged their own incessant war against soldiers of both sides, and, unfortunately for the humans, they achieved a high kill ratio.

Crammed into camps, soldiers were liable to be attacked by dysentery, measles, smallpox, malaria, and other diseases. In some regiments between 30 and 50 percent of men suffered from measles; these epidemics usually lasted for one to two months and killed some 5 percent of afflicted individuals.[31] Overall, in the course of the war a Confederate soldier was sick or wounded, on average, six times. Unlike in peacetime, the disease mortality rate in the army was strikingly high. According to the U.S. Census, while in the year preceding the war it was 6.3 per 1,000 males between the ages of fifteen and fifty, it grew to 48.7 in the first year of the hostilities, only to skyrocket to 65.2 in 1862.[32]

Diseases and epidemics would long continue to present a much more serious risk to soldiers' lives than enemy firepower. Not until the First World War did twice as many combatants die from battlefield injuries as from diseases (excluding the victims of the Spanish flu that broke out in 1918–1919 and caused several dozens of millions of deaths).[33] Eventually, a decisive change in the patterns of the mortality ratio occurred during the Second World War, when more casualties were inflicted by actual fighting than diseases.[34] The famous American bacteriologist Hans Zinsser even went so far as to argue provocatively that, unlike microbes, soldiers have rarely won wars.[35] In short then, from a military medical point of view, what statistically mattered more was ultimately not surgery and helping the wounded but the pharmacological treatment of diseases.

The Salutary Opium and Morphine

The most common afflictions among soldiers during the Civil War were gastrointestinal disorders, particularly acute diarrhea, from which as many as 995 in 1,000 men suffered in the Union forces. These diseases were prevalent and frequently fatal (288 deaths per 1,000 cases). The aftereffects of war were equally disturbing for those who survived, since an estimated 63,000 veterans suffered from chronic diarrhea, which sometimes dragged on for years. This lingering and debilitating condition was commonly treated with opium or morphine which, in turn, usually quickly resulted in addiction.[36]

The most lethal soldiers' diseases were typhoid, dysentery, and pneumonia.[37] Opium was already considered the best cure for these afflictions well before the war. The drug was widespread also in the treatment of tuberculosis (opium suppresses chronic cough); rheumatism (because no effective remedies were available, the only obtainable measure was to reduce the pain); malaria (from which over one million soldiers suffered in the Union forces alone, and for which opium was administered simultaneously with quinine); and other lesser disorders like toothaches, headaches, or stomach pain. Because, as mentioned, the etiology of diseases was then not yet known (bacteria were still waiting to be discovered), opium and morphine were regarded as the universal medicament. They were readily and easily available as poppies were cultivated across the North and South alike; the main growing states were Virginia, Tennessee, South Carolina, and Georgia.[38] And physicians did not realize, or did not want to realize, their highly addictive potential. When injection was introduced in the United States as a new method of morphine administration in the late 1850s and early 1860s, the belief which widely prevailed was that, as opposed to ingestion, it would not cause a greater appetite for morphine. Thus went the false argument: remove the act of swallowing, and you eliminate the hunger for the drug.[39]

Before Silas Weir Mitchell, a noted American physician and writer, turned to writing at the age of fifty-one, he had been one of the very first—and one of the leading—American neurologists; the coauthor of the classic textbook *Gunshot Wounds and Other Injuries of Nerves* (1864); and a founder of an American clinic for patients with mental disorders, established in 1861. In his novel *Characteristics* (1892), he told a story of morphine being used to subdue pain: "Then I yielded, and my doctor gave me a hypodermatic injection of morphia. I lay awake all night in perfect comfort, heedless of the passage of time, and wondering at the bliss of relief. It was heaven bought with hell, for the next day I was doubly tormented."[40] There is another striking passage, which concentrates more on the psychological than the medical reasons for taking morphine:

> None who have not known long chronic illness can conceive of the misery enforced idleness inflicts on a man used to active life. This intensity of ennui, comparable only to that which some children suffer, is eased by morphia. The hours go by almost joyously. Misfortunes trouble no longer. One drifts on an enchanted sea. This death of ennui is the most efficient bribe which opium offers.[41]

Apart from being used for a range of physical afflictions and as a painkiller, opium and morphine were also issued to mitigate mental disorders caused by severe anxiety, flashbacks, and recurrent traumatic images of war. Stress, fear, and psychiatric breakdowns are the products of every military conflict, but during the Civil War they took on an extra charge compared to earlier wars, due in particular to its modern and almost total character. Killing in the war zone, an experience of death and dying, and the fear of suffering and death are the decisive factors producing psychiatric disorders. Consider the bloodshed at Gettysburg, where the battlefield was littered with thousands of injured soldiers, lying surrounded by piles of the mutilated bodies of their fallen comrades and dead horses. Such would be a truly horrific sight, even for the most insensitive observer. All-encompassing death and the decaying corpses of lifeless men grievously damaged the psyches of those who survived the battle. The great American writer Walt Whitman, who served as a corpsman and took care of injured soldiers in the Washington area, provided us with the following vivid description:

> Then the camps of the wounded—O heavens, what scene is this?—is this indeed *humanity*—these butchers' shambles? There are several of them. There they lie, in the largest, in an open space in the woods, from 200 to 300 poor fellows—the groans and screams—the odor of

blood, mixed with the fresh scent of the night, the grass, the trees—
that slaughter-house! . . . One man is shot by a shell, both in the arm
and leg—both are amputated—there lie the rejected members. Some
have their legs blown off—some bullets through the breast—some
indescribably horrid wounds in the face or head, all mutilated, sicken-
ing, torn, gouged out—some in the abdomen—some mere boys . . .
Such is the camp of the wounded.[42]

Inevitably, such harrowing experiences often caused war trauma, a condition
which since 1980 has been called "posttraumatic stress disorder" (PTSD) but
at the time of the Civil War was commonly referred to as "nostalgia."

It manifested itself in an array of symptoms, including numbness, madness,
depression, insomnia, partial paralysis, gastrointestinal disorders, epilepsy,
shortness of breath, chest pain, and heart palpitations. Jacob Mendez da Costa,
a physician and surgeon, after investigating the condition of cardiac neurosis
and chronic asthenia among soldiers, contended that it was rather psychiatric
than physical. To describe it he coined the term "soldier's heart," yet it later
came to be known after him as "Da Costa's syndrome." Whereas in the first
year of the war 5,000 soldiers were diagnosed with "nostalgia," at the end of the
conflict among the Union troops alone there were 10,000 confirmed cases.[43]
William Hammond, the Union physician who pioneered research on nervous
and mental disorders among the troops, insisted that the main cause of such
widespread "nostalgia" was the immaturity of soldiers. Some recruits were only
sixteen, and we now know that the younger the age the greater the likelihood
that an individual will develop trauma-related problems. Thus Hammond reasonably called for an increase in the minimum age of draftees to twenty years
of age. This was, however, beyond reach given the total character of the war
and the demand for a constant supply of fresh manpower.

But what of drugs? Alcohol, opium, and morphine turned out to be the
most common means of coping with the symptoms of war trauma. Intoxicants
enabled soldiers and then veterans to ease the pain of the invisible wounds
and the suffering inflicted by the gruesome experience of modern total war.
In his book *The Opium Habit, with Suggestions as to the Remedy* (1868) Horace
Day noted, "Maimed and shattered survivors from a hundred battlefields, dis-
eased and disabled soldiers released from hostile prisons, anguished and hopeless wives and mothers, made so by the slaughter of those who were dearest
to them, have found, many of them, temporary relief from their sufferings in
opium."[44] Day's is also the first major account of the relationship between the
Civil War and drug abuse. He estimated the number of opium and morphine
addicts living in the United States from 80,000 to 100,000 and contended that
the war significantly contributed to higher rates of addiction.[45]

A particularly telling example of the liberal, uncontrolled, and careless administration of opiates to troops is the story of Major Nathan Mayer, the Union surgeon of the 16th Connecticut Infantry Regiment. He did not trouble to dismount from his horse to diagnose soldiers but dispensed morphine from horseback. In his reminiscences Mayer recalled:

> It was my duty to stop with those who fell out and see whether they were sick, or played out, or malingering. In one pocket I carried quinine, in the other morphine, and whiskey in my canteen. The hospital steward was behind, if I wanted further stores. But ordinarily, when on horseback, I could inquire and judge without dismounting, and I got entirely practiced to dispense from the bottle into my hand and know the exact quantity. The quinine—Weightman's—was cottony, the morphine a fine powder. They licked from my hand and the men carried water in their canteens to wash it down.[46]

What is especially striking about this account is not only the highly unhygienic way of issuing medicines it describes but also the routine carelessness in distributing morphine. Inevitably, such practices meant that opiate addiction among soldiers and veterans hit hard. Who would, however, have bothered about the potential side effects of drugs when highly important strategic objectives were at stake? What matters in war is the ability to quickly rebuild military capabilities and effectively restore manpower.

The Myth of the "Soldiers' Disease"?

The opinion that the Civil War gave rise to the "soldiers' disease," that is to say the social problem of a devastating epidemic of opium and morphine dependence among veterans, has become widely popular, but it has also triggered some controversies. One of the best known critics of the idea is Mark A. Quinones, whose objections, put forward in 1975, can be summed up in four points.[47] First, there is no evidence in the sources to support the assumption that veterans constituted any special or separate category of addicts. Second, the highly addictive route of intravenous morphine administration was still rare during the war. Instead, the drug was generally used in powdered form, either taken orally or rubbed into wounds. Third, the statistics do indicate an increase in opium imports to the United States, yet not in the 1860s (50,000 kilograms), as the soldiers' disease thesis would imply, but in the following decades (87,000 kilograms in the 1870s, 149,000 kilograms in the 1880s, and 233,000 kilograms in the 1890s).[48] At this point, however, Quinones's counterargument is rather flawed because, actually, this historical dynamic only points to the development of the opium problem in postwar America. Fourth, as discussed, in the second half of the nineteenth century the majority of addicts in the United States were not men but women.

A leading contemporary critic of the assumption that the Civil War resulted in a dramatic increase in the rate of addiction in American society is Jerry Mandel. He sees the soldiers' disease as a useful myth for politicians, created a long time after the war was over in order to justify the introduction of the first federal antidrug law.[49] So this false image was built, Mandel claims, to validate and legitimatize the position taken by the proponents of the restrictive Harrison Act, which was passed by Congress in December 1914 and became the basis of the American federal drug control policy well until the 1970s. The Act banned the possession and sale of drugs except for their medical use. Francis Burton Harrison, the representative who proposed the act, and his supporters needed an appealing justification to introduce new regulations; it was vital to demonstrate that drugs were responsible for grave social problems. The logic of the argument, which grew into a kind of paradigm, could be summed up in the following formula: the availability of drugs leads to their use; the use results in abuse; a habit turns into addiction; which eventually becomes an acute social problem. The Civil War and its aftereffects, namely the prolific consumption of opium and morphine, were thought to be a perfect illustration of this dynamic in action. The case was exploited for a reason—to create the modern myth of the soldiers' disease, which could be employed to threaten society with the nightmarish vision of the inevitably catastrophic consequences of uncontrolled access to psychoactive substances. Not coincidentally, the image of the soldiers' disease allegedly contracted by the veterans of the Civil War came into being and circulation at almost exactly the same time as the struggle for the Harrison Act. It came, moreover, to be deeply rooted in the popular consciousness. Thus in the article "The Course of Narcotism in America—A Reveille," published in 1915 in the *American Journal of Public Health*, Yale professor Jeannette Marks warned:

> Did you know that there is practically no old American family of Civil War reputation which has not had its addicts? Did you know that it was called "the army disease" because of its prevalence? Did you know that with the war which now hangs over us, the drug evil will spring into a giantism of even more terrible growth than the present?[50]

In the nineteenth century the issue of soldiers' disease or army disease did not exist at all, because—as Mandel encourages us to believe—there was simply no such problem. He goes so far to argue that the "soldier's disease is a fanciful reconstruction of the past by writers one hundred years or more after the Civil War."[51] The pervasive consumption of drugs during the war did not, Mandel insists, give rise to narcotism as a social problem. Medical statistics on the use of opium and morphine apart, no official report concerning drug addiction among soldiers and veterans was written in 1861–1865. And this tells a story. In 1871 a Boston druggist remarked, responding to a survey, that "veteran soldiers who contracted the habit in the army hospitals are still addicted to the use of opium." Another pharmacist observed that "veteran soldiers, as a class, are addicted to it."[52] Such records are, however, few and far between. Thus Mandel raises a disturbing question: "Why?" If there were so many addicts, as the notion of the soldiers' disease implies, why had this not been officially recorded anywhere? How could such a major social problem have gone unnoticed? In addition, as Arnold Trebach points out, the New York Times index for the years 1853–1874 did not contain any mention of the word "opium."[53] Mandel reminds us that references to soldiers' disease began to appear in literature only about a century after the end of the Civil War. From 1964 until the end of the 1980s it had already been mentioned in some hundred publications. One of the most telling descriptions of the phenomenon can be found in the 1971 article by Gerald Starkey, who claimed that during the Civil War military doctors

> injected the young wounded veterans with huge amounts of Morphine daily (every four hours) to kill their pain . . . It was necessary for the surgeons to do full-quarter amputations—literally take the arms and legs off right at the start of the body, usually to stop infectious gangrene. In 1865 there were an estimated 400,000 young War veterans addicted to Morphine . . . The returning veteran could be identified because he had a leather thong around his neck and a leather bag (with) Morphine Sulfate tablets, along with a syringe and a needle issued to the soldier on his discharge . . . This was called the "Soldier's Disease."[54]

Mandel does not deny that the war left many veterans addicted. What he does challenge, however, is the common view that it was a large-scale phenomenon with profound social and public health consequences. David Courtwright, a prominent writer on the history of drugs, has also not found any evidence to support the thesis about the epidemic narcotic problem among Union and Confederate soldiers and veterans. He, nonetheless, contends that the rates of dependence must have been high, arguing that because the prevalence of drug consumption had already been reported before the outbreak of the war, the conflict itself had been but one of the sources of morphine and opium habits in the United States. The three other major factors were the liberal administration of intoxicants by careless and often incompetent physicians, self-dosage, and the growing nontherapeutic use accelerated by the rising popularity of the hypodermic syringe.[55] It should be remembered again that it was not the veterans, and not even males, who constituted the majority of addicts in the second half of the nineteenth century, but unhappy, frustrated, socially restricted, or simply bored American women.

It seems to me that Quinones, Mandel, and Trebach tend to present the view that if a problem was neither documented by military or government reports nor covered by the press, it simply did not exist. They do not, however, take into account at least two important things. First, during the war no attention was given to the side effects of therapeutic agents because a more burning issue was to save the lives of the many injured and sick. Overall, the main goal of military medicine was to restore soldiers' combat readiness and return them to the frontline as soon as possible. Second, veterans are generally reluctant to talk about their wartime experience and any consequent problems. On their return home they usually feel, and often are, isolated from society at large. Civilians do not know the reality of war and find it difficult to understand veterans and their struggle to adapt to civilian life. In order not to distance themselves further from the society, they talk little about their own problems, particularly substance abuse and addiction.

There are two other points that require attention when analyzing the arguments of those authors who challenge the notion of the soldiers' disease. The first is that the Civil War veterans deliberately hid their addiction problems because they feared losing their pensions. Thomas Davison Crothers noticed this issue writing in 1902, "Many veterans of the Civil War became morphinists to relieve the pain and suffering following injuries received in the service, and the addiction is often concealed to prevent the possibility of imperilling their application for pension."[56] The second point is that the lack of reliable official sources documenting the soldiers' disease does not necessarily mean that the problem was nonexistent, as it could have remained present in social consciousness and oral history. Given the controversies over the army disease in postwar America, it is worth keeping in mind Paul Valéry's observation, made in his *Regards sur le Monde Actuel* (*Reflections on the World Today*, 1931):

> History is the most dangerous concoction the chemistry of the mind has produced. Its properties are well known. It sets people dreaming, intoxicates them, engenders false memories, exaggerates their reflexes, keeps old wounds open, torments their leisure, inspires them with megalomania or persecution complex, and makes nations bitter, proud, insufferable and vain.[57]

Despite all the controversies, doubts and arguments raised by skeptics, I think David Courtwright has a point that the Civil War must have increased the rates of addiction.[58] Even a short-term use of opium and morphine, no matter whether for strictly medical or nonmedical purposes, can lead to the development of dependence. So how would it be possible that the long-term use of opium or morphine by injured and ill soldiers would not have made them habitual users?

The wave of addiction among veterans, even if it did not develop into a social problem, was most acute between 1865 and 1900. The spread of the morphine and opium habit brought about by the war was particularly alarming in the South. This was due to two factors—one was physical and the other psychological.[59] First, in relation to population size, the Confederacy suffered more casualties than the Union, including the injured who in the course of medical treatment became dependent on powerful painkillers. Second, the psychological effects of the defeat were profound owing not merely to the fact of the defeat but because of its social consequences. The breakdown of the lifestyle based on slave labor caused a sort of trauma among the plantation owners, and depression often made them seek escape and consolation in drugs. Opium and morphine offered quick and effective but deceptive relief.

To sum up, a veteran of the Civil War was but only one type of addict in postwar America, next to women, pharmacists, and opium smokers. And the war was but one source of the higher rates of opium and morphine dependence in the second half of the nineteenth century. According to divergent, because impossible to verify, but conservative estimates, in 1914 there were between 200,000 and 300,000 habitual opium users in the United States.[60] And between the 1840s and the 1890s, the number of addicts jumped sixfold.[61]

The epidemic of the soldiers' disease was soon to take its toll also in Europe. The Prussian army showed a keen interest in the developments in pharmacology, particularly in the synthesis of morphine and the technique of its intravenous injection. We should not be surprised, then, that the opiate-based management of pain in the treatment of gunshot wounds among the Prussian army during the wars of German unification, that is, with Austria (1866) and France (1870–1871), led to addiction among the ranks of truly alarming proportions. The reckless administration of a wonderful liquid painkiller typically ended in the "morbid appetite for morphine." Further, the habitual use of opiates was not only the problem of combatants but also of their families. Let me quote one example of a Dresden woman who in 1865 was given morphine for gallstones and "resorted to the injections again during the war of 1870–1871, to try to overcome her anxiety about the daily dangers to which her male relations were exposed."[62] After all, the German "Iron Chancellor" Otto von Bismarck, privately a person with a very fragile psyche, was a regular morphine user, like many other individuals of the era.[63] Perhaps inevitably, soldiers also increasingly turned to morphine to shield themselves from the sorrows and suffering of combat.[64]

In short, war, especially in its modern incarnation, was a significant factor that greatly prompted the consumption of intoxicants. While the most prevalent drug during the American Civil War was opium, during later conflicts—notably the European wars of Prussia, the Spanish–American War (1898), and the First World War—it was morphine that became the most common drug.[65]

The Colonial Wars
and the Terrifying "Barbarians"

The next best thing to a good friend is a good enemy.
—John Glenn Gray, *The Warriors: Reflections on Men in Battle*

During the colonial wars of the nineteenth and early twentieth centuries, forces of local tribes, who in many places had to face technologically and organizationally superior invading imperial armies, fueled themselves by chewing, smoking, drinking, or eating a wide and disparate variety of stimulating and hallucinogenic psychoactive drugs.[1] Intoxicants, then, played (or may have played) a key role in transforming indigenous warriors into rabid, fanatic, ruthless, and terrifying killers who posed a considerable challenge to the Western professional militaries. In this chapter I examine two specific cases: the Zulu warriors in the 1879 war with the British, and the Moro warriors in the Philippines during their rebellion against the Americans in 1899–1913. While the Zulus went to battle hopped-up on plant drugs, the way the Moros fought suggested that they might have been heavily intoxicated; yet, as we now know, they were not.

The Zulus

We spared no lives and did not ask for any mercy for ourselves.
—K. Gwabe, a Zulu warrior quoted in Edmund Yorke,
"Isandlwana 1879: Dividing Your Forces"

An independent Zululand and its army of 50,000 men stood in the way of the British colonization of Southern Africa and the empire's plan to set up a confederation of resource-rich provinces. When the British high commissioner for Southern Africa, Sir Henry Bartle Frere, insisted that the Zulu King Cetshwayo dismantle his military system, Frere probably knew he was making an unacceptable demand. Disbanding the army would, in fact, mean the eradication of Zulu culture and identity, and thereby the destruction of a society which was, as Eileen Jensen Krige put it, "a great military camp with war the only thought of the people."[2] The Zulus were highly belligerent men, and their kingdom was strikingly similar in character to ancient Sparta.

When the British decided to subdue them, they did not expect to encounter the extremely determined resistance they did. In the most famous battle, of Isandlwana on January 22, 1879, the Zulu army of 20,000–25,000 warriors decisively defeated in hand-to-hand combat a British force of 1,700 men. The battle took the lives of 1,300 British soldiers and between 1,000 and 3,000 of the Zulus.[3] It was a catastrophic debacle for a European army, and perhaps one of the most humiliating defeats in British military history, a disaster that deeply shocked the English government, press, and public.

A number of factors contributed to this great victory for the Zulus, which built up their image as savage, fierce, and bloodthirsty warriors. The first was the haughtiness of the British, who disregarded the potential and skills of their enemy and, worse still, made scores of tactical errors. The second was the Zulus' well-organized, centralized military structure and the very character of their society, which was deeply formed by a belligerent culture. The third was the customary ritual of preparation for war, because contacts with supernatural forces were an important psychological means of raising courage and facilitating the almost unlimited endurance of the warriors. The fourth, most interestingly for us, was intoxication, through which the Zulus made themselves into fiercer and tougher fighters.

The shamans, who served as tribal and army doctors, had at their disposal a wide range of psychoactive herbs, which they eagerly dispensed to the regiments. Before battle they performed special preparation rituals intended to strengthen the army and inspire courage in the warriors.[4] Like other premodern peoples, the Zulus sought supernatural assistance in war. They did so through a series of ceremonies, the principal one was eating special psychoactive plants and herbs given by their shamans. Carefully selected "magic" plants induced ritual communal vomiting that aimed not only to purify warriors and make them ready for a ceremonial meal eaten before battle but also to bring men together "as a strong fighting force."[5] Further, warriors were provided with various herbs to eat, drink, or inhale. They were, for example, administered an extract of *intelezi*, a traditional plant commonly taken in purifying rites to get rid of evil spirits and used to boost the morale of the troops.[6] While *intelezi* was believed to make the Zulus fearless warriors, a specially medicated beer was thought to provide them with extraordinary protection, allegedly making them more resistant to enemy attacks and fire.[7]

In addition, the warriors received rations of *dagga*, the South African vari-ety of cannabis, which initially after taking has a stimulating rather than sed-ative effect. Prior to combat they got drugged as a group either by smoking *dagga*, inhaling its fumes, or drinking a cannabis broth. Alfred T. Bryant, one of the greatest early twentieth-century authorities on Zulu history and cus-toms, observed that the young warriors smoked *dagga* before an attack so that they were capable of accomplishing almost any feat.[8] They aroused themselves also during fighting, since they carried a good stock of cannabis with them into battle. So *dagga* gave the Zulus extraordinary bravery and emboldened them to fight recklessly.[9] Members of the special "commandos," whose task was to breach the enemy lines to enable the regular troops to flow and carry out a rapid encircling maneuver called the "horns of the bull," received a spe-cial drug that both sharpened their senses (particularly sight and hearing) and enhanced concentration and alertness. They were probably given, though here we can only speculate, *Amanita muscaria* because the fungus occurs in Africa, the properties of which I have discussed. The shaman doctors also had at their disposal a special remedy for the wounded—a potent painkiller and halluci-nogenic. It was most likely produced from the bulb of *Boophane disticha*. This poisonous native flowering plant of the Amaryllis family, commonly known as "killer plant" or the "Bushman Poison Bulb," was used in traditional medi-cine in South Africa for the treatment of anxiety. It contains buphanidrine, a toxic alkaloid with highly hallucinogenic but also anesthetic properties very similar to codeine or morphine. The dosing of the bulb required great skill and experience because, as Ben-Erik van Wyk, a botanist from Rand Afrikaans University in Johannesburg, notes, the dosage of buphanidrine necessary to reduce pain is perilously close to a toxic dose.[10]

The Zulus fought with fanaticism, dedication, and fury. Armed and fortified by their shaman doctors with potent intoxicants, they went into battle utterly without fear; they believed they were protected by their deities and thereby impervious to the British bullets. Even when injured they did not stop fighting because their bodies were rendered insensitive to pain through the use of pow-erful anesthetizing plant remedies. The Zulu warriors seemed immune to the enemy rifle fire, so they readily launched almost suicidal massed charges and incredibly easily retained their combat effectiveness. The commander of the British troops, Lord Chelmsford (Frederic Thesiger), noted in his correspon-dence how terribly astonished his men were by the sheer raw courage, desper-ate fighting spirit, and resilience of the enemy.[11] And we have to acknowledge that it was Zulu pharmacopoeia, their potent traditional medicine, that con-tributed extensively to making them truly fearless warriors.

The Zulus' traditional belligerence, their vicious methods of fighting, and pharmacologically raised courage and stamina counteracted the technological edge of the British military (notably the rifles, machine guns, and cannon) as well as their finer organization and training. For the British, the Zulu warriors were dangerously unpredictable, specifically as they employed various irregular methods of fighting, particularly the "hit and run" tactics that enabled them to track and destroy individual enemy units.[12] Sir Henry Bartle Frere described the Zulu warriors as the members of a "frightfully efficient man-slaying machine."[13] Eventually, however, they were outnumbered and had little chance of winning facing the overwhelmingly technologically superior British forces. Hence, in the end, these highly disciplined and honorably proud warriors were defeated when the imperial troops captured the Zulu capital of Ulundi in July 1879. The Zulu pharmacopeia could not compensate for the technological advantages of the British.

Interestingly, the perception of the Zulu people by the British changed fundamentally over time. At first they regarded them as primitive, savage, and belligerent, but after their defeat a sort of fascination developed for those "noble, heroic and proud" African warriors who were said to embody the ideal of male brotherhood. Certainly, this idealization of the Zulus should be seen for what it was: an imperial propaganda campaign dressed in romanticizing interpretation. Thus the British soldier faced "a worthy and courageous adversary—a noble savage," and, of course, triumphed in the end.[14]

In the nineteenth century the Zulu people were probably the best known tribe of African warriors to the West, but they were not the only ones who went into battle intoxicated. Take, for example, another South African tribe, the Sotho, whose warriors regularly used cannabis, which they called "mutokwane." As David Livingstone, the Scottish explorer of Africa and one of the celebrities of Victorian Britain reported, they "sat down and smoked it, in order that they might make an effective onslaught."[15] The warriors of the Massai people, who inhabited Eastern Africa, prepared themselves for fighting by drinking a highly intoxicating drink made of the bark of the *thorny olkiloriti* tree.[16] Or take the case of the peoples of West Africa who traditionally used cola nuts, which contain two stimulating alkaloids—caffeine (2–4 percent) and theobromine (1–2.5 percent), as well as vitamins, microelements, and nutrients.[17] Cola has similar mild stimulating effects to coca leaves. In the nineteenth century during the colonial wars in Africa, the French soldiers became familiar with cola nuts and the ways of using them. Impressed by the results of a series of experiments conducted by its army in 1885, the French command staff acknowledged the highly desirable boosting effects of the plant and opted for distributing cola nut extract to the units as a refreshing and energizing drink.[18] The result was amazing, as the supplement enabled a battalion to make fifty-five kilometers a day under the scorching African sun.[19] Thus the Western militaries often learned from their "barbarous" adversaries diverse ways of using pharmacology to enhance the performance of their troops.

The Moros

> The fighting was the fiercest I have ever seen. They are absolutely fearless, and once committed to combat they count death as mere incident.
>
> —Captain John Pershing quoted in Richard K. Kolb,
> " 'Like a Mad Tiger:' Fighting Islamic Warriors
> in the Philippines 100 Years Ago"

In 1884 the American pharmacist John Pemberton began selling a tonic of his own invention made of wine and extracts from cola nuts and coca leaves. He created the drink to help the morphinists in breaking their habit, and Pemberton himself was a morphine addict who developed a drug problem as a result of the treatment of his wounds received in the Civil War. Thus when in 1899 the American soldiers arrived in the Philippines to suppress the anti-American rebellion, they could perhaps already refresh themselves with Pemberton's coca-cola, though unfortunately, from 1886 it was based on water instead of wine.[20] In the Philippines the Americans had to confront an exceptionally formidable and unpredictable enemy—the Moro people. Fighting with great courage and grim determination these indigenous Muslims, who inhabited the southern islands, had previously successfully resisted all Spanish attempts at conquest. They were so brave and belligerent that the Spanish, who had ruled the Philippines from the sixteenth century, had never managed to establish full control over their land, so the Moros preserved their independence. After the United States took over the Philippines following the Spanish–American War of 1898 and succeeded in suppressing the anti-American rebels in 1902, the Americans, in turn, had to face the fierce resistance of the Moro. These Muslim warriors posed a daunting challenge until as late as 1913.[21]

The fearless Moro swordsmen, who traditionally fought hand to hand, carried out frenzied ritualized attacks known as *juramentado* (from the Spanish *juramentar* meaning the one who takes an oath to kill the infidels), which often ended in their martyrdom. In the local Tausug language they were called *pagsabils*, roughly meaning "suicide warriors."[22] The Moro warriors were true religious fanatics who, just like the Assassins, believed that they would go to heaven by killing white Christians, and that the more enemies of Islam they eliminated the more houris they would possess.[23] Hence every *pagsabil* sought to kill as many opponents as possible in a single strike. The boys selected for the *juramentado* entered the path to paradise, and their journey there was preceded by a whole range of rituals. They prayed, took a ceremonial bath, and shaved their whole body. Before putting on a white robe and white turban, they firmly wrapped a strong band around their waist and put cords around ankles, knees, upper thighs, wrists, elbows, and shoulders. This served to restrict the blood flow and prevent the warriors from bleeding too heavily from injuries. They also tightly bound the genitals with wet cords, which upon drying and shrinking cut off the blood flow to the penis and testicles.[24] This, in turn, caused such an intense pain that it fueled a towering rage. Thus the Moro warriors behaved as if they entered an altered state of consciousness and at the same time, paradoxically, they felt less pain from battle wounds. They seemed to be anesthetized by self-inflicted pain. Peter Gowing provided a good summary of the Moro tactics: "With the possible exception of Japan's kamikaze pilots in the closing days of World War II, warfare has rarely known a more frightening phenomenon than the *juramentados*."[25]

The Americans inherited from the Spanish a stereotypical image of the Moro as ferociously cruel and backward barbarians. For example, the ruthless policy of repression and pacification carried out by Major General Leonard Wood, the military governor of the Moro province that was established by the Americans in 1903, is hardly surprising given his view of the Muslims as "religious and moral degenerates." The Americans perceived the Moro in exactly the same way as the British initially saw the Zulus and, in fact, there were striking similarities between the Zulu and Moro warriors. It can therefore be said that the Moros were the United States' Southeast Asian equivalent of Great Britain's South African Zulus. Both were fierce and savage fighters. And what frightened the Westerners most was their resistance to bullets, as after being shot several times they still kept fighting, causing further death and terror. Killing them was not an easy task; they were like zombies. The bullets pierced their limbs and torsos, scratched their bodies, but astonishingly the Moro did not drop dead, just like the Zulus. Captain Cornelius C. Smith reported that "in hand-to-hand combat our soldiers are no match for the Moro. If our first shot misses the target, we rarely have time to get off another."[26] The Americans, therefore, came to the conclusion that to successfully fight the Moro, soldiers needed a weapon of heavier caliber than the Colt .38 revolver, a standard sidearm of the American forces adopted in 1894. This demand for a more powerful firearm that could stop the ferocious Moro fanatics was the primary catalyst for designing, constructing, and developing the Colt .45 caliber semi-automatic pistol. Paradoxically, however, the American troops in the Philippines did not receive the new weapon before the ultimate suppression of the Moro rebellion in 1913. Hence the Colt .45 was never used for its original and most urgent purpose.[27] A similar story, although based on anecdotal evidence, is associated with black people in the southern American states in the early twentieth century. The myth holds that cocaine gave them such superhuman power that they were essentially impervious to .32 caliber police balls, so that the police had to switch to the Colt .38 caliber.[28] While this story came from whites' fear of blacks and reflected segregationist attitudes, the Moro warriors' extraordinary immunity to bullets was actually fact. Regrettably, the Moro problem was reduced to the caliber problem. The only solution to the ferociousness of the enemy that the Americans could come up with was technological superiority. Inevitably, then, war against the Moros turned out to be utterly brutal: between 10 and 20 thousand Moros were killed, as compared to 130 Americans.[29]

Contrary to some press reports, gossip, and stories, the Moro probably did not get drugged before battle; or it is at least very difficult to find any evidence in support of this claim. They fought like "mad tigers" and seemed to be heavily intoxicated, yet it was not drugs that got them high but something else. Self-inflicted pain apart, it was also honor, pride, and, above all, religion. As Robert Fulton notes, they "were propelled by will and naked belief, not chemicals."[30] They came from a typical warlike culture in which surrender was considered dishonorable and in which faith and social values left no room for the fear of death. They fought not only to defend their land, independence, and unique style of life; but, most importantly, they also resisted the infidels who sought to deprive them of their autonomy and spiritual identity. The Moro waged their own jihad. History teaches us that religion has indeed often been a particularly potent social intoxicant.

From Coca to Cocaine

The First World War

Rumours are circulating that the factory's [Nederlandsche Cocaïne Fabriek's] deliveries during the war were misused to enhance soldiers' performance on the battlefield. Cocaine wasn't just used as an anaesthetic, but as an instrument of war!
—Conny Braam, *The Cocaine Salesman*

The Early Experiments with Coca and Cocaine in Europe

The newest born of all drug cravings is that for cocaine.
—T. Clouston, Edinburgh psychiatrist, 1890 quoted in Richard Davenport-Hines, *The Pursuit of Oblivion: A Global History of Narcotics*

Only in the early nineteenth century did the Europeans begin to seriously consider the possibility of using coca to improve the physical endurance and raise the fighting spirits of troops. General William Miller, an English-born soldier who in the 1820s fought alongside the Peruvian army during Peru's war of independence, realized that chewing coca leaves was an essential and effective means of increasing soldiers' strength and resilience. During a campaign in 1824, he ordered his men to use coca and later reported his observations in a book entitled *Memories of General Miller in the Service of the Republic of Peru.* Miller, who greatly contributed to the popularization of the plant among the English, described the role of coca in Andean society in the following way:

Their every day pedestrian feats are truly astonishing. Guides perform a long journey at the rate of twenty or twenty-five leagues a day ... A battalion, eight hundred strong, has been known to march

thirteen or fourteen leagues in one day, without leaving more than ten
or a dozen stragglers on the road.[1]

In Europe it was Paolo Mantegazza, an Italian neurologist and physiologist,
who conducted the first research on the stimulating effects of coca leaves.
During his visit to Latin America, he carefully watched the Indians using
coca, and in 1859 when back in Italy he experimentally confirmed its boosting
properties. Most significant for the popularization of coca in the West were,
however, the trials carried out by the distinguished Scottish toxicologist Sir
Robert Christison from the University of Edinburgh. In 1870 he investigated
the effect of coca on fatigue with two of his students, who tired themselves
by walking sixteen miles. After they were given between six and eight grams
of leaves, hunger, thirst, and fatigue vanished, so they could continue walking for another hour.[2] The overall effect, then, was remarkable. Five years
later, after obtaining another batch of coca leaves, Christison could repeat his
experiment. He again asked students to perform walking exercises, and this
time they managed to cover a longer distance up to thirty miles. Eventually,
in May 1875, at the age of seventy-eight, Christison tested the effects of coca
on himself. The results of his experiments were published in 1876 in the influential *British Medical Journal*. He was very enthusiastic about the potential use
of coca as a highly effective means of mitigating exhaustion caused by strenu-
ous physical exertion.[3] This being so, the plant could perhaps also be used to
improve performance of soldiers. After all, William Hammond, the former
surgeon general of the U.S. Army, publicly admitted using a stimulating coca
tonic on a daily basis and "found it constantly refreshing, and never suffered
any subsequent depression."[4]

In France, also in the 1870s, Qiarles Gazeau tested coca on himself and
came to the conclusion that its potent appetite-reducing property could be
crucial in sustaining troops in the field. The French *Dictionnaire encyclopedique
des sciences medicales*, published in 1876, recommended the use of coca in both
army and industry.[5] And in Britain in 1893 Field Marshal Sir Henry Hvelyn
Wood tested the military value of coca on British soldiers and described the
results in a document entitled *Reports on Army Manoeuvres in Berkshire and
Wiltshire*. The following excerpt is particularly illustrative:

> The experiment was made of the use of coca leaves to allay thirst.
> About 1/8th ounce of leaves was issued at a time to each of those
> making the experiment, and they were chewed with a small quantity
> of slaked lime. The men, except for a few who objected to the taste,
> declared that they found great benefit from the leaves, the feeling of
> thirst at once being allayed.[6]

Thus the European armed forces slowly began to recognize the unique properties of coca and its potential military applications. Theodore Aschenbrandt,
a Bavarian army physician, was familiar with the discovery made in 1859 by
Friedrich Wöhler and his student Albert Niemann, who were the first to syn-
thesize cocaine from the coca plant. Their invention was announced the following year, and in 1862 Merck of Darmstadt, an old German pharmaceutical
company established in 1668, launched the manufacture of cocaine. Merck
advertised its new product as "a stimulant which is peculiarly adapted to
elevate the working ability of the body, without any dangerous effect."[7] So, in
1883 Aschenbrandt carried out an experiment in which soldiers on maneuvers
were given cocaine dissolved in water. He summed up the results of his trials
by remarking:

> I hope that with this study, which certainly is not complete nor entirely
> exact as to dosage and which certainly does not claim to be final proof
> of the properties of cocaine, I have drawn the attention of the military
> and inspired them to further research. I believe I have given sufficient
> evidence of its eminent usefulness.[8]

At that time, the overall military utility of the drug was recognized not in its
boosting but rather its appetite-reducing effect. Hence it was first and foremost
seen as a potential effective means of lowering by an estimated 15 to 20 percent the costs of army food supply.

Aschenbrandt's experiment caught the attention of Sigmund Freud, a
twenty-nine-year-old student of medicine. In a letter to his fiancée he wrote:
"A German has tested this stuff on soldiers and has reported that it has really
rendered them strong and capable of endurance."[9] In 1884 Freud bought one
gram of Merck's cocaine, a huge investment for a student because it cost the
equivalent of one month's average salary, and he began to conduct his first
experiments on himself.[10] What motivated him was a desire to help his friend
and scientist Ernst Fleischl von Marxow, a morphine addict who developed
the habit after the amputation of his thumb when doctors treated him with
morphine to alleviate phantom pain. Freud somehow believed that cocaine
could be a perfect drug in overcoming morphine addiction.[11] The initial results
of his work were so promising that in July 1884 he published an essay entitled
Über Coca.[12] It should be kept in mind that Freud saw cocaine as a good opportunity to promote himself and gain esteem in the medical profession, to garner
publicity, and to make money. In 1885, after testing cocaine to cure facial neu-
ralgia, he confessed: "I am so excited about it, for if it works I would be assured
for some time to come of attracting the attention so essential for getting on
in the world."[13] Freud not only formed hasty and untested opinions on the

medical effects of cocaine but also sometimes even slightly falsified research results. But he did not, in fact, hide his desire to make a quick and successful career at any cost, through fraud if necessary. And his dreams came true partly due to cocaine. He could not, however, forgive himself for the consequences of his intervention; although his experiments helped Fleischl von Marxow out of morphinism, they turned him into a lifelong cocaine addict.[14] For in the late nineteenth century it was not yet apparent that cocaine was a strong habit-forming drug. Now, of course, we know that by blocking neurotransmitters it increases the dopamine level in the regions of the brain associated with pleasure; in other words, it triggers a wave of euphoria, which inevitably results in the rapid development of dependence.

Unlike Freud, others pursued more rigorous and reliable research. Many European and American doctors experimented with cocaine in the search for new breakthrough applications. They found these not only in medicine (for example, in anesthesia and the treatment of fever) but also in sport, which explains why the early history of cocaine and the history of doping in sport are joined at the hip. In 1876 the American walking champion Edward Weston, who covered 109 miles in twenty-four hours, was accused of chewing coca leaves. He admitted that on the advice of his physician he had, indeed, chewed coca before the competition but discontinued the practice during the race because it had a sedative effect on him, just like opiates.[15] Weston's explanation seemed strange, not to say incredible, given the refreshing and invigorating effects of coca, but nevertheless the path for the use of cocaine by athletes was paved.

At the time of the revival of the Olympic Games in 1896, sport was actively promoted and enthusiastically supported by states. Organized sports were important for a reason; as Martin van Creveld reminds us, everywhere "they had a distinct militaristic flavor, allegedly serving to steel bodies and prepare spirits for the coming great struggle."[16] Sport proved to be an extremely useful instrument of state policy, since it prepared young boys for their future role as soldiers. Speaking of the connections between sport and war, it is important to remember that cocaine, one of the first true doping substances in modern sport, also found new applications in the great competitive game played by the major powers. Aschenbrandt's prediction concerning the future military utility of cocaine was proven correct by the First World War, during which the drug amply demonstrated its overall battlefield effectiveness.

The Wartime Cocaine Boom

Despite the fact that many of the hundreds of thousands of First World War soldiers who were exposed to morphine when treated for their war-related injuries developed severe addiction, it was not morphine but cocaine that dominated the discourse on this war.

Although demand for cocaine remained rather low until well into the late 1880s, its production increased steadily. The statistics available from Merck, the leading pharmaceutical company in the market, vividly illustrate this dynamic: while in 1879 it manufactured a total of 50 grams of cocaine hydrochloride, between 1881 and 1884 it produced 1.4 kilograms and almost 30 kilograms of the drug in 1885 alone.[17] In 1913 production reached nearly 9,000 kilograms. The war interrupted international trade and impeded the supply of European factories with Peruvian coca leaves. The halt in exports of coca and crude cocaine from Peru seriously affected the manufacture of cocaine in Europe. By late 1915 Merck's annual production fell to only 500 kilograms.[18] Paradoxically, the First World War created an increasing demand for cocaine, but at the same time it caused a great disturbance in international trade, which significantly reduced the supply of raw materials and thus hampered the production of the drug. However, the decline of international trade in coca and cocaine made for the rapid development of one pharmaceutical company: Nederlandsche Cocaïne Fabriek Ltd. (NCF). Established in March 1900 in Amsterdam as a joint venture of the Koloniale Bank and coca-plantation owners in the Dutch East Indies, the factory produced cocaine from coca leaves grown in the colony. Back in 1878 the first coca plant seedlings had been imported to Java from Peru. The plant thrived in the local soil and climate so well that, interestingly, the Javan coca turned out to be of higher quality (containing 2 percent of cocaine alkaloid) than its original Peruvian variety (containing "only" 1.2 percent of cocaine).[19] The cultivation of the coca plant in Java flourished so much that soon the Dutch East Indies emerged as the leading supplier of leaves, outpacing Peru. Javan coca exports grew from twenty-six metric tons in 1904 to 800 metric tons in 1912, a more than thirty-fold increase in just eight years.[20]

The Dutch writer Conny Braam tells a narrative history of NCF in her novel *The Cocaine Salesman*. The historical background of the book is based on detailed research conducted by the author in numerous Dutch, Belgian, British, and German archives and libraries. Lucien Hirschland, the protagonist of the story, is the titular "cocaine salesman" who travels across Europe to negotiate contracts for NCF-manufactured cocaine. Owing to his outstanding sales results, the company earns huge profits from exporting the drug to many countries, mostly to Austria, Belgium, France, Germany, and Britain. Only after the war does he realize that the armies of the warring parties were supplied by their national pharmaceutical companies with Dutch-produced cocaine. And that the drug was issued to soldiers not only as a medicine for pain relief but also as a potent stimulant.

During the war NCF, which eagerly sold the high-quality cocaine to both the Central Powers and the Allies, developed into the world's leading manufacturer, producing an average of 14,000 kilograms of white powder a year. The war gave the company the perfect opportunity to choke off its competitors and make enormous profits. As production increased the factory modernized and nearly doubled in size. A huge growth in demand from the military led to a sharp rise in the production, which went up to between 20,000 and 30,000 kilograms per year.[21] But unavoidably, this high supply resulted in a considerable drop in cocaine's price. Once exorbitant and unaffordable, it became cheap and accessible, even abundant. Its price slumped from 280 dollars an ounce in 1885 to a mere 3 dollars an ounce in 1914.[22] The neutrality of the Netherlands during the war fostered the enormous expansion of NCF, once a small and little known company.[23] In Braam's novel a British contractor is outraged by finding out that NCF is supplying not only the Allies but also Germany and Austria, so Lucien Hirschland explains to him:

> The Netherlands is neutral, you know. As a manufacturer of pharmaceuticals we do what we can. Everyone has free access to our help. Every wounded soldier has the right to the best anesthetics. The Dutch government takes the view that we can't assist one warring party to the detriment of another. See us as the Red Cross.[24]

Of course, what was at stake here was not humanitarianism but business. From the very beginning NCF greatly benefited from not being bound by treaty obligations to honor the patent on cocaine, which expired anyway in 1903, bringing in several new German manufacturers.[25] In addition, the war severely hit the competitors, because under the international blockade the export ban on coca leaves from Java cut off European pharmaceutical companies from raw materials from the Dutch East Indies. Hence the rivals in neighboring countries became dependent on Dutch cocaine. Moreover, what also favored the rapid development of the Amsterdam factory was the Netherlands' geographical location, relatively close to the frontlines. It could deliver in short order even large quantities of cocaine almost directly to the war fronts. And it was precisely at the line of fire that the demand for the drug was highest.

The rate of cocaine use by soldiers remains unknown, and there is no way to estimate the figures. What is certain, however, is that never before and never after did the military consume such large amounts of this drug as it did in 1914–1918, not only for medical purposes but also for the enhancement of performance. There were three major factors that contributed to such a prevalence of cocaine. The first was the character of the war, which required the deployment of huge armies. The second was the severe battlefield conditions, especially in the trenches of the Western Front, conjoined with the alienating and dehumanizing effects of military technology, which caused unprecedented levels of injuries and war-related trauma. The third was that cocaine was not a controlled substance; it was legally and easily available and widely used as an ingredient in various popular medicaments.

The armed forces of the warring parties dispensed cocaine to keep the combatants energized and fuel their fighting spirit. It usually helped soldiers with shattered nerves calm down a little and improve performance. The drug was taken during long-distance flights by German fighter pilots. Also, French records reveal that the early airmen were particularly keen on using the upper: "Cocaine infused into the few duellists of the air who made use of that cold and thoroughly lucid exaltation which—alone among drugs—it can produce . . . at the same time it left intact their control over their actions. It fortified them, one might say, by abolishing the idea of risk."[26] But cocaine was certainly much more popular among the infantrymen than airmen. For example, shortly before an attack at the battle of Gallipoli (April 1915–January 1916), the Australian soldiers were administered significant amounts of the drug. Further to that, the wounded and sick soldiers of the Australian and New Zealand army corps were treated by not overly competent medics, who routinely prescribed the easiest and most effective treatment, that is to say, the two potent pain medications: morphine and cocaine.[27] Unsurprisingly, many patients developed an irresistible appetite for these substances; many became addicted and continued to self-administer drugs long after their recovery. Such was the grim reality among the armies of European great powers.

The British Army used extensively a medicine available on the market from the beginning of the twentieth century under the trade name "Tabloid" or "Forced March." The drug contained cocaine and cola nut extract and was manufactured by Burroughs Wellcome & Co., a well-known London pharmaceutical company and also the first one to launch the production of cocaine in tablet form. This development marked a "pharmaceutical revolution" of a kind, as it allowed the shelf-life of the drug to be extended and enabled its more convenient storage and intake as well as improved hygiene standards. The advertising slogan for Tabloid said that it "allays hunger and prolongs the power of endurance." The recommended dosage was one tablet "to be dissolved in the mouth every hour when undergoing continued mental strain or physical exertion."[28] Forced March was successfully used in long and exhausting polar expeditions, for example during the failed race to the South Pole led by Ernest Shackleton (1907–1909) and the successful 1912 polar trek of Robert Falcon Scott, who reached the South Pole only a month after its first conqueror, the Norwegian Roald Amundsen. And the latter, too, invigorated himself with the Burroughs Wellcome upper pills.[29] Because Forced March worked so well during these extremely wearying expeditions, it is hardly surprising that the command of the British Army decided to try it out on the soldiers of the expeditionary force in Europe.

Given the addiction of epidemic proportions among the veterans of the First World War, there are reasons to believe that the conflict left hundreds of thousands of men addicted to cocaine. The combatants, particularly on the Western Front, were in all probability usually unaware of being given a white "boosting" powder mixed with food or drink. Based on her research Conny Braam concludes that British soldiers "got a cup of rum before they went over the top and the cocaine might have been in the rum, because with alcohol it works doubly well. I think a lot of these soldiers had no idea."[30] One of the characters in her novel, Robin Ryder, wears a mask which hides his face, half blown away by a German grenade in Flanders in 1917. But Ryder carefully hides from the world still another secret of his war experience: his cocaine habit. When the time comes when he can no longer keep his harrowing secret, Ryder begins to tell his story of

> how they'd coerced him into taking cocaine in the trenches, to help overcome his mortal fear. How objecting almost landed him in front of the firing squad for insubordination and cowardice. That he was hooked, no matter how hard they'd tried to shake it, he and his pal Charlie, who'd also got addicted at the front. . . . It only got worse after I was wounded. Life was unbearable. The depression was appalling.[31]

This is, of course, a literary account but a very plausible one. Ryder epitomizes the fate of the lost generation of soldiers of the Great War who were physically mutilated, suffered from war trauma, felt socially rejected, and became addicted to drugs, mainly morphine and cocaine. Lucien Hirschland wonders why the demand for cocaine did not decline despite the ending of the war, for there were no more crippled bodies of soldiers who needed to be desensitized. The traveling cocaine salesman appears to be naive, and one of his interviewees bluntly reminds him that

> [t]he massive cocaine use in the trenches had created an entire army of addicts. Thousands, hundreds of thousands . . . If you think about how much our firm [NCF] alone supplied, you can work it out. Everywhere—in England, France, Belgium, Austria, the United States, even in Australia and Canada—they're having huge problems with addicted veterans.[32]

Indeed.

The Great War and the Cocaine Panic in Britain

Although the French accused the Germans of smuggling cocaine in order to deliberately weaken the French race, it was in Britain that the truly nationwide drug panic broke out. The hysteria was largely generated by the media, politicians, and military establishment. The *Times*, for example, hailed cocaine as a grave danger even "more deadly than bullets." The problem was grossly exaggerated and presented as a threat not only to the British troops on the front but also to the British Empire. The panic ensued mainly because of the Canadian soldiers temporarily stationed on the Isles waiting to be deployed to the Western Front. In 1914–1915 between 200,000 and 250,000 Canadians passed through London. In January 1916 a Canadian major based near Folkestone in Kent discovered the source of the supply of cocaine to his units. He carried out what today would be called a "sting operation" by buying a packet of cocaine from a man named Horace Dennis Kingsley and a London prostitute called Rose Edwards. They both admitted obtaining the drug in a West End pub from a man who supplied all local women of easy virtue. Kingsley and Edwards were sentenced to six months' hard labor for "selling a powder to members of HM Forces, with intent to make them less capable of performing their duties."[33] In the course of their trial it emerged that some forty men in a local camp had developed a drug habit. This widely publicized incident became a true bombshell and the grist to the mill of the proponents of bringing addictive substances under tight governmental control. Other minor incidents, such as robbery and a fatal beating, which also involved the Canadians, only confirmed the public belief in the already well-established but false media myth that it was the Canadian troops who had brought the cocaine habit to Britain.[34] In the period 1906–1910 politicians, clerics, officials of the judiciary, and various social activists in Canada frequently raised the problem of the increasing consumption of cocaine. The issue was widely discussed in parliamentary debates as well as in the professional medical journals.[35] The Canadian soldiers had not, however, created the cocaine problem in Britain; they merely aggravated it by fueling the demand for the drug that already existed.

Before the war cocaine was a common ingredient in medicines and tonics for hay fever as it cleanses the respiratory track by reducing swelling of the mucosa and nasal discharge. The most popular American drug, called Ryno's Hay Fever, the content of which was 99.9 cocaine, was touted as the best cure for a clogged, reddened, and sore nose, to be used when it gets "stuffed-up."[36] Also the British Burroughs Wellcome & Co. manufactured the already mentioned Tabloid cocaine tablets marketed as perfect for singers and public speakers longing to improve their voices.[37] Overall, mass-produced cocaine, which was believed to be as harmless as tobacco, had become widespread well before the war, and soldiers were but a minority of its users. Thus, if the consumption of drugs in Britain developed into a problem, it was a problem not so much of the army alone but of society at large. Cocaine's presence in literature might be illustrative of the extent of its nonmedical use; one of the finest examples is Sherlock Holmes. He is an eccentric character and a cultural icon whom Arthur Conan Doyle made a habitual user who takes cocaine to combat boredom and boost his mental faculties. The world's most famous detective is, in fact, a regular recreational cocaine-taker. Holmes's habit is directly observed in the novel *The Sign of the Four* (1890) and in the short story *A Scandal in Bohemia* (1891).[38] At the very beginning of the novel Holmes injects into his arm a 7 percent solution of cocaine in front of Dr. Watson, contentedly sighs with pleasure, and relaxes in his armchair. He dopes himself for intellectual stimulation, as his mind revolts against apathy and stagnation. Conan Doyle is a moralist here, for he makes Dr. Watson express his own anxiety about the harmful effects of cocaine use:

> But consider! Count the cost! Your brain may, as you say, be roused and excited, but it is a pathological and morbid process, which involves increased tissue change, and may at least leave a permanent weakness. You know, too, what a black reaction comes upon you. Surely the game is hardly worth the candle. Why should you, for a mere passing pleasure, risk the loss of those great powers with which you have been endowed?[39]

Watson's concerns were loudly echoed in wartime Britain. In February 1916 many pharmacies were fined for selling soldiers cocaine and morphine without observing the restrictions of the 1868 Pharmacy Act. Among those punished were not only the famous London store Harrods but also Savory & Moore, a well-known Mayfair pharmacy with a long tradition. In a December 1915 edition of the *Times* Savory & Moore advertised a small mail-order medical kit in a handy case containing, among other items, cocaine and heroin. And Harrods offered small packages of morphine and cocaine complete with syringe and spare needles, which was recommended as "A Useful Present for Friends at the Front."[40] Girls often brought to the train station a cocaine kit as an ideal gift for their loved ones leaving for war. Despite itself advertising cocaine products, the *Times*, like most other papers, created alarm by suggesting that supplying soldiers with this drug would inevitably undermine the combat effectiveness of the British Army. In the February 12, 1916, issue, its journalist expressed no doubt that

> [t]o the soldier subjected to nervous strain and hard work cocaine, once used, must become a terrible temptation. It will, for the hour,

charm away his trouble, his fatigue and his anxiety; it will give him fictitious strength and vigor. But it will also, in the end, render him worthless as a soldier and a man.[41]

The *Daily Chronicle*, too, contributed to heating up the cocaine hysteria by reporting, for example, that soldiers were literally crawling into chemists' shops to get the drug. Readers were informed that the habit "is driving hundreds of women mad. What is worse, it will drive, unless the traffic in it is checked, hundreds of soldiers mad."[42] The consequences of cocaine taking were said to be terrifying, as crazed soldiers turned aggressive, insubordinate, and sometimes even committed murders. It was suggested, in essence, that the armed forces were plunging into confusion and anarchy. Moreover, in the first months of 1916 the police confirmed that a well-organized underground market for cocaine existed in London. Drug dealers in the West End used Soho prostitutes, popularly known as "cocaine girls" or "dope girls," to distribute cocaine to military personnel. The press and public opinion immediately linked cocaine with sex, hedonism, moral decay, and enemy subversion. Because in the popular imagination drugs were clichéd and commonly associated with hostile foreign influences, they were easily portrayed as a tool of war employed by the scheming enemy to undermine the spirit of Britannia. And the wartime conditions only favored the rise of numerous conspiracy theories and xenophobic narratives. As we know, however, the world's largest cocaine manufacturer and supplier was not in hostile Germany but the neutral Netherlands.

The politicians, particularly Sir Malcolm Delevingne, the undersecretary of state at the Home Office; military commanders; and the media promoted and reinforced the view that intoxicants were a secret or unfair weapon (today we would perhaps call it "asymmetric") deployed by the Central Powers, mostly Germany, which was, after all, a pioneer country in the production of cocaine. The drug covertly supplied by the Germans was believed to get British soldiers addicted, thus eroding their combat performance, undermining military discipline, and ultimately causing a rapid decay of the army. Sir Francis Lloyd, a general in command of the London district, accurately captured the essence of the cocaine panic that seized public opinion: "I am told that this evil practice is exceedingly rife at the present time. It is doing an immense amount of harm, I am told. They say that it is so ingrained that once you take it you will not give it up."[43] The drug plague was therefore allegedly destroying the British military. Sir William Glyn-Jones, the secretary of the Pharmaceutical Society, warned with regard to morphine, though he could well have been, to an extent, talking about cocaine, "It was an exceedingly dangerous thing for a drug like morphine to be in the hands of men on active service . . . It might have the effect of making them sleep on duty or other very serious results."[44] Of course, cocaine could not make troops sleep on duty, though it was claimed it had other debilitating effects. With politicians and media playing on the paranoid fears of enemy subversion, the moral panic around cocaine was spreading at lightning speed and turning into mass hysteria not only over cocaine but over drugs in general.

Given such an explosive social climate, with public opinion highly suscepti-ble to manipulation, the military command could not stay idle. It seemed that it was high time to take emergency action in defense of the army and Britain's fighting power. Hence, under intense and relentless public pressure, on May 11, 1916, the Army Council issued an order banning any unauthorized sale or supply of psychoactive substances—mostly cocaine, but also codeine, hemp, heroin, morphine, and opium—to any member of the armed forces, except for medical reasons and only by prescription.[45] All violations would constitute an offense punishable by six months' imprisonment. Further regulations were introduced under the Defence of the Realm Act (DORA), which was already in force having been passed four days after Britain entered the war in August 1914. DORA served as the cover for various wartime regulatory schemes and social control mechanisms, including censorship and a limited prohibition on alcohol. The Act allowed the executive to create criminal offenses through regulation, hence under DORA regulation 40B, passed on July 28, 1916, the sale of cocaine and opium-based products to military personnel without a nonreusable prescription was prohibited for anyone except for medical prac-titioners, pharmacists, and veterinary personnel.[46] Soldiers could face court-martial if accused of violating the ban. The historical importance of DORA 40B lay not so much in its scope, since it was limited to cocaine and opium and covered neither marijuana nor heroin, but in the essence of the prohibi-tive principle, that is, putting particular substances under strict state control and criminalizing their sale and use. The subsequent Dangerous Drugs Act of 1920 retained most of the provisions of DORA 40B, thereby transforming the wartime regulation into a peacetime law. The drug control regime was sig-nificantly widened to cover not only military personnel but also all citizens. Moreover, the list of controlled substances was extended to include cocaine, heroin, morphine, raw opium, and also, to an extent, barbiturates. The Act brought Britain in line with national control regimes introduced earlier by the United States (under the Harrison Act of 1914) and the Netherlands (under its opium act of 1919) and, above all, with the demands put forward by the Versailles peace conference on the need to impose restrictions on the interna-tional trade in opium. Therefore, the overblown problem of cocaine use in the military resulted in the adoption of strict government drug control regulations in Britain. Thus the war not only favored the rise of cocaine and morphine taking but was also critical in fostering the introduction of a comprehensive substance control regime, for the implementation of which the issue of servicemen's use and abuse of intoxicants was merely instrumental. So, similar to the opium and morphine problem and the "soldiers' disease" in the aftermath of the American Civil War, the cocaine crisis in Britain was widely exaggerated and grossly overestimated. The findings of the Select Committee on the Use of Cocaine in Dentistry unequivocally debunked the myth that cocaine addiction was hitting hard in the British forces:

> We are unanimously of opinion that there is no evidence of any kind to show that there is any serious, or, perhaps, even noticeable prevalence of the cocaine habit amongst the civilian or military population of Great Britain. There have been a certain number of cases amongst the oversea troops quartered in, or passing through, the United Kingdom, but there is hardly any trace of the practice having spread to British troops, and, apart from a small number of broken-down medical men, there is only very slight evidence of its existence amongst the general population.[47]

The new dimension of state control spread also into the realm of art. The film director Graham Cutts experienced this firsthand, when the Board of Film Censors tried to ban the distribution of his 1922 movie under the telling title *Cocaine*. The film sent a clear warning against the dangers of cocaine use by showing an underworld of night clubs and drug gangs, in which the stimulant is omnipresent, and ultimately brings death to a young character. Yet the authorities feared that the movie might actually encourage cocaine taking.[48] Moral panics preclude rational interpretation and sound judgment.

To conclude, the character of the First World War with its totality, brutality, anonymity, and harsh conditions on the frontline, propelled the military demand for cocaine, and not merely for its medical value. Along with alcohol, tobacco, and morphine, it allowed for temporary escape from the terrifying reality of modern warfare. Although cocaine would never again achieve such popularity among combatants, it soon emerged as a highly fashionable intoxicant among bohemian artists and in the world of popular culture. It was the war indeed that was in part responsible for the rise of cocainism in European societies. If the First World War brought cocaine to the frontline, the drugs of choice during the Second World War would be amphetamines.

The Second World War

> During the Second World War, amphetamine and methamphet-
> amine were adopted in the military services on all sides, in quasi-
> medical efforts to tune mind and body beyond normal human
> capabilities.
> —Nicolas Rasmussen, *On Speed: The Many Lives of Amphetamine*

The Speed

Although amphetamines have been available on the market since the late nineteenth century (phenylpropylmethylamine, the derivate of amphetamine, was
first synthesized in 1887 while methamphetamine was obtained in 1919),
their dynamic history began on June 3, 1928. On that day in Los Angeles
the chemist Gordon Alles tested on himself a new substance, which he had
created the previous year when working on a cheaper equivalent for ephedrine. He called it "beta-phenyl-isopropylamine," yet it has come to be known
as "amphetamine." His friend, a doctor called Hyman Miller, injected him
with fifty milligrams of the new drug, which was five times what would later
become the standard dose in medical treatment.[1] Alles watched his body carefully and took detailed notes. He felt well and was so strongly stimulated that
he had a sleepless night full of racing thoughts but, surprisingly, he felt exceptionally well the next morning. Additional visible effects of the drug were high
blood pressure, unusual talkativeness, and uncongested nose in spite of sniff-
ing. Above all, Alles experienced an overall "feeling of well-being." In 1932 he
was granted a patent on amphetamine sulphate as a chemical, which he transferred in 1934 to the Philadelphia pharmaceutical company Smith, Kline &
French (SKF, today GlaxoSmithKline). SKF launched the production of the
Benzedrine inhaler for nasal congestion. The applications of amphetamine
were later widened to include asthma, hay fever, and slimming therapy, and by
1946 its medical use was generally accepted in the treatment of almost forty
afflictions, such as schizophrenia, low blood pressure, narcolepsy, epilepsy,

Parkinson's disease, seasickness, obesity, chronic hiccups, and dependence on morphine and caffeine.[2]

Soon its nonmedical use also became widespread. Truck drivers in the United States, who traveled long distances between the East and West Coasts, discovered that they did not get sleepy or experience lapses in concentration if every few hours they took a Benzedrine pill. Thus "truck drivers" became one of the popular names for amphetamine, next to such slang terms as "speed," "pep pills," "wake-ups," "eye-openers," and "lid-poppers." By stimulating both central and peripheral (specifically the sympathetic division) nervous systems, amphetamines enhance alertness and cognitive functioning while at the same time suppressing appetite. Like cocaine they trigger the release of dopamine, the leading neurotransmitter that regulates the reward system in the brain, and inhibit its reuptake. The enhancing and energizing effect of Benzedrine caught the lively interest of the American armed forces. It was, however, the Nazis who were the first, in 1938, to pioneer the military use of amphetamines. In the course of the Second World War the British, Americans, Japanese, and Finns followed suit in authorizing the distribution of speed to their military services.

The Nazis

The Third Reich fought bitterly against the social consumption of intoxicants. Addiction was considered shameful, and Nazi propaganda portrayed cocaine as an evil drug of the demoralized European bohemians. It was in Germany in the Weimar period, writes Henry Hobhouse, that sex and cocaine taking were bound closer than anywhere else.[3] Cocaine was commonly associated with lechery, prostitution, hedonism, and the underworld—in short, with all the immoral things disgraceful for true Aryans. The Nazis, by the way, saw and treated "perverse jazz music" similarly, seemingly managing to eliminate it by 1933.[4] According to the Nazi Party's doctrine, any psychoactive substance (*Rauschgifte*), be it alcohol, marijuana, cocaine, or opium, was not so much a drug but rather "inebriant poison" that drained the vitality of the Aryan master race.[5] Put differently, intoxicants were assumed to destroy the spirit of "national unity." Paradoxically, all this did not prevent the Nazis from drugging their glorious soldiers and turning a blind eye to heavy alcohol and methamphetamine abuse in the ranks. Purity and abstinence were, therefore, to be confined to the society of civilians, because entirely different standards applied to the armed forces and high-ranking Nazi officials. Take, for example, Joseph Goebbels or Hermann Göring, who were both heavy morphine addicts. The latter developed his lifelong habit after the First World War, in which he got wounded as a pilot, was treated with morphine, and quickly became dependent on the narcotic. When cocaine was used to drag him out of morphinism it made him, in turn, a cocaine addict.[6] To conclude, the double standards applied to most aspects of life in the Third Reich and, unsurprisingly, also to drug use.

High Hitler

Although Adolf Hitler himself did not smoke, was a staunch opponent of drinking, and was an eager vegetarian, he was heavily hooked on medicines, particularly psychoactive substances. His was a paradoxical attitude to say the least. On the one hand, "the chief reason for Hitler's abstinence," writes Alan Bullock,

> seems to have been anxiety about his health. He lived an unhealthy life, with little exercise or fresh air; he took part in no sport, never rode or swam, and he suffered a good deal from stomach disorders as well as from insomnia. With this went a horror of catching a cold or any form of infection. He was depressed at the thought of dying early, before he had had time to complete his schemes, and he hoped to add years to his life by careful dieting and avoiding alcohol, coffee, tea, and tobacco. In the late-night sessions round the fireplace Hitler never touched stimulants, not even real tea.[7]

On the other hand, "under the stress of war . . . Hitler began to take increasing quantities of drugs to stimulate his flagging energies."[8] His great passion for healthy food and hygienic living did not preclude pharmacological self-poisoning. Was it a contradiction, an absurd inconsistency, or irony? One does not need to try hard to find the answer. Consider his appearance; Hitler was not the embodiment of masculine virtues but sharply diverged from the Nordic pattern that he so fervently extolled and promoted. Let me unpack this paradox by referring to the German philosopher Max Schelling, who was once asked why he did not follow the rules which he praised, and he answered that no one would expect a signpost to follow the path that it indicates.

We know that methamphetamine was only one among many other drugs taken by the führer. Theodor Morell, a regular house doctor who specialized in venereal diseases, was from 1936 until Hitler's suicide his most trusted private doctor. He perfected the method of making Hitler feel good by administering potent pharmacological substances. Usually, these were intravenous injections aimed at combating fatigue or alleviating depression.[9] Because the führer had a fear of pills, Morell injected him with most of the medicines. When Hitler needed a strong stimulus, for example, before delivering a demagogic and inflammatory public speech, he was given injections of strychnine, hormones, and methamphetamine. Think of June 22, 1941. That day, before Hitler left the Chancellery to go to the Reichstag to declare war on the Soviet Union, Morell administered him an injection.[10] Thus he gave a rousing speech pharmacologically enhanced. Many observers have wondered about the source of Hitler's great inherent ability to influence the masses. His trenchant critic Otto Strasser's diagnosis, for example, was that

> Hitler responds to the vibration of the human heart with the delicacy of a seismograph, or perhaps of a wireless receiving set, enabling him . . . to act as a loudspeaker proclaiming the most secret desires, the least admissible instincts, the sufferings, and personal revolts of a whole nation. . . . I have been asked many times what is the secret of Hitler's extraordinary power as a speaker. I can only attribute it to his uncanny intuition, which infallibly diagnoses the ills from which his audience is suffering.[11]

Allan Bullock reminds us that some likened this unique gift to "the occult arts of the African medicine-man or the Asiatic Shaman; others have compared it to the sensitivity of a medium, and the magnetism of a hypnotist."[12] But something else was involved too: well into the war the potent mixtures of drugs increased his self-confidence and self-mastery, induced intense bursts of energy, and got him steamed up. Hitler's charisma was, therefore, in part pharmacologically induced.

As the Nazi leader was a great hypochondriac, Morell dispensed different sorts of medications to him as a cure for his numerous afflictions both real and imaginary.[13] Hitler was prescribed about eighty-two different medicines during his rule of Nazi Germany. Some drugs were created by Morell himself, such as, for example, a mixture of sulphonamide, a compound banned by the pharmacological department of the University of Leipzig for having a detrimental impact on the human nervous system. Another "supplement" of Morell's design was Vitamultin, a performance-enhancing combination of various vitamins.[14] The tablets were known as Morell's "golden pills," ("Novel-Vitamultine") for they were wrapped in gold foil. Hitler's otolaryngologist Dr. Erwin Giesing recalled that the führer blindly believed in the overall effectiveness of the medications prescribed by Morell, keenly took some 150 pills a week, and received plentiful additional injections, including Testoviron for sexual potency.

Morell also made Hitler glucose and testosterone injections (a primitive Viagra) and prescribed synthetic opiates—especially Eukodal, a near-cousin of heroin—and probably cocaine as painkillers.[15] Dr. Karl Brandt, one of the führer's attending physicians, who was sentenced to death in the Nuremburg trials as a war criminal, reported that

> Morell took more and more to treatment by injections, until in the end he was doing all his work by this method. For instance, he would give large doses of sulphonamides for slight colds, and gave them to everyone at Hitler's headquarters. . . . Morell then took to giving injections that had dextrose, hormones, vitamins, etc., so that the patient immediately felt better; and this type of treatment seemed to impress Hitler. Whenever he felt a cold coming on, he would have three to six injections daily, and thus prevent any real development of the infection. Therapeutically this was satisfactory. Then Morell used it as a prophylactic. If Hitler had to deliver a speech on a cold or rainy day, he would have injections the day before, the day of the speech, and the day after. The normal resistance of the body was thus gradually replaced by an artificial medium.[16]

By the end of the war, Hitler was receiving up to several injections every day. Their boosting effect was further enhanced by the large quantities of Morell's golden pills.[17] Taking potent doses of uppers on a daily basis caused severe insomnia, but still even without pharmacological stimulation Hitler suffered from sleep disorders. So to make him able to sleep at night, Morell issued equally potent doses of sedatives and hypnotics, mostly barbiturates and bromine. The result was that oftentimes Hitler was extremely hard to wake up in the morning, a fact that can help explain some events that continue to puzzle historians to this day. Take, for example, the delayed German reaction to the Allied landing in Normandy on June 6, 1944. The lag resulted not only from utter strategic surprise, not only from Hitler's ill-fated order requiring all major military decisions to be referred to him for approval, but also from the mundane fact that he could not be woken up that day. Hence Hitler's dependence on drugs can be seen as one of the reasons for the Germans not seizing the initiative in the first hours of the Allied D-Day landing.[18] When Hitler was under the too-powerful influence of sedatives, Morell dispensed him boosting medications. Thus was a junkie führer persistently artificially stimulated and quieted with uppers and downers.[19]

Having said above, Hitler's use of psychostimulants remains a contested topic. In 2015—when my book was already in the production at OUP—a German writer and novelist Norman Ohler published a seminal book *Der Totale Rausch: Drogen im Dritten Reich* (*Total Rush: Drugs in the Third Reich*). Based on his reading of private records of Theodor Morell on his treatment of Hitler and archives of the Nazi state in Germany and Washington, Ohler calls into question that the führer was given methamphetamine. He found that only once, on December 19, 1944 Morell mentions this drug. Instead, Hitler was addicted to Eukodal, a strong opiate closely related to heroin and steroids (animal hormons). Eukodal made Hitler feel invulnerable and euphoric even when the reality wasn't looking euphoric at all. The generals kept telling him, "We need to change our tactics; we need to end this; we are going to lose the war, and he didn't want to hear this. He used Dr. Morell give him the drugs that made him feel invulnerable and on top of the situation."[20]

Ohler's recent reading of Morell's records suggest that the story of Hitler being regularly given methamphetamine is to be treated as a rumor. Nevertheless, he was still heavily addicted to various other pharmaceuticals. In a word, he was a junkie führer who received daily a dizzy array of drugs, mostly injected. In an interview for *Deutsche Welle* Ohler was asked: "What came as the biggest surprise to you during your many years of research for this book?," and he answered: "I found Hitler's excessive drug abuse to be the most astonishing."[21]

Already in the 1930s, as noted by observers, Hitler exhibited symptoms similar to Parkinson's disease, and there are authors who have even tracked this in the movies. In *The Triumph of the Will*, a 1934 propaganda film by Leni Riefenstahl, some notice that the forty-five-year-old Hitler, addressing the Second Annual Nazi Party Congress in Nuremburg, displays a severely limited movement of the left hand, which he keeps clamped against his side.[22] Even if this interpretation might be somehow exaggerated, in the course of the war his symptoms became so acute that eventually the führer was thoroughly examined. In January 1945, Dr. Max de Crinis, a professor from the University of Berlin, provided a diagnosis, which remained undisclosed to the patient: *paralysis agitans*, or Parkinson's disease. On September 10, 1944, SS-Obersturmbannführer Otto Skorzeny attended a party at the führer's headquarters and was truly horrified by Hitler's physical condition. Skorzeny saw a hunched and oldish man with weak voice. His left hand trembled so much that he had to clamp it down with his right hand. So when on April 30, 1945, Hitler committed suicide, he was an exceptionally weak, mopish, and ailing man. "Though he suffered from no organic disease," writes Trevor-Roper, Hitler "had become a physical wreck."[23] And what of his armed forces?

The Wehrmacht on Meth

Despite the Nazis' near unanimous condemnation of the social use of drugs, not only the führer and his close collaborators but also the German military were significantly pill-popped. Pharmacology played a crucial, though largely untold, role in the German war effort, especially in the initial stage of the conflict. Nicolas Rasmussen put it particularly well: "The German Blitzkrieg was powered by amphetamines as much as it was powered by machine."[24] Pharmacology became a built-in feature of the blitzkrieg to such an extent that it should be seen equal to other recognized parts of the German revolution in land warfare, that is, tanks, planes, radio communication, and armored infantry. Speed and the extraordinary mobility of the panzer divisions were essential in translating tactical advantage into operational success. The blitzkrieg owed its speed not only to technology and military organization, but also to methamphetamine available on the market under the trade name Pervitin. The blitz as we know it would not only not have happened without fuel to drive tanks but also without pharmacological boosters to fuel the troops. To illustrate this claim let me take the popular nineteenth-century metaphor of war as energy. By unlocking the internal energy of soldiers, methamphetamine can be seen as one of the engines that powered the ultrafast blitzkrieg. In the initial phase of the war, the Wehrmacht emerged as the first army "on meth" in military history, and the speediest one at that. The invigorating effects of methamphetamine perfectly corresponded with the Nazi cult of endurance, efficiency, and obedience—in short, with the superhuman features and abilities of the Herrenvolk. What was not allowed for ordinary citizens was allowed for the Aryan warriors in their pursuit of Lebensraum.

Three-milligram Pervitin, manufactured by the Berlin-based pharmaceutical company Temmler-Werke, reached the market as an easily available drug at the turn of 1938 and 1939. It was the early version of what we know today as crystal meth. The effects of methamphetamine are more intensive and last longer than those of amphetamine, and are similar to adrenaline, a hormone and neurotransmitter produced by the body, although the effects are also much more potent. How does the body respond? The drug increases self-confidence and willingness to take risks; sharpens concentration; enhances alertness; and significantly reduces hunger, thirst, pain sensitivity, and the need for sleep. All these properties, highly desirable for the military profession, made Pervitin a perfectly appealing stimulant for the German troops, particularly in the opening stages of the Second World War. (At the 1936 Olympic Games in Berlin, Hitler had already directly ordered the Third Reich to pursue a deliberate policy of pharmacological doping by giving its athletes both steroids and methamphetamine to increase their competitive edge.[25]) For the first time in combat, methamphetamine was used on a trial basis as a performance enhancer during the Spanish Civil War (1936–1939).[26]

The incredible properties of the drug were brought to the attention of Otto Ranke, a military doctor and director of the Institute for General and Defense Physiology at Berlin's Academy of Military Medicine. In September 1938 and in April–May 1939 he tested Pervitin on university students and came to the amazing conclusion that it could help the Third Reich win the war.[27] Ranke's opinion was further supported by military physicians who dispensed the drug on their own to the soldiers during the seizure and occupation of Czechoslovakia in 1938. Reports on these trials were optimistic, indeed enthusiastic.[28] Pervitin, it was thought, would be one of the means of improving stamina, physical endurance, and the morale of the troops. It was hoped to turn the Luftwaffe pilots, Wehrmacht soldiers, and Kriegsmarine sailors into superhuman warriors or, in a word, to produce an army of true Aryan *heroes.*

Therefore, during the German invasion of Poland in September 1939, Pervitin became a popular German "assault pill." From April to December 1939 the Temmler company supplied the army with twenty-nine million tablets.[29] The Wehrmacht soldiers used the "boosting pills" pervasively, and in the peak months of the blitzkrieg, in April, May, and June 1940, the military consumption of methamphetamine was truly excessive. For in the course of the conquest of the Netherlands, Belgium, Luxemburg, and France, German soldiers were issued over thirty-five million pills of Pervitin and its modified version called Isophan, manufactured by the Knoll pharmaceutical company.[30] A German commentator observed that those units to which methamphetamine were administered "are very useful in modern battle conditions when used in mass attacks."[31] Methamphetamine was dispensed in the form of chocolate bars too—as *Fliegerschokolade* (flyer's chocolate) for pilots and as *Panzerschokolade* (tanker's chocolate) for panzer crews. Oftentimes soldiers also received Pervitin by intravenous injection.

German forces would never again consume such vast amounts of uppers as they did in the spring of 1940 during the conquest of France, when thousands of soldiers regularly went into battle propelled by the methamphetamine issued by their commanders. Many men developed an addiction during this period. When combatants experienced shortages of Pervitin or serious delays in its supply, they would obtain the drug on their own, as it was easily available on the market in Germany. In a letter, dated November 8, 1939, to his family in Cologne, a twenty-two-year-old soldier stationed in occupied Poland wrote: "It's tough out here, and I hope you'll understand if I'm only able to write to you once every two to four days soon. Today I'm writing you mainly to ask for some Pervitin . . . Love, Hein." A few months later, in a letter dated May 20, 1940, he asked again: "Perhaps you could get me some more Pervitin so that I can have a backup supply?" And writing on June 19, 1940, from Bromberg he asked again: "If at all possible, please send me some more Pervitin."[32] This is a strikingly laconic form of correspondence, given that this young soldier who could hardly live without the wonder drug was Heinrich Böll, the 1972 Nobel Prize winner for literature. Böll had been drafted only after completing the first semester of his studies in classics. Yet in the years to come, he was, it seems, to be intoxicated not so much by the great works of classical literature as by methamphetamine.

The military leadership adopted a careful approach to Pervitin in response to some disturbing effects of the stimulant that were observed relatively early. A day after the ingestion of the drug soldiers were generally in a much worse physical condition, some experienced health problems like excessive perspiration and circulatory disorders, and in a number of isolated cases death was reported. Also, the number of accidents among the Luftwaffe pilots increased noticeably. A soldier going to battle on Pervitin usually found himself unable to perform effectively for the next day or two. Suffering from a drug hangover and looking more like a zombie than a great warrior, he had to recover from the side effects of methamphetamine—very much as a berserk would have recovered from the intoxication induced by fly agaric several centuries earlier. At times, the effect of Pervitin was extremely aggressive behavior, which might, to some extent, help explain why Wehrmacht soldiers turned into ruthless murderers, often committing the cruelest massacres of civilians. It also happened that soldiers on speed resorted to violence against their superior officers, which constituted a serious threat to army morale. Drawing on this experience the Germans began to see the drug as a useful performance enhancer, not necessarily for the regular troops but rather for elite special units. Therefore, the military went on to discourage its large-scale use. Responding to reports of Pervitin's harmful effects, by December 1940 its consumption was significantly reduced, from 12.4 million to only 1.2 million pills a month.[33] Its use was further decreased in 1942, after German doctors officially recognized the addictive potential of amphetamine and methamphetamine, and their side effects, which sometimes resulted in death from circulatory system failure.

More importantly still, Pervitin was also identified as having a negative effect on tactical combat performance. Nicolas Rasmussen tells the following story. During the siege of Leningrad an SS infantry company of one hundred men surrendered to the Soviets without a fight. On taking them prisoner the Russians noticed that the Germans appeared oddly nervous and jumpy and discovered that they had completely run out of machine gun bullets. This was extremely strange for a well-trained elite unit, but as Rasmussen explains, "Apparently the men had used up their ammunition the night before, when they fired it all in a collective methamphetamine-induced delusion that they were under attack."[34] Although the story is undocumented, it seems highly probable. It is also illustrative of the most serious negative effect of Pervitin—methamphetamine psychosis. Unsurprisingly, the German command did not want its troops to take Pervitin too freely and without proper control, as this could have disastrous consequences for the operational effectiveness of the units. Certainly, the Leningrad-like scenario was by all means deemed highly undesirable.

This does not, of course, mean that the Wehrmacht ceased to drug its members; the Luftwaffe, however, abandoned the regular use of methamphetamine soon after the beginning of the war. Reich health leader Leonardo Conti believed that the problem of the massive military use of Pervitin must be approached with reasonable caution. On March 19, 1940, in a speech at a conference of the National Socialist Association of German Doctors in Berlin, he openly expressed his view:

> If you fight fatigue with Pervitin, you can be sure that the collapse of fitness must follow one day. Giving it to a top pilot who must fly for another two hours while fighting fatigue is probably right. It may not, however, be used for every case of tiredness where fatigue can in reality only be compensated by sleep. As physicians this ought to be clear to us immediately . . . In principle, the indication is identical to that for opiates. I can only wish that these thoughts will penetrate to all physicians. Those who have not understood them have not, as far as I am concerned, grasped the true nature of medicine, and are and remain simple laborers.[35]

Conti's attitude was that of a responsible doctor. In a letter dated December 1940 he wrote:

> My current standpoint on the prescription of Pervitin is that I cannot approve of it at all, except in certain clearly defined cases where, for a short period of time, an improvement in performance is necessary, which has to be attained under exceptional conditions of war. . . . I have considered whether a harsher policy of prescription for Pervitin could not be introduced, for example by declaring it a narcotic and prescribing it under clearly defined conditions.[36]

Eventually Conti succeeded in pushing through tough regulations that limited the distribution of Pervitin in the military by proclaiming in June 1941 that the drug was subject to the opium law. However, because these restrictive measures were introduced at exactly the same time as the German invasion of the Soviet Union began, the grim reality of combat in the Eastern Front hindered the stringent enforcement of the new rule. For in harsh, often extreme conditions of the winter of 1941–1942, the Wehrmacht managed to fight the Red Army largely due to regular supplies of methamphetamine. The military historian Shelby Stanton captured the importance of Pervitin in the German war effort in Russia:

> They dispensed it to the line troops. Ninety percent of their army had to march on foot, day and night. It was more important for them to keep punching during the Blitzkrieg than to get a good night's sleep. The whole damn army was hopped up. It was one of the secrets of the Blitzkrieg.[37]

Although military doctors became slightly more cautious in administering Pervitin, in the first half of 1942 the Wehrmacht medical services still sent to the Eastern Front some ten million tablets of this wonder assault drug. Hence, since it was very difficult to enforce the prohibitive measures, the military authorities attempted to more precisely regulate the rules governing the use of the stimulant. On June 18, 1942, a new instruction booklet called the "Guidelines for Detecting and Combating Fatigue" was issued. It resembled the previous documents of this type but it mentioned the risks of Pervitin's possible side effects and its addictive potential. Overall however, the general guidelines remained unchanged: "Two tablets taken once eliminate the need to sleep for three to eight hours, and two doses of two tablets each are normally effective for 24 hours."[38] The more rigorous rules, which aimed at limiting the availability and consumption of the drug, could not, nevertheless, prevent many cases of Pervitin addiction among soldiers and veterans. Gerd Schmückle of the 7th Panzer Division, later a four-star general, shared his observations on the effects of the stimulant after the fighting around Zhytomyr in Ukraine in November 1943:

> I could not sleep. During the attack I had taken too much Pervitin. We had all been dependent on it for a long time. Everyone swallowed the stuff, more frequently and in greater doses. The pills seemed to remove the sense of agitation. I slid into a world of bright indifference. Danger lost its edge. One's own power seemed to increase. After the battle one hovered in a strange state of intoxication in which a deep need for sleep fought with a clear alertness.[39]

Although it is difficult to measure the number of pills issued to German soldiers fighting in Russia, some reports reveal that an Army group consumed as much as 30 million tablets of Pervitin over a few months.[40] Methamphetamine's boosting effect conformed to the Nazi cult of power, obedience, endurance, efficiency, and superhuman might. For as Hitler declared: "We don't need weak people, we want only the strong!" Whereas the social consumption of intoxicants was regarded as a very non-German activity, enhancing soldiers' performance with methamphetamine, which could help Germany win the war, was by contrast seen as very German.

The result of the Second World War, the most total war in history, was to depend on the mass mobilization of societies and states, whose economies were entirely converted to military production, and particularly on the general mobilization of human resources—the physical energy and the fighting spirit of the soldiers in the field and workers in factories. Therefore, late in the war, when the Reich called for all available manpower resources both on the home and war fronts, and when the Allies carried out carpet bombings of German industrial and urban centers, "there were plants," writes Grunberger, "which—with official approval—included sedatives in their employees' pay packets, though at the same time the authorities tried, without much success, to curb over-consumption of medicines and pills, which some people used as substitutes for food in the later stages of the war."[41]

On becoming aware of the negative side effects of Pervitin, the Germans admittedly attempted to limit its military consumption. This did not, however, mean that they discontinued research on new and even better uppers that could bring them tactical advantage and, ultimately, longed-for victory. Although the information that the Wehrmacht units were given steroids to create stronger, more violent, less compassionate soldiers is sometimes found in the literature, there are no reliable sources to support this claim, which should as such be taken as a rumor or a myth.[42] What has been confirmed though is the story about secret research on a new wonder stimulant. In 1944 the Nazis began working on a magic bullet that they hoped would become one of Hitler's brilliant weapons. In March 1944, during a meeting with pharmacists, chemists, and army commanders in the seaport of Kiel, Vice-Admiral Hellmuth Heye commissioned the invention of a drug "that can keep soldiers ready for battle when they are asked to continue fighting beyond a period considered normal, while at the same time boosting their self-esteem."[43] A few months later a team of scientists under Professor Gerhard Orzechowski came up with a new stimulant codenamed D-IX. It was an extremely potent cocktail of five milligrams of cocaine, three milligrams of methamphetamine (Pervitin), and five milligrams of Eukodal.[44] The first test of the new drug, which was carried out on the crewmembers of a small submarine in Kiel Bay, was very promising. In order to further test the effect of D-IX Otto Skorzeny, a Waffen-SS colonel and a special commander of the Marine commandos who was involved in the search for new fighting methods, ordered a thousand tablets for his troops. The upper seemed to be the desired secret weapon that could bring victory to the Third Reich. But it had to be tested further before being put to use in combat. What was its potential for unleashing the power of the human body? For how long could it fuel a man undergoing a physical ordeal? In essence, what were the limits of strength and stamina it might foster? To provide the answers, in November 1944 the Nazi doctors began testing high dosages of cocaine and methamphetamine, but not the real D-IX, on eighteen inmates at the Sachsenhausen concentration camp, who were forced to march for twenty-four hours without rest carrying twenty-kilogram backpacks. Some of these guinea pigs managed to walk up to ninety kilometres a day before falling to the ground dead or barely alive.[45] D-IX increased a man's active ability and will, supplied him with an almost machine-like endurance, and preserved the body's energy. It was hoped that it would become a fantastic weapon that could turn the Wehrmacht soldiers into near-robots, propel them forward, and enable the Nazis to inflict an ultimate defeat on the Allied forces. Yet before the magic bullet went into mass production, Germany lost the war.

To conclude, if we want to understand the psychological aspects of the Nazi political and military program with its power, dynamics, and appeal, we need to consider—apart from many other factors such as its racist ideology and occultism—the substantial role of methamphetamine. Uppers, which improved soldiers' endurance and fueled their aggression and ruthless determination but simultaneously made them addicts, emerge as a link connecting murderous ideology and war, conquest and genocide. This connection is well illustrated by the title of the seminal book edited by Werner Pieper: *Nazis on Speed* (2002).

The British

At roughly the same time as the Germans were reducing the consumption of methamphetamine among their troops, the British approved the use of amphetamine for combating fatigue. In June 1940 some mysterious tablets were found with the Luftwaffe pilots who were shot down during the bombing raids on Britain. The Royal Air Force (RAF) commissioned research by the famous physiologist Henry Dale, under the auspices of the Flying Personnel Research Committee, to find out what these tablets were. In September 1940 Dale identified them as methamphetamine and went further to strongly suggest that its value for the British Army should be explored. Thus the earlier, unverified information obtained by the intelligence that the German pilots were given powerful uppers was now unequivocally confirmed.[46]

There was an important reason for the official British interest in amphetamines. To protect the sea convoys coming from the United States, which carried supplies under the Lend-Lease program, the British long-range planes flew routine patrols over the Atlantic, tracking and combating German submarines. These were lengthy missions as the Whitley bomber was able to stay in the air for eleven hours, and the Catalina flying boat could remain aloft for up to thirty-six hours. Pilots had already begun taking Benzedrine amphetamine tablets on their own initiative in order to stay alert during these exceedingly monotonous flights, which were conducted mostly at night. This basically explains why amphetamine became widely known as a "co-pilot" in both Britain and the United States. Faced with unauthorized stimulant use by its crews, the RAF had to take a position; it therefore commissioned research into the effects, risks, and operational utility of amphetamine. The study was carried out by R. H. Winfield, a medical officer from the RAF's physiological laboratory, who from April to October 1941 accompanied the Costal Command crews on fourteen missions testing the in-flight effects of amphetamine (Benzedrine, purchased from the American company SKF) and methamphetamine (Methedrine, available from the British firm of Burroughs-Wellcome). Based on Winfield's report, the RAF ultimately approved the routine dose of two five-milligram Benzedrine tablets on long air missions.[47]

Although the convoy patrol flights were severely draining and stressful missions, the bombing raids over Germany proved to be much more risky and demanding. The primary objective of the strategic air offensive was, as laid down in a directive approved at the Casablanca Conference in January 1943, "the progressive destruction of the German military, industrial and economic system, and the undermining of the morale of the German people to a point where their capacity for armed resistance is fatally weakened."[48] The attempt to achieve this goal was made at a high cost to the air crews. To avoid being shot down, pilots had to fly at night at high altitudes. Military aviation technology enabled this type of mission while at the same time confronting man with a formidable challenge. Dr. Charles Stephenson, an American naval officer stationed in London, expressed this problem very succinctly; in aviation, he said, "the machine has far outstripped the man."[49] The acceleration of aircraft speed brought a higher gravity load, colder conditions, and a more rarefied atmosphere in the cockpit, which endangered not only pilots' performance but also their health—in extreme cases causing loss of consciousness. With military technology reaching a new level of development, traditional logic had been reversed: it was no longer the tools of war that had to be adjusted to man, but man had to be fitted to these increasingly advanced, faster, and more powerful machines. Research on heating, oxygen supply, pressurized cabins, and eventually special suits preventing the loss of consciousness due to high centrifugal forces was but one response to this challenge. The efforts to improve man's "cover" came along with the attempts to improve his body from within. To that end, the military utility of special vitamin supplements and steroid hormones, particularly testosterone, was explored. So at this point, amphetamine could have served a dominant role as a powerful performance enhancer for pilots.

To check its utility, Winfield was commissioned to undertake further experiments. Between August 1941 and July 1942 he flew twenty missions with the Whitley and Stirling bomber crews, including the raids on Kiel, Hamburg, Cologne, Essen, Rostock, the Ruhr valley, and Lübeck. The results of his research on pilots proved highly promising—the drug not only boosted vigilance on the return flight but also improved the overall performance of aircrews. For instance, a pilot on the mission over Cologne dropped from 15,000 feet down to less than 8,000 so the crew could identify targets and release their bombs below the heavy cloud layer. "Although the aircraft was hit just before the bombs were released," the crew managed to deliver a direct hit on the target.[50] Overall, it was reported that the Benzedrine-enhanced pilots were highly determined to accomplish their task, willing to run more risks, and displayed greater courage. Amphetamine seemed not only to improve physical capacities and invigorate pilots by overcoming fatigue but also to modify their mood and behavior.

Benzedrine fostered all the qualities that were recognized to be the most desirable for creating a perfect pilot. In addition, it mitigated the fear and anxiety associated with long and hazardous sorties. The statistics showed that about 5 percent of the bombers did not return from their mission. Many accidents occurred during the return flights, when after completing an assignment tension gave way to relief and relaxation, which frequently proved treacherous because a state of lowered alertness often resulted in fatal errors during landing. Amphetamine offered an almost perfect solution.

To sum up, Winfield concluded that half the men who had been supercharged with amphetamine performed much better than the unassisted ones. He found that by generating the right combination of optimism and aggressiveness, uppers induced in airmen a state that enabled them to achieve "peak efficiency" in combat.[51] Because the attitude induced by Benzedrine was exactly the kind that armed forces expect of their members, Winfield suggested making amphetamine pills available to all air force crews. On adopting his recommendations in 1942, the RAF Bomber Command established the guideline for using the drug: two five-milligram Benzedrine tablets (one taken when the plane entered the enemy's airspace and another for the return flight) for all air crews, subject to ground testing prior to the operational use of the drug to identify any potential side effects and unexpected individual body responses.[52]

Most of the results of academic research on amphetamine conducted in Britain were not published until after the war because of national security concerns. And even though amphetamine's superiority over caffeine as a military enhancer had not been proved scientifically, in terms of subjective experience, that is, its positive behavioral and emotional effects, it was seen as both vital and irreplaceable. Although at first pilots saw Benzedrine as a "funny" way of boosting performance and remained rather suspicious and skeptical, with time they got on the drug not only because it improved mood, increased self-confidence, and facilitated courage, but because it fueled the moderate aggressiveness that is the essential quality in combat.

It is precisely for these reasons that, even with no definite scientific confirmation of its special effectiveness as a stimulant (no evidence was found "that it enabled a tired man to perform his work to a high capacity"), amphetamine became popular in both the aviation and ground forces.[53] In his book *The Sharp End of War*, John Ellis writes that "many rear-echelon troops with demanding jobs, especially those who sometimes had to work days and nights at a stretch, were issued with liberal quantities of amphetamines."[54] Ellis quotes a paper prepared by Brigadier Q. V. B. Wallace, the deputy director of Medical Services of the 10th Armoured Corps, which provided the following evidence of the widespread use of amphetamines in the British Army:

> "Pep" tablets, i.e. benzedrine tablets, were used for the first time in the Middle East on a large scale. 20,000 tablets were issued to the ADMS [Assistant Director Medical Services] of each division ... who was responsible for their distribution and safe custody. The initial dose was 1 1/2 tablets two hours before the maximum benefit was required, followed six hours later by another tablet, with a further and final tablet for another six hours, if required ... I consider that "Pep" tablets may be very useful in certain cases, particularly where long-continued work is required over extended periods, i.e., staff officers, signallers, lorry drivers, transport workers, etc. The tablets must only be used when an extreme state of tiredness has been reached. The tablets have practically no ill-effects, and an ordinary night's sleep restores the individual to his original working capacity.[55]

As we know, Brigadier Wallace would be proved wrong about the lack of negative effects of amphetamines, and the Germans were the first to learn of them.

In Africa, General Bernard Montgomery, who in August 1942 took command of the 8th Army, carried out his own informal field research on the effectiveness of Benzedrine. Its results were so promising that Montgomery enthusiastically authorized his troops to use it on a regular basis. He hoped that uppers would invigorate soldiers sufficiently to overcome the skepticism of officers toward his idea of a bold tactical maneuver—an all-out armored attack on the German positions at El Alamein, followed by fierce infantry assaults. Montgomery pinned his hopes on Benzedrine, which could, he believed, compensate for the weaker determination of his army compared with Erwin Rommel's fearless and relentless Afrika Korps. It was hoped that amphetamine would lift the fighting spirit of the British troops, which was flagging at the time, and help them defeat the enemy forces led by the famous Desert Fox. Montgomery planned to throw all his men, fortified with pep pills, into a single offensive against the German positions. For the initial attack, which began on October 23, 1942, he allocated 100,000 Benzedrine pills.

The battle of El Alamein proved to be a turning point of the war in North Africa. It brought the first major victory to the British and the title of "the 1st Viscount Montgomery of Alamein" to Montgomery. It is difficult to accurately assess the role played by amphetamine in the British triumph. One of the reasons is that the drug does not always work as intended. In his Pulitzer Prize–winning book *An Army at Dawn*, Rick Atkinson describes the rather slow advances of the 8th Army after El Alamein, an army which "lumbered like 'a dry horse on a polo field,' in the British historian Correlli Barnett's phrase, despite an enthusiasm for the amphetamine Benzedrine, which was issued in tens of thousands of tablets 'to all Eight Army personnel' on Montgomery's order."[56] There were numerous cases of amphetamine-induced numbness and hallucinations among soldiers, especially tank crews, which jeopardized their fighting efficiency. Therefore some considerable controversy regarding the general combat effectiveness of amphetamine stimulants at the battle of El Alamein persists.

Overall, in the course of the Second World War, the British armed forces used about seventy-two million Benzedrine tablets.[57] With time and the growing totalization of the war, the initial reason for the pharmacological enhancement of the troops moved from the "mundane," combating fatigue and increasing alertness, to improving endurance and efficiency.

The Americans

The early history of the military use of amphetamine in the United States was similar to that of Britain. Beginning in mid-1940, intensive work on the effects and medical use of various pharmaceuticals was conducted under the auspices of the National Council for Scientific Research. The Americans, like the Germans, drew on the results of research on techniques for enhancing performance in sports. In 1941 Peter Karpovich, in cooperation with Frances A. Hellebrandt, published in the journal *War Medicine* an article which summed up the state of research on the "methods used for improving the physical performance of man."[58] The authors recognized similarities in fatigue patterns in sports, labor, and military training, thus recommending that the lessons for enhancing performance with stimulants be adapted from athletics to the field of warfare. For Karpovich and Hellebrandt, wartime conditions and the state of emergency justified extensive research on doping drugs. The stakes of total war loosened the brakes of ethics. The victory of democracy and freedom over the dark forces of totalitarianism and enslavement had to be given priority over the dilemmas concerning the potential harmful effects of psychoactive substances. Research that aimed at extending the boundaries of human performance could not be overly inhibited by ethical considerations.

In mid-1941 the National Council for Scientific Research set up a team of medical experts to serve as an advisory body for the armed forces. But even before it managed to formulate its final recommendations the American air force began in late 1942 to procure large amounts of Benzedrine from Smith, Kline & French. Nicolas Rasmussen is, I think, right in speculating that in such circumstances Andrew C. Ivy—a physiologist from Chicago, who played a chief role in the research on the use of amphetamine to reduce combat fatigue—found himself under tremendous pressure to provide the military with what was in fact an ex post facto justification for a decision already made. In an article coauthored by Louis Richard Krasno and published in 1941 in *War Medicine* he noted: "Amphetamine in most persons certainly promotes wakefulness and the feeling of well-being and decreases the sense of fatigue and boredom in performing tedious work over rather long periods. The drug tends to improve psychomotor activities in the majority of subjects."[59]

Further, in December 1942 the *New York Times* published a report that summarized the research findings of Dr. Maurice Tainter, a professor of pharmacology at Stanford University. According to Tainter one-ten-thousandth of an ounce of methyl-benzedrine (a derivate of Benzedrine) would suffice to "keep a man so stimulated and alert that sleep would be impossible for at least eighteen hours" and would allow him to "think more clearly and react faster."[60]

Following the air force's example, the army authorized the operational use of Benzedrine, popularly known among servicemen as "benny." From 1943 soldiers' medical kits included amphetamine tablets, with the recommended dosage being one five-milligram pill every six hours.[61] It is impossible to precisely assess the amount of Benzedrine consumed by American troops in the Second World War. The estimates vary considerably. Based on the government contracts with SKF amounting to 877,000 dollars, Rasmussen assumes that the military services purchased at least 250 million Benzedrine sulfate tablets. This is, however, the most conservative calculation, and the real figure might well be more like 500 million pills.[62] What we do not know is the government procurement price for Benzedrine, which was certainly much lower than the market price. It is difficult to estimate the scale of amphetamine consumption by the American military because of the veil of silence over this politically controversial issue. Research conducted at the end of the war in an American military hospital revealed that 25 percent of the patients abused amphetamine and 89 percent had taken it regularly during their tour of duty.[63] Overall, in the course of the war some 15 percent of American servicemen took Benzedrine routinely. A military-commissioned study on a group of pilots revealed that 15 percent of those who used the drug regularly did not follow the recommended dosage instructions and abused it.[64] As we know from the aforementioned British experience, no objective scientific evidence confirmed amphetamine's positive effects on physical endurance, but what mattered most was the overall subjective perception that the stimulant worked well. It did wonders for morale, elevated mood, increased fortitude, and fueled aggression—in other words, it improved all the most desirable qualities in combatants. Simply put, it made men fight harder. Rasmussen captures the essence of this ambiguity surrounding the use of amphetamine by concluding, "The drug was simply too useful for the military to do without, regardless of what science had to say."[65]

The case of the fierce and bloody battle at Tarawa, fought from November 20 to 23, 1943, over an atoll occupied by the Japanese, demonstrates well the massive use of speed among American troops. The cruel and uncensored face of this most brutal of battles in the history of the U.S. Marine Corps was movingly depicted by Louis Hayward in his short documentary *With the Marines at Tarawa* (1944). Not only was this the first time in the Pacific War that an American landing met with such ferocious Japanese resistance, but probably also for the first time the Marines were administered immense amounts of amphetamine. American casualties amounted to 1,204 killed and missing in action and 2,282 injured, while the Japanese lost 4,800 men, almost their entire garrison.[66] The Americans painfully experienced the non-Western way of warfare. The limitless readiness of Japanese soldiers to die was truly terrifying, and their fierceness called for great endurance on the part of the Marines. On the night of November 22–23, the Japanese carried out a banzai charge, in which 325 Japanese and 173 Americans were killed. Faced with a hopeless situation, the Japanese infantry units would surge en masse toward the enemy, running in a human wave attack under heavy American fire. The psychological effect of such ferocious suicide tactics was enormous, as Samuel Hynes comments, "No American soldier would do that, nor any Briton or Frenchman or German, or could even imagine doing it; such behavior came out of a state of mind that seemed so alien as not to be human."[67] Severe combat conditions and a bitter enemy required extreme physical and mental exertion. All of this would seem to indicate that amphetamine *may* have helped the Marines to defeat the formidable and fanatic enemy at Tarawa.

The image of the American soldier using bennies made its way into movies and literature. Take just two examples. The first is Anatole Litvak's 1951 film *Decision Before Dawn*, which tells the story of German POWs recruited in

1944 by American intelligence to undertake a spy mission in Germany. We see one of them, the Benzedrine-assisted Karl Mauer, aka "Happy," as played by Oskar Werner, being parachuted into enemy territory. The second is the book *Cryptonomicon* (1999) by Neal Stephenson.[68] This science fiction/cyberpunk novel is set in two different time periods. One is during the Second World War and tells the story of American and British cryptanalysts and the frontline soldiers with whom they cooperate. The other is in the late 1990s and shows their descendants during the Internet boom. We see a few of the characters, mostly the frontline soldiers, regularly boosting themselves with Benzedrine. Thus the pill popping of soldiers was so prevalent that it was lodged in the popular consciousness.

Although fighting "on speed" became the practice in the British and American ground units, it was the air forces that remained the largest consumers of amphetamine until the end of the war. New aerial technologies, which allowed for greater speed and higher altitudes, posed considerable challenges to American pilots in exactly the same ways as they did to the RAF crews. The huge B-29 superfortresses were capable of flight at up to 31,850 feet, but the concentration of oxygen in the air at such altitudes is too low for the human body. Specially designed cabins maintained constant pressure, yet the pilots were still exposed to exceptional physical and mental exhaustion. Amphetamine was seen as one of the countermeasures that could help overcome these obstacles. By 1943 pep pills were widely distributed among the crews on long missions, and the packages of five-milligram "Benzedrine pills were in the emergency kits in every American bomber."[69] The use of speed by air crews came to be not only customary but also discretionary, since despite the official guidelines for the recommended doses of amphetamine, it was usually the pilots who decided whether they wanted to get stimulated.

Strategic bombing raids over Germany and Japan were therefore often carried out by pilots "on speed." Yet the destruction and casualties they inflicted were by no means a form of drug-induced hallucination, though the atrocious consequences of carpet bombing might have looked horribly surreal. But they were all too real. By razing to the ground or seriously damaging Hamburg, Berlin, Dresden, Tokyo, and many other cities, the Allies sought to undermine not so much the industrial infrastructure but the spirit of resistance in enemy societies. To this end, pharmacologically boosted "superpilots" flying "superfortress" bomber aircraft dropped thousands of tons of bombs, which brought about "superdestruction." Psychoactive substances, then, played a crucial role in violating the Western, Judeo-Christian ethics of war and burying under the ruins of bombed cities the centuries-old principles of the just war tradition. In the course of the war, the warring parties, contrary to the customary *ius in bello*, used all available means. Pharmacology was one of them.

An article entitled "With a B-29 over Japan—A Pilot's Story," published on March 25, 1945, in the *New York Times*, described how the use of bennies had become an utterly normal part of bomber missions on long-duration flights of a dozen or so hours. Readers learned that the navigator "just rubs his tired eyes, takes some more Benzedrine and goes to work again."[70] In a word, amphetamine had emerged as intrinsic to strategic bombing campaigns. In this context one might provocatively ask, as a logical conclusion, whether Paul Tibbets the pilot and commander of the B-29 superfortress *Enola Gay* and other members of his crew had taken a Benzedrine "super pep pill" before delivering the "absolute weapon" that brought about the atomic destruction of Hiroshima. Or did they perhaps take it on their way back after completing the mission? Or maybe no amphetamine was involved in the nuclear destruction of Hiroshima, as the crew had been made sufficiently hopped-up by the invigorating nature of the task. Whichever was the case "hibakusha," the survivor-victims of the atomic bomb, must had been overwhelmed by the sensation of an acute hallucination on experiencing the scope and character of the destruction and injuries inflicted by the bombing and the latter horrible symptoms of radiation sickness. By the way, an interesting though willfully perverse question that might be asked here is: "How many victims were at the time of their death or mutilation under the influence of intoxicants?"

The Japanese

Obscene as it may sound, the question is not entirely unfounded, because the Japanese extended the practice of performance enhancement through methamphetamine from the military to the whole society. Thus every civilian working in a sector relevant to the nation's war effort was obliged to take a proper dose of the "wonder drug." This, in fact, might be seen as a new aspect of the totality of the Second World War, especially given that Japan broke with a traditional and core principle: the historically sacred and strictly enforced prohibition on the use of intoxicants.

The Shift in Japan's Drug Policy

In that respect, Japan had for centuries followed a rational policy aimed at the protection of its culture, tradition, spirituality, or, broadly speaking, security. Japan's drug policy had been two-dimensional. On the one hand, beginning in the fifteenth century, the consumption of mind-altering substances had been strictly controlled. On the other hand, the Japanese supported and promoted the sale and trade of drugs in the neighboring countries and occupied territories, in China in particular.

Opium smoking and its nonmedical use had been banned as early as the seventeenth century, and in 1868, the first year of the Meiji period, a severely prohibitive anti-opium law was introduced. Opium was restricted and used for medical purposes only, and physicians and druggists were required to file special reports on each occasion they distributed opium-based medicines. "Anyone who sold opium to smokers or who tempted others to smoke was subject to execution," writes Bob Tadashi Wakabayashi.[71] The great success of the Tokugawa and later Meiji regimes in protecting society from disastrous consequences of opium taking had an additional outcome, as it facilitated the centralization of power. For it was the state that maintained full and effective control over the use of intoxicants, thereby providing domestic security and protecting the life, health, and dignity of its population. In spite of the forced "opening" of Japan to the West imposed in 1854 by the United States, under the Treaty of Amity and Commerce signed in 1858, Japan managed to secure a ban on the American export of opium. The agreements signed later with other states, namely the Netherlands, France, Russia, and Great Britain, included similar provisions. The smuggling of drugs was punishable by death as it was considered a hostile act that endangered public security.[72] Thus the protection against the import of intoxicants appeared to be one of Japan's vital national interests.

How can we account for this hard-line and consistent stance on drugs? Well, the Japanese were resolutely determined never to share the tragic fate of the Chinese, who had free trade in opium imposed on them as part of their subjection to exploitation and colonization. China, being ravaged by the Opium Wars, served as a stark warning for Japan in reference to which it framed its politics in order to avoid the mistakes and shameful fate of its larger, yet powerless, neighbor. While Japan drew important lessons from the Opium Wars, in the late nineteenth century it gradually began to take over from Great Britain the role of the imperial drug dealer in China, thus joining the club of Western states that made huge profits by taking advantage of the Chinese weakness for opium smoking. Japan, therefore, pursued a twin-track policy, for in the occupied territories it strongly supported trafficking in opium and opiates, which served as both a substantial source of revenue for the state budget and a means of keeping the controlled and increasingly addicted populace weak and docile.[73] Shortly after the Second World War, Sir Thomas Russell of the Central Narcotics Intelligence Bureau in Egypt expressively captured the essence of this approach by observing that "Japan had decided upon heroin addiction as a weapon of aggression and deliberately converted the territories she conquered from China into one huge opium farm and heroin den."[74]

Japan's use of drugs as an instrument of imperial policy was, however, punished. After the end of the war, on October 12, 1945, General Douglas MacArthur's General Headquarters issued a memorandum to the Japanese government entitled "Control of Narcotic Products and Records in Japan," which introduced a strict ban on the cultivation, manufacture, import, and export of intoxicants.[75] At the same time the Allies were preparing for the trial of Japanese officials accused of drug trafficking in China. From August 30 to September 6, 1946, the International Military Tribunal for the Far East (the Tokyo Tribunal) heard the case of Japan's opium policy in China. Eventually, the Tribunal declared it to have violated the international anti-opium treaties (i.e., the two opium conventions of 1912 and 1925 both ratified by Japan) and sentenced the accused leaders as Class A war criminals for crimes against peace.[76] Additionally, a number of Class B and C war crimes trials were held in China, while the Kuomintang government executed 149 imperial Japanese subjects on drug-related charges.[77]

We must now turn to the question of where to find the roots of Japan's imperial drug policy, which brought some of its prominent politicians, generals, and businessmen before the International Military Tribunal. Japan's first experience with the "opium problem" was in Taiwan, which it gained in the war with China (1894–1895). The Japanese quickly learned that the opium trade could be immensely lucrative and discovered "the irresistible power of opium to accumulate capital."[78] So Japan's first opium regime was created in Taiwan, and the next was soon established in Korea, annexed by Japan in 1910 following its victory over Russia in the war of 1904–1905.

The largest area for the expansion of the drug trade was of course China, where Japan's opium regime developed in three stages.[79] The first lasted from the 1890s through to 1933. During this period drugs were smuggled into the Chinese treaty ports by Japanese imperial subjects under the guise of extraterritoriality. Unscrupulous carpetbaggers known as "continental adventurers" saw the smuggling of drugs as a quick and easy way to line their pockets while the authorities turned a blind eye to their activities.[80] Fujiwara Tetsutarō, a Kwantung government-general official, estimated in the 1920s that in the city of Tiencin, northern China's economic heartland, about 70 percent of the 5,000 Japanese were involved in the distribution of opium. He insisted that it was difficult to find a Japanese bar, restaurant, pharmacy, or simply a store that did not deal in illicit drugs.[81] In the second stage, which lasted until the turn of 1938 and 1939, the civilians who smuggled drugs were joined by Japanese corporations (zaibatsu), such as Mitsubishi and Mitsui, which started selling Iranian opium. And the third stage lasted until the end of the Second World War and was marked by the Japanese state itself taking over the leading role in the manufacture, import, and export of drugs. These activities were conducted mainly by the army and organizations created especially for this purpose. Kumagai Hisao, the acting director of Shōwa Trading, a company established by the army in July 1939, observed that "the army used opium as a 'treasured pharmaceutical' to pacify conquered areas and acquire food and other goods from the populace."[82] The Japanese saw intoxicants as a social weapon suitable for turning addicts into degenerates, for tearing the social fabric, and facilitating conquest and occupation. By the end of the 1930s nearly 10 percent of China's population, or some forty million people, were hooked on opium.[83] Civilian dealers continued to smuggle the drug with the army's support and protection. Unlike Britain, Japan went even further to distribute not only opium (imported largely from Iran and Korea) but also other purified drugs, often of its own manufacture, mainly morphine, heroin, and cocaine. For example, cocaine was produced by a factory in Taiwan, while the processed opium was manufactured in Mengjiang (Mongol Border Land), a puppet state set up in 1936 in controlled Inner Mongolia.[84] By promoting trade in intoxicants in the occupied territories and the neighboring countries, the Japanese enabled gangs, which were often closely associated with the armed services, to dominate the market in mind-altering substances. It was precisely these circumstances that greatly facilitated the expansion of the Japanese mafia (Yakuza).

The government of Manchukuo, a puppet state set up in the aftermath of the Japanese invasion of Manchuria in 1931, made a lot of money from the illicit production of and trade in opium. Pu Yi, the last Qing emperor of China, who was forced to abdicate in 1912 and later installed by the Japanese as the head of Manchukuo, recalled that about one-sixth of its budget revenues came from opium and opiates.[85] In the 1930s Japan earned more than 300 million dollars a year from Manchurian opium and heroin.[86] The Manchukuo authorities followed Japan's example and used opium also as an instrument of racial segregation. The manual of the Kwantung army read: "The use of narcotics is unworthy of a superior race like the Japanese. Only inferior races, races that are decadent like the Chinese, Europeans, and East Indians, are addicted to the use of narcotics. This is why they are destined to become our servants and eventually disappear."[87] In Japan opium was plainly seen as a source of great evil, both to the individual and the group. Therefore, the fact that the Japanese people proved resistant to the drug plague was considered evidence of their remarkable racial superiority over the nations affected and ravaged by addiction.

The intensification of Japan's expansionist policy and later its deteriorating position in the course of the Pacific War significantly increased the regime's heavy reliance on the drug trade, thereby deepening the ruthless exploitation of China's resources. Japan used a barter exchange system, acquiring the commodities necessary for the conduct of the war in exchange for intoxicants. Motohiro Kobayashi captured the essence of this matrix of drugs and war well by remarking, "Indeed, Japan depended on opium to wage 'total war.' "[88] In other words, without its extensive drug regime and intense trade in intoxicants Japan would not have been able to wage war on such a scale and for as long as it did. But mind-altering substances played yet another crucial role in Japan's war effort.

Nippon's two-faced drug policy—a strict prohibition of intoxicants at home and their promotion for profits abroad—began to be transformed in the second half of the 1930s and changed dramatically in the course of the Pacific War. Under considerable pressure of the reality of total war, the government succumbed and not only allowed its citizens to use stimulants but in many instances demanded and coerced them to do so. In 1941 the Japanese launched the production of Philopon, an upper whose trade name was coined by the combination of two Greek words: "philo" (love) and "ponos" (labor). This drug, which was thought to instill a love for work, was methamphetamine, which had a long history in Japan, the country where it was first synthesized— by the chemist Akira Ogata in 1919. Much earlier however, in 1888, Nagayoshi Nagai, during his research on the Maou plant (*Herba Ephedrae*), discovered one of its extracts, which he initially called "M33N." His discovery sank into oblivion for over half a century, and only in the 1940s did scientists begin to search for medical applications for "M33N."[89]

The Imperial Army on Meth

Not only did methamphetamine become the leading stimulant used by the Imperial Japanese Army, but the authorities eagerly supported research on new performance-enhancing drugs. In wartime Japan, as in other countries, amphetamines were seen as an absolutely marvelous remedy for different afflictions—from asthma to low blood pressure. At the time of the attack on Pearl Harbor in December 1941 as many as twenty-four patented medicines containing amphetamine or methamphetamine were available on the market in Japan.[90] A radical "paradigm shift" in drug policy meant not only the routine administration of uppers to the troops but also a strong and deliberate promotion of the liberal use of potent stimulants in the society. Thus every man and woman working in the arms industry or any other sector relevant to the war effort was obliged to take pharmacological helpers for greater productivity.[91] What is important in total war is the maintenance of production capacity and the ability to supply forces in the field. The "armies of workers" at the home front are equally important for waging war as are the troops at the war front. For total war goes far beyond battlefields and "enlists" workers at the end of the production line. It was Ernst Jünger who earlier, writing on the new symbiosis of the worker and the soldier, remarked: "Just as the life of the soldier transformed itself ever more into the life of a worker, a technician of war working under very dangerous conditions, so too has the life of the worker formed itself at home into a soldierly life."[92] Hence methamphetamine issued to the Japanese workers came to be the instrument for boosting their performance, thereby allowing for their greater contribution to the war effort.

The Japanese called stimulants *senryoku zokyo zai*, which means the drugs to inspire the fighting spirit.[93] Michael Vaughn, Frank Huang, and Christine Ramirez particularly well summed up their crucial role in the Japanese war machine:

> Pilots were expected to flight planes for many hours beyond their physical capacity; soldiers were expected to fight as long as days at a time with no rest; submarine commanders and midshipmen were required to endure months of maritime service on meager rations; factory workers labored in subhuman conditions with deteriorating and broken equipment. Taking stimulants to enhance performance was a mark of patriotism.[94]

Soldiers on guard were administered pills called *Nekomo-Jo* (cat-eye tablets). The Japanese Imperial Army also had at its disposal an injectable methamphetamine, which, as we know, acts much more rapidly than a dose taken orally but is quickly habit-forming.[95]

The most famous methamphetamine users in the ranks were the kamikaze. The pilots of the special forces leaving for a special one-way *tokkōtai* (kamikadze) mission were, however, supplied with special pep pills called *Totsugeki-Jo* or *Tokkou-Jo*, meaning "storming tablets." These were ceremonially stamped with the emperor's crest and consisted of methamphetamine blended with green tea powder.[96] These tablets increased the courage and improved the stamina of the kamikaze much more than a ritual drinking of rice wine. Methamphetamine, in short, assisted the young tokkōtai pilots in accomplishing their mission. From a reading of kamikazes' dairies and the recollections of those pilots who survived (usually by making an emergency landing because their plane malfunctioned), we know that, contrary to government propaganda, most of them were not volunteers. Air force squadrons were converted into special tokkōtai units from day to day, and pilots were left with very little choice. Formally they could opt out; this would, however, bring the stigma of cowardice upon them and their families and a disgrace which, in a culture contemptuous of an unhealthy and shamefully excessive attachment to life, was equivalent to committing "social suicide." The refusal to volunteer was

considered inimical to the principles of the emperor-centered state nationalism and Shintoism that required every Japanese to be willing to lay down his
life for the divine emperor, who was believed to be "the incarnation of the self-
less wisdom of the universe."[97] Opting out was not, then, a realistic option.
Therefore, coerced by culture, tradition, and social pressure, the kamikaze did
not generally face their imminent death with happiness or enthusiasm. In most
cases they were not true volunteers and, generally speaking, "the tokkōtai
operation was a 'forced' voluntary system."[98]

Inevitably, before and during their last mission the boy pilots were torn by
doubts, dilemmas, and fear. Methamphetamine helped mitigate these emotions a bit. By empowering them with greater confidence and energy, the drug
might also have fostered the irrational belief that they might fulfill their duty,
survive, and somehow return home in glory. We can, by the way, ask whether
the aforementioned banzai tactics were grounded merely in a distinct strategic
culture based on the principle of the dominance of spirit over matter. Was it,
then, only fierce patriotism and samurai honor transplanted into the modern
national military that empowered the Japanese soldiers to die? Or were they
embarking on their suicidal missions also in an altered state of mind, invested
with artificial courage, and having rational thinking impaired by methamphetamine? The latter is not improbable, but one must be careful here not to
overstate the pharmacological factor. For both the kamikaze phenomenon and
the banzai tactics were the expression of the Japanese way of fighting, which
was rooted deeply in Japanese history, culture and, most importantly, in the
samurai ethos called bushido. Honor was in Japan inextricably bound up with
the fight for life and death. Without Confucianism we cannot grasp the basic
principle of fighting to the very end and the "no-surrender" doctrine. In *The
Analects*, Confucius remarked: "To see what is right and not to do it is cowardice."[99] Thus the Japanese samurai and then soldiers of the Imperial Army
adhered to the rule that "it is a true courage to live when it is right to live, and
to die when it is right to die."[100] Hayashi Ichizō, a tokkōtai pilot who died in
April 1945 off Okinawa, expressed the same in his diary: "Within two or three
months, I will die. If my death is a glorious battlefield death, then, I will welcome my fighting. . . . Our ancestors' wish was to die beside the emperor. Loyal
individuals wished to do so."[101] Yet there is something else worth adding, for
suicide was customarily an honorable way out of a hopeless situation. It was
the way of the samurai, a true warrior, because taking his own life, writes Ruth
Benedict in her seminal study of the Japanese character, *The Chrysanthemum
and the Sword*, "was only a choice of means; death was certain."[102] With the end
of centuries-old feudal system in 1868, the samurai tradition was adapted to
the reality of the newly created modern nation-state. The officer corps of the
newly established armed forces included some of the best former samurais

who passed the principles and values of bushido down to their enlisted men. In this way bushido had been extended over the whole nation and adapted to the needs of the nation-state and later to its militaristic ideology. In short, after abolishing the samurai class, Japan needed to produce an entire nation of "modern samurais." All of which can lead to the conclusion that we should always bear in mind that sometimes culture is an equally potent "dope," fueling and sustaining men in the field as well as pharmacological uppers of various kinds.

Despite the highly destructive American carpet bombing of Japanese cities and the atomic annihilation of Hiroshima and Nagasaki, the immense stocks of methamphetamine, carefully gathered in preparation for war by the armed forces and pharmaceutical companies, survived Japan's surrender. The American occupation authorities managed to seize but a tiny part of this stockpile. Not only did the manufacturers sell out their stocks of stimulants, but the Yakuza also handled the distribution of methamphetamine among the desperate and depressed residents. The trade in drugs, in fact, became the Yakuza's main source of income and propelled its later expansion both at home and abroad.[103] Before long the Japanese mafia was to derive between 35 and 50 percent of its annual revenues from dealing in amphetamines.[104]

The pharmaceutical industry advertised stimulants as a perfect means of boosting the war-weary population and restoring confidence after a painful and debilitating defeat. In addition, soldiers returning home carried with them considerable stocks of unused uppers, which they later found particularly useful for "staying awake while studying or working through the night."[105] Hence veterans contributed to the increasing social popularity of intoxicants. Drug abuse rapidly spread from the cities to the countryside. The years of 1945–1955 are referred to as the "first epidemic period" in the history of drugs in Japan. At its peak in 1954 the Japan Association of Pharmacists estimated that there were 1.5 million drug abusers; but more alarming still, other sources placed the number at 2 million or 2.2 percent of the total population.[106] Whereas in 1951 some 17,500 people were arrested for abusing amphetamines, by 1954 the number had jumped to 55,600.[107] Most crucially of all, for a long time methamphetamine was not popularly associated with anything appalling or unsafe but was rather seen as an exceptionally attractive and advantageous supplement. It was only in 1948 that the authorities declared methamphetamine, though still legally available, a "dangerous drug." This was in response to the tragic high-profile deaths of people who were known for using Philopon regularly, like the famous comedienne Miss Wakana in 1946 and the popular novelist Sakunosuke Oda in 1947. Incidents such as these and the popular notion that many brutal crimes were committed by people in the grip of methamphetamine psychosis made people realize that Philopon might, in fact, be highly dangerous.[108] Although the 1951 Stimulant Control Law prohibited the

possession of methamphetamine, it was only with the passage of its amendment in 1954, which imposed heavier punishments for violations, that a true
campaign for the eradication of the drug was ultimately launched. As a result,
the consumption of methamphetamine began to fall very quickly, so that by
1957 the early postwar drug problem was basically overcome.

The example of Japan shows how the military use of intoxicants can morph
into a social issue in the aftermath of war. Japan was not, of course, the only historical example of a country experiencing higher rates of substance addiction
after the fighting stopped, as the problem had crossed the barriers of culture
as well as time. Previously such a dynamic had been observed, apart from the
aforementioned case of the United States after the Civil War, in Russia in the
aftermath of the Crimean War, in Prussia in the years following the Franco-
Prussian War (1870–1871), and in France in the aftermath of the First World
War (1914–1918).[109]

The Finns: A Special Case

It may seem surprising or hard to believe, but in the late 1930s and in the 1940s
Finland was the country with the highest per capita consumption of legal
(i.e., medical) heroin in the world.[110] The Finns in general used large quantities of various drugs. As an example consider one of the few references in
the Finnish literature. The protagonist of *Suuri illusioni* (*Grand Illusion*, 1928),
the first novel by a famous twentieth-century Finnish writer, Mika Waltari,
goes with his friend Hellas to buy cocaine directly from a German ship in
the port of Helsinki. Hellas talks enthusiastically about cocaine as a modern
Western drug, unlike the dull "old fashioned" opium, describing it to be pure
reason, concentrated sunshine, and a glimmer on steel.[111] Before the 1920s the
Finnish drug scene had been rather vague and had no long-standing tradition,
except for alcohol, a well-established intoxicant of choice. In the early 1920s,
like in most other European states, a cocaine craze swept through Finland,
which became a major transit country for smuggling the drug to the Soviet
Union. Part of that cocaine remained in Finland for domestic illicit consumption.[112] Generally, however, recreational drug use in Finland was fairly rare and
certainly did not develop into a social problem. Heroin was taken mostly for
medical purposes because it was a valuable, effective, and cheap medicine for
coughs, tuberculosis, insomnia, and stress. It was available in pharmacies in
the form of the popular syrup Pulmo and as pills, which, although a prescription was required, were issued quite liberally by physicians. Yet interestingly,
the massive consumption of heroin in the 1930s did not lead to an increase in
the number of addicts. The main explanation for this is that the plethora of

mixtures and concoctions containing heroin as an ingredient had a rather low concentration of the drug, which effectively hampered its abuse.

The consumption of psychoactive substances for therapeutic purposes, particularly heroin but also cocaine, opium, and morphine, was so common-place in Finland that when in 1934 the League of Nations urged its members to prohibit the use of heroin, the government of Finland, based on the rec-ommendations of the Finnish Medical Board, flatly and expressly refused.[113] Defying the trend toward the criminalization of drugs and the imposition of regimes of state control, Finland opposed the idea of introducing any regula-tion of substance use whatsoever. In the late 1940s the League's successor, the United Nations, investigated the fact that the annual consumption of heroin in Finland (whose population was less than four million), was as high as other nations with much larger populations (for instance, Great Britain, Italy, or Sweden) used over a twenty-five year period.[114] Because at that time Finland was not yet a member of the UN, it could afford a vague, not to say insolent, response: according to the Ministry of Interior the country would not only keep using heroin but, for the very sake of the "public health," would need even more of it because the stocks were emptying after the Second World War. In line with this statement, in 1946 the Finnish people used some ninety-nine kilograms of prescription heroin, and the drug remained available from phar-macies up until 1957.[115]

In 2009 Mikko Ylikangas published the first major history of drugs in Finland from the beginning of the nineteenth century until the mid-twentieth century. This seminal work, based on archival research, was awarded the best science book of the year in Finland in 2009 by the Federation of Finnish Learned Societies. Ylikangas admits being astonished on discovering how prevalent the use of intoxicants in his country had been. How does he explain this pervasive consumption of drugs, heroin in particular? He points to three factors. First, heroin was an effective panacea, especially for upper respiratory tract infections, which were very common among the Finns due to the cold cli-mate they lived in. Second, in the conditions of the economically and socially difficult 1930s, heroin was simply much cheaper than other medicines, and thus it was affordable and easily available for all people.[116] Third, its use was primarily therapeutic, was kept under control, and thereby had neither turned into abuse nor developed into a social problem of addiction.

When Stalin decided to attack Finland to seize the territories that would secure the city of Leningrad for a probable future confrontation with Hitler, he had no reason to suspect that a war with this Nordic country would last three and half months (from November 1939 to March 1940), take the lives of between 230,000 and 270,000 Russian soldiers, damage the health of a fur-ther 200,000 to 300,000 men, and, most importantly, severely jeopardize the reputation of the Red Army. Stalin thought of the campaign against Finland as a glorified "police action" that would take no longer than two weeks, and the estimates of the demand for artillery ammunition were actually based on the assumption that "the entire Finnish operation would last twelve days, no more."[117]

The apparent weakness and clumsy efforts of the Soviet troops convinced Hitler to hasten his invasion of the Soviet Union. The Russo-Finnish Winter War is an example of asymmetric confrontation at its most profound. The Soviet Goliath suffered serious losses from the confrontation with the Finnish David. The weaker Finnish army played according to its own rules by waging a kind of guerrilla warfare, using agile military units of skiers wearing white camouflage uniforms, employing deadly sniper commandos (the most famous sniper was Simo Häyhä who holds the record in any major war with 505 confirmed kills, which is an average of over five kills a day), and using Molotov cocktails.

Both the familiar terrain and harsh weather worked in favor of the Finns. The winter of 1939–1940 was the coldest since 1828, when records in Finland began; the temperature remained below –34°C but in some places it went as low as –41°C. The Red Army sought to imitate the German blitzkrieg, a tactic that was totally misplaced in the Nordic terrain and climate. Moreover, the Soviets came up with the idea of soldiers and tanks using white camouflage in the snow only in the third month of the ongoing operation. Overall, the Red Army was not prepared for a war waged in extreme winter conditions, on rough terrain, and with an enemy who fought in a highly unconventional way. And in Finland—William Trotter reminds us—"unconventional tactics—ambushes, long-range ski patrols, deceptions, raids—were enshrined as doctrine and refined until they fitted into the overall national strategy."[118] Immobility, the biting cold, and serious disruptions in food supplies further weakened the Soviet forces. When Finnish units had to retreat they mined abandoned villages, roads, and fields. Writing about booby traps and mines, the Soviet *Pravda* characterized the Finish combat techniques as "barbaric and filthy tricks."

The remarkable endurance and persistence of the Finnish troops came from their strategy of exhausting the enemy—of wearing down the opponent by a variety of means—combined with perfect adaptation to the harsh climate, drilling, and extraordinary mobility. But something else was involved, too. The Finnish army used significant amounts of drugs, namely heroin, morphine, and opium. While preparing for the Soviet attack the armed forces extended and strengthened the defensive Mannerheim line, built stone roadblocks designed to stop Soviet tanks, mined all the strategic areas that the Red Army would have to pass through, and created reserves of armaments. They also sought to accumulate huge stockpiles of drugs, mostly opiates. Under government contract the Orion Pharmaceutical Company in Espoo committed itself to maintaining permanent stocks of raw opium equivalent to 150 kilograms of pure morphine.[119] In November 1939 the Medical Department of the General Staff ordered from the Swiss pharmaceutical company Hoffmann-La Roche fifty kilograms of morphine (the main pain medication) and thirty-five kilograms of heroin (an amount enough to produce some seven million five-milligram tablets). Nonetheless, when the war broke out in November 1939, the military medical services had, in fact, shortages of all major drugs other than heroin. Most of the substances and raw materials ordered from abroad arrived in Finland but only when the Winter War was over. Thus, for example, over 1.5 tons of raw opium to produce morphine and heroin from Sweden and the American Red Cross were supplied by as late as the end of 1940. The army could not, therefore, use pharmaceuticals as widely as it had expected. Only in December 1940, the military pharmacy was full of drugs, having stockpiled 117,500 five-milligram heroin tablets and 469,500 one-milligram morphine pills. In addition, it stored 917 kilograms of opium and 351 kilograms of morphine.[120]

Heroin was used extensively—almost like aspirin—as the best remedy for cold, and infections and diseases of the respiratory tract to which soldiers fighting in extreme winter conditions were heavily exposed. Ylikangas remarks, "To my knowledge, no country involved in a war had distributed heroin in such large amounts."[121] Cheap and effective, it became the most important medicine in military pharmacopoeia. Frontline military pharmacies received heroin in boxes containing 500–1,000 five-milligram tablets wrapped in five- or ten-pill paper tubes. The company medics had large amounts of them at their disposal and issued the pills quite liberally. Soldiers going to the outpost for a watch received "a package of five heroin pills to suppress coughing and to unwind the nerves."[122] With the Winter War progressing, the consumption of heroin became increasingly rampant. There was little control and concern about the risks of overdose. As one veteran recalled, "They gave you right away a handful to the bottom of your pocket."[123] Another veteran reminisced about heroin: "The shelves in the dugouts and the bags of the medics were full of it. When you had cough or when something was aching they throw heroin pills to your hand and said to take that. You did not understand what it was."[124]

Morphine and heroin were also routinely administered to wounded soldiers with medics not following the recommended dosage, particularly when treating severely injured patients in tormenting pain. Reino Naavasalo, a medical officer, thus explained the humanitarian value of morphine: "When a badly wounded soldier was kept all the time in a strong morphine 'tipsy' the fear of death did not bother him. He felt good and he knew that he could receive a new injection if necessary."[125] It was more important to ease the suffering than to follow the dosage instructions for painkillers.

The Finnish soldiers fought heroically and with great devotion over the course of 105 days of the Winter War because they were a brave nation, wholeheartedly determined to defend their freedom. For the Finnish soldiers had *sisu* in their blood. The little word *sisu* is difficult to translate adequately, but it means something like "'guts,' 'spunk,' 'grit,' or 'balls,' or a combination of all these words."[126] In other words, it stands for the strength and courage to continue against all odds, fortitude and fighting spirit, or, broadly speaking, the morale or even the national characteristics of the Finnish people. Carl Gustaf Mannerheim, Marshal of Finland and commander-in-chief, said in his farewell order on March 14, 1940: "Soldiers! I have fought on many battlefields, but never have I seen your like as warriors! . . . [A]s before we must be ready to defend our diminished Fatherland with the same resolution and the same fire with which we defended our undivided Fatherland."[127]

Thus they continued fighting the Soviets during the Continuation War (June 1941–September 1944), in the course of which the Finnish armed forces distributed 250 million tablets of heroin and morphine (although the latter was used mostly in liquid form). For example, from June to October 1941 the 10th Division, which fought in the northern areas of the Karelian Isthmus, consumed 15,653 heroin pills.[128] Every year the troops were also administered between seven to nine million tablets of a popular painkiller called Antineuralgin, which included five milligrams of heroin.[129] Heavy amounts of narcotic analgesics were administered particularly during the Finnish offensive in autumn 1941, which left many wounded. Medical officers at each company were equipped with bags containing the following psychoactive substances: two ampuls of liquid cocaine, four ampuls of morphine, thirty three-milligram opium pills (used mainly in the treatment of bad diarrhea), and thirty five-milligram heroin tablets.[130] Having at its disposal much greater stockpiles of various drugs than in the course of the Winter War, the military liberally dispensed them to the troops, the wounded in particular. The massive medical use of narcotics, in turn, inevitably led to the development of dependence. One veteran who was injured in 1944 admitted: "When I got morphine the roses started to blossom. There was no pain: Morphine, methadone, heroin . . . in 1944 I was already a total junkie."[131]

While during the Winter War drugs were mainly used for medical purposes, in the Continuation War they were also employed, though rather selectively, to enhance performance of the troops. For, in addition to heroin, morphine, opium, and cocaine, the army also began administering methamphetamine. Following the Winter War, after Finland became cobelligerent with Germany and joined them in the fight against the Soviet Union, in the summer of 1941 the Third Reich started supplying it with considerable amounts of Pervitin. It may well be that one of the explanations for such generous German assistance was not only close military cooperation but also their aforementioned attempt to reduce the use of methamphetamine by the Wehrmacht due to its undesired side effects and offload massive stocks of Pervitin. So, in 1941 the Finns had already at their disposal 850,000 tablets of Pervitin, which they issued to special commandos and also to regular units on particularly heavy missions, such as rapid retreats, evacuations of the wounded, or the patrols and raids of the ski snipers. According to army instructions, methamphetamine was to be used to combat fatigue or raise the stamina of the troops and galvanize them to action when great physical endurance was required. The use of Pervitin by regular infantry units was somewhat selective and methamphetamine was never, unlike heroin, consumed much like aspirin. Its use was usually limited to emergency situations, as, for example, the large-scale Soviet offensive in 1944 during which infantrymen were dispensed methamphetamine quite liberally. For there were cases when, for example, a battalion surrounded by the Soviets had to defend itself in harsh winter conditions, and the medical officer issued Pervitin to his exhausted, cold, and wet men.

The main consumers of methamphetamine were, however, special commando units. From October 1941 the personal medical kit of each commando included one tube containing twenty five-milligram pills of heroin (with the recommended dosage of up to three tablets a day taken in divided doses for cough and pain, or two to three tablets to be taken at once if wounded, but no more than six pills a day), three-milligram opium pills, and three-milligram Pervitin.[132] Special commandos used methamphetamine on a regular basis during demanding raids, which often required soldiers to walk or ski long distances chased by the enemy. The opening of a skiing track was a particularly demanding and exhausting mission. A commando Urho Ylitalo remembered:

> We had crossed many enemy tracks and we were tens of kilometres in the rear of the enemy where its strongest units were located. The snow cover was one meter deep and when the track was opened the ski sank each time to the moss. The front man was able to proceed only a mere one hundred meters at a time and then the front man had to be changed to the next one. When we had skied constantly almost two days and nights we were starting to exhaust. . . . We were, however, prepared for situations like this as we had received Pervitin pills from the Germans. When a fatigued man took two pills he was high for several hours, full of increasing strength. . . . The group leaders kept the tablets and distributed them to the men, because the pills had to last for many more days. . . . We crossed man lakes where melted water

was half way up the leg. Arms and legs felt reckless but Pervitin gave us incomprehensible vigor and optimistic willpower. . . . Without Pervitin we would have never returned from there.[133]

In essence, as we already know, Pervitin could do marvels with human performance. One commando quoted by Ylikangas recalled that the drug "was a peculiar lunch. It was such a small trifling but when you took it, you felt like you could do anything."[134] Thus in a way, by providing vigor, reducing hunger, and subduing pain, stimulants worked toward improving the *sisu* of the members of the special commandos.

Of course, methamphetamine has also serious side effects and overdosing might be dangerous. So, to get acquainted to the drug and check men for its possible side effects, special ski units took methamphetamine during training for the next patrol or raid. The drug was thus tested in advance to identify any individual undesired reactions. Pervitin could enable the men to complete a mission and return to base but still its adverse events, such as disorientation, hallucinations, overexcitement, and bravado, could put the whole unit at risk. There are many examples of battlefield hazards caused by Pervitin. Take the following particularly telling stories. A commando member recalled the hallucinations he experienced on the way back from a long ski patrol:

> We were chased by the Russians and I felt that my strength was running out. I remember that Honkanen gave me Pervitin. . . . When we reached Lake Ohta I realized that something was not right. I saw strange things. . . . I started to talk and said to Ohtonen that why do we need to go back now to the base and to our tents. Let's go instead to that two story stone house where those girls in white dresses are dancing in the bright light of crystal chandeliers.[135]

The same man remembered another ski patrol during which his fellow man sat in the snow after taking Pervitin and said: "What the hell do we ski here totally in vain! Let's call a taxi and drive to Kettunen [a popular bar in the town of Kajaani]."[136] Pauli Savinainen, another member of a special commando, observed that when a unit opened a ski track, it was best to give Pervitin but only to the front man. Issuing it to all soldiers at the same time was quite undesirable for the risk of the men getting overactive and so hopped-up that they could lose "the patience to ski in a row and start skiing in a trance, competing with each other, every man opening his own track in the deep snow."[137] Such a Pervitin-induced "skiing competition," which threatened to jeopardize the whole mission, was sometimes reported.

Pervitin was also used by military commanders but much more widely by medical personnel. Medical officer Reino Naavasalo recalled how during the Autumn 1941 offensive in Soviet Karelia

> [w]ounded soldiers are brought in constantly. The yard is packed of ambulances, all beds and corridors are full. . . . The policlinic and the surgery are working day and night. The wards are crowded with patients. We are tired, we drink black coffee all around the clock and Pervitin is given also to the nurses in the policlinic and the surgery. . . . I haven't slept at all for three days, my head is humming, my eyes burn, I have lost my appetite. I have the notion that I am too important, that I may be needed in any moment.[138]

Overall, Pervitin was distributed extensively among the personnel of military hospitals to propel high performance and enable continuous surgeries despite the acute lack of sleep and rest. Thus by assisting doctors and nurses methamphetamine helped save lives of the injured. At the time people were, however, not fully aware of Pervitin's highly addictive potential, so that taking it was commonly seen as, to quote one nurse, "more or less like drinking strong coffee."[139]

War memoir literature shows that methamphetamine was also taken recreationally, especially when soldiers wanted to take the maximum advantage of their short leaves. Pervitin, colloquially called by the Germans "the holiday pill," allowed for greater fun, even more so as it was also known to increase male potency. Overall, in the course of the Continuation War, methamphetamine tablets proved so valuable and gained such a good reputation that a cold medicine introduced to the Finnish market after the war was branded "Pervitin," even though it had nothing to do with amphetamines.[140]

As happened in many other military conflicts in which troops have been pharmacologically assisted, we will never be able to accurately assess the true role of intoxicants in the entire Finnish war effort. What is certain, however, is that while heroin was used in large quantities, neither the scale of methamphetamine consumption was massive nor its role vital.[141] Therefore, we must again be careful not to overestimate the "drug factor."

One consequence of the Second World War was a sort of egalitarianization of nonmedical use of psychoactive substances in Finland. Before the war the recreational consumption of drugs was a problem but mostly of the higher social classes, and opiate addiction was in fact referred to as "upper class morphine dependency." This, however, changed. For once they had been tested and taken on the frontline, intoxicants ceased to be reserved only for the crème de la crème of the Helsinki's elite. In this regard, the Continuation War proved a powerful democratizing force, which inevitably led to the higher, yet not alarming, rates of addiction in the years following 1945. "Getting hooked on opiates," notes Miska Rantanen, "in the midst of war was seen as something of a routine event in the heat of war."[142] Given the prolific use of heroin, liberal administration of opiates in treating the wounded, and the distribution—though much more restrictive—of methamphetamine, the fact that not many veterans developed substance dependence is indeed truly surprising. A major medical study conducted in 1956 revealed that as little as 13 percent of male drug addicts who were hospitalized in the postwar period had developed their drug problem during treatment of their combat wounds.[143] What is beyond doubt, however, is that many postwar addicts had learned the use and effects of drugs, mostly heroin pills and Pervitin, in the course of combat.

The Russians

Was the Red Army, which for three and a half months could not break the determined Finns, enhancing the performance of its soldiers with drugs such as amphetamines during the Second World War as the Germans, British, Americans, Japanese, and Finns were? The answer is "no." The Russians remained faithful to their traditional means of fueling strength, increasing fortitude, combating fatigue, and preventing war trauma among the troops. These were vodka and valerian.[144] Alcohol had an added invigorating advantage as it supplemented poor food rations with a good amount of extra calories. The Red Army was the only great power army during the war that did not make use of stimulants, except maybe for a popular yet not commonly used drink called the "trench cocktail"—a mixture of vodka and cocaine. In addition to being used as a performance enhancer, the cocktail was employed as an anesthetic during surgery.[145]

The Krasnoarmeet fought with great devotion because the Russian soldier had always fought with commitment and tenacity. During the Winter War, the Finns were sometimes astonished to watch the enemy troopers who charged with what Mannerheim characterized as "fatalism incomprehensible to a European."[146] Consider, for example, the method for demining an area to clear it for incoming tank divisions. The infantrymen formed close-order rows and "marched stoically into the mines, singing party songs and continuing to advance with the same steady, suicidal rhythm even as the mines began to explode, ripping holes in their ranks and showering the marchers with feet, legs and intestines."[147] Such human waves were repeated until the goal was accomplished. Tanks were more valuable than humans. Incredible as it seems, the Krasnoarmeets cleared the mines with their bodies, because they had no other choice. And ironically, the chance of a soldier surviving such a mission was higher than it would have been if he refused to obey the order or fled the action, since such behaviors would mean a bullet in the head. A survivor of one such Russian attack against minefields recalled, "There was no fear, only a dull apathy and indifference to impending doom pushed us ahead."[148] Was it dazed automatism or rather liquid courage? Probably it was both. Given the harsh winter conditions and the irrational fatalism mentioned by Mannerheim, the Soviet soldiers numbed themselves heavily with vodka. Alcohol rendered the perception of a brutal and desperate reality a little more bearable.

Conclusion

In the course of the Second World War, armed forces were the greatest consumers of amphetamines. During this conflict, both the Nazis and the Allies eventually violated the last remnants of just war doctrine. It is hardly surprising then that ethical dilemmas over the routine administration of intoxicants to the troops were not of much concern. Plutarch had observed in the first century AD that *Inter arma silent leges* (In times of war, the law is silent). Let us also bear in mind that in the 1930s and 1940s amphetamines were legally available in most Western countries as prescription medicines, commonly used for medicinal purposes, and were by no means considered the "hard" drugs they are today.

It is difficult to overestimate the role of the performance enhancement of troops with speed for the development and popularization of amphetamine doping also in sport, especially cycling, in the 1940s and 1950s. As a result, between 1948 and 1970 amphetamine was the most common doping agent in sports in the United States, used under the guidance and with the connivance of coaches and physicians. The end of the war in general marked the beginning of the period during which amphetamines spread through the war-weary societies. It was actually the homecoming soldiers who popularized speed. Amphetamine was widely available, and by the 1950s its use had spread to college students, athletes, truck drivers, nightclub musicians, and housewives in the United States. Lots of people who wanted to keep themselves awake or needed extra energy reached for it. Unsurprisingly, in many countries the consumption and production of amphetamine increased significantly in the decade following the war.[149] It is important to keep in mind that the drug was not seen as a form of doping but was rather considered an established and legal cure; after all, people knew that it was liberally dispensed to soldiers during the war. Overall, stimulants, writes Paul Dimeo, "had a positive aura in the immediate post-war period."[150]

PART TWO

THE COLD WAR

From the Korean War to the War Over Mind Control

We must be engineers of the human soul.
—Vladimir Lenin quoted in Robert Jay Lifton, *Thought Reform and the Psychology of Totalism. A Study of "Brainwashing" in China*

The Korean War

But once war is forced upon us, there is no other alternative than to apply every available means to bring it to a swift end.
—Douglas MacArthur, Address to Congress, 1951

It could be argued, provocatively, that in the Korean War one of these "all available means" was not nuclear weapons, as MacArthur had wished, but amphetamine pep pills. Although, as we have seen, they had been in circulation since the Second World War, it was in Korea that uppers were allowed to be used on a routine basis by American military personnel.[1] It was during the Korean War, too, that soldiers were given intravenous amphetamine injections and issued a more potent methamphetamine.[2] Overall, "speed" proved to be highly valuable as it enabled the troops to endure long, often nighttime, intense fighting, particularly against the fierce attacks launched by Chinese "volunteers."

In the Second World War, Benzedrine was usually issued to American pilots on long-haul and exhausting missions, to the infantrymen fighting in harsh combat conditions and to the navy men who had to stay alert on lengthy night voyages. Despite its widespread use amphetamine was not, as had been the case previously with alcohol, dispensed automatically as a standard ration to every serviceman. Instead, its use was formally limited to special circumstances. This changed profoundly during the Korean conflict, when amphetamine, and to a lesser extent also methamphetamine, came to be administered almost routinely, with the SKF company regularly meeting the demand for Dexedrine under contract to the government.[3]

Such a universal and near-excessive use of speed was by no means surprising given that amphetamine had been as popular as vitamins in the United States well until the 1950s. In the 1940s and 1950s it was an easily available ingredient of many medicines. Only in 1951 did amphetamine tablets become a prescription drug (but one issued by physicians both willingly and widely). Benzedrine inhalers, however, remained commonly available until 1965, when the Drug Abuse Control Act limited retail sales and the prevalence of medical use of amphetamines. While in 1958 an estimated three and a half billion tablets of amphetamine were manufactured in the United States, less than a decade later annual production skyrocketed to eight billion pills, rising to ten billion in 1970.[4] Amphetamine was cheap and readily obtainable, for it was still believed to be safe and have no harmful side effects. Take, for example, a contemporaneous study which argued: "As experience with the amphetamines has ripened they have become firmly established as versatile and helpful remedies given to millions of people and under such conditions as to offer remarkably low potential for causing them harm."[5] In the *Dexedrine Reference Manual*, published in 1953, the SKF drug manufacturing company adamantly denied that amphetamine had any potential to be habit-forming.[6] An on-board service menu from an early Pan American World Airways Flight dated circa 1950 included Benzedrine inhalers as a free service item next to chewing gum, tooth brushes, electric razors, sewing kits, and medical kits.[7] Amphetamine was thus available in the sky at passengers' fingertips, recommended to minimize the discomfort during take-off and landing. So, it was not only American Air Force pilots who could experience the other meaning of the phrase "flying high" but also the passengers of commercial airlines, though of course to a limited extent. Therefore, the saying "flying high on high" took on a double meaning. Certainly, when compared with soldiers, civilian passengers could feel a very moderate effect of amphetamine as the inhaler was designed to decongest a stuffy nose.

In the United Kingdom, too, the 1950s was a decade of great "speed mania," which was fueled largely by the postwar demobilization of soldiers who had experienced the invigorating effects of pep pills in wartime. Until the 1960s amphetamine was a commonly prescribed remedy for diverse afflictions from moderate depression to obesity.[8] It was fairly popular also among politicians; Adolf Hitler was not the only speed-boosted leader of the era. For example, amphetamine proved very beneficial to Winston Churchill; he used it, along with barbiturates, on prescription from his private physician Lord Moran, and reported that the drug cleared his head wonderfully and gave him great confidence.[9] Churchill's successor as prime minister, Anthony Eden, confessed that in 1952, at the height of the Suez crisis, the only thing that kept him alive was regular doses of Benzedrine.[10] Another telling example is that of John

F. Kennedy, who took an injection of Dexedrine on many occasions, such as just before his historic televised debate with Richard Nixon during the 1960 presidential campaign. The drug was administered to him by Max Jacobson, a New York physician who was famous of giving his patients injections of vitamins, steroids, placenta, and amphetamines, a therapy which earned him the nickname "Dr. Feelgood." Jacobson administered Kennedy, who suffered from an assortment of health problems, his "feel good injections" regularly, usually twice a week. He also assisted the president on some of his foreign trips, for example, to Europe in 1961. We know that Kennedy was "on speed" at the time of his first meeting with the Soviet leader Nikita Khrushchev and in the course of the Cuban missile crisis in October 1962.[11]

As has been mentioned, as early as 1940 the Germans were the first to learn about the undesired harmful effects of amphetamines. Yet in the United States it was only at the turn of the 1960s and 1970s that the overly positive cultural, social, and medical perception of the drug had changed fundamentally. A previously widely accepted and universally used remedy and stimulant was now transformed into a reviled and controlled substance. This radical change was summed up well by one of the most successful and well-known antidrug slogans in American history: "Speed kills."[12] It is, I believe, only in this broader sociohistorical context that the use of amphetamines by the American forces in Korea can be properly assessed and understood.

To return, then, to the 1950s and the Korean War, the easy accessibility of amphetamine resulted in the first major wave of drug abuse among active duty servicemen. Apart from the controlled consumption of the pep pills distributed by the authorities to boost the combat performance of the troops, recreational drug use thrived among American soldiers in Korea. In addition, they discovered the method of multiplying the effects of amphetamine by mixing it with heroin, which was incredibly cheap as one dose cost eighty to ninety cents. This injectable cocktail came to be colloquially known as a "speedball," though today the term is usually used to describe a mix of heroin and cocaine.[13]

From a reading of the Army's official statistics one would not conclude that American forces in Korea struggled with a drug problem. For example, the 25th Infantry Division reported only twelve cases of illegal drug use, while the 3rd Infantry Division confirmed just two cases in an eight-month period. Nonetheless, the problem existed and over time became increasingly acute, with even a small number of deaths from heroin overdoses recorded. In 1952 the Department of Defense was forced to admit that since 1949 the number of soldiers arrested for substance abuse in the Far East Command had more than tripled, from 201 to 715.[14] And these were only the detected cases.

When in 1952 the army command finally realized the severity of the problem, it linked drug abuse to the subversive methods employed by the communists. Intoxicants were perceived as a danger not only to the physical health of the troops but most of all also to their morale. They threatened, it was assumed, to weaken the body's resistance to communist ideology. Soldiers usually scored drugs in North Korea when on leave in Japan, mostly in brothels and night clubs. Consequently, "the brothels," writes Callum A. MacDonald,

> were considered undesirable by the high command, not only because they were a source of infection, but also because they supplied nar-cotics. . . . It was suspected that the brothels were at the center of an international communist conspiracy to subvert American youth. "Every drug addict" was "a potential communist."[15]

This might have seemed so because between 30 and 40 percent of dealers arrested in Japan and South Korea had run drugs from communist China.[16] Thus the country from which the substance was largely sourced was associated with hostile ideological activities, and the logic of this thinking was later advanced on the wave of the "Second Red Scare" and anticommunist hysteria. The report by the Senate subcommittee investigating the drug problem in the United States, headed by Price Daniel (the Daniel Subcommittee), reflected this peculiar "drug McCarthyism." In 1956 the committee declared that the number of addicts in the United States exceeded the total number of addicts in other Western countries. The main explanation for this was that it resulted from the dirty war waged by the communists against American society and culture. The Daniel Subcommittee concluded, "Subversion through drug addiction is an established aim of Communist China. Since World War II, Red China has pushed the exportation of heroin to servicemen and civilians of the US and other free nations of the word."[17]

When the army launched efforts to limit the consumption of intoxicants in Korea, it soon discovered that the issue was much more complicated than it seemed at first sight. In order to effectively handle the problem a close coop-eration with the local South Korean police force was necessary. The police were, however, actively involved in trafficking in women and smuggling them to brothels, thus providing cover and protection for the entire underground sex and drug trade economy. Further, the antidrug initiatives met with a cold response in Japan. More important still, it turned out that most heroin arriving in the Japanese Islands was delivered by the American airline Civil Air Transport (CAT). It was a supplier to American military bases, which remained excluded from Japanese custom control under the principle of extra-territoriality. CAT, which later in 1959 changed its name to Air America, was the property of the CIA. The company was sometimes called "Air Arlington" (from the CIA's headquarters in Arlington, Virginia) because it was used by the agency for its clandestine operations in East and Southeast Asia.[18] The CIA gave considerable assistance to the local anticommunist gangs, mafias, and warlords by supplying them with equipment, providing logistical support, and helping in the distribution of drugs. Thus the agency largely helped foster the growth of the Golden Triangle (Burma, Thailand, Laos, and Vietnam), which by 1963 had developed into the world's largest poppy-growing area. CAT also transported drugs for the Chinese Kuomintang nationalists in exile in Northeast Burma and North Thailand, who were seen as a potential anticommunist guerrilla force to be used in the future to undermine the Maoists.[19] In short, to keep the anticommunists in power, concludes Martin Booth, "the CIA became inextricably entangled with the Golden Triangle opium trade, handling opiate consignments, flying drug runs and tolerantly turning a blind eye to the affairs of their criminal allies."[20] So, in part due to the American actions and commitments in the region and the lack of willingness on the part of the armed forces to take decisive action, drug abuse among American soldiers in Korea proved an insurmountable problem. The army itself limited its antidrug activity to the penalization of offenders, so that most servicemen caught abusing psychoactive substances were punished either by the extension of their tour of duty or by imprisonment.

After the units of the Chinese People's Volunteer Army (the "volunteers") crossed the Yalu River on October 19, 1950, entering Korea and engaging in the war against the South Korean and UN forces, Western soldiers painfully experienced the strikingly different strategic culture of the Orient. The 300,000 man strong Chinese army, made up largely of peasants, was poorly equipped and badly trained. But the huge manpower and resolute soldiers compensated for the grave shortcomings in armaments and equipment. Above all, the Chinese commanders sought to deny the American technological superiority by fighting according to their own rules. In general, the Chinese had a very low opinion of the condition and combativeness of their opponent. In the aftermath of the first clash with American troops near Unsan on October 25, 1950, the People's Liberation Army issued and circulated a pamphlet in which it warned its soldiers of the great enemy firepower, but at the same time depreciated the courage of the individual American soldier. The paper observed: "Their infantrymen are weak, afraid to die, and haven't the courage to attack or defend. . . . They will cringe when, if on the advance, they hear firing."[21]

The tactics adopted by Mao Tse-Tung assumed that a decisive defeat of the Republic of Korea Army (ROKA) would create a panic among American troops, who would be then harassed, drained, and eventually forced to retreat.[22] The Chinese attacked to produce a terrible psychological shock, leaving the enemy stunned and demobilized. They moved en masse, screaming shrilly and charging like a wild wave washing through the battlefield, and were decimated by the firepower of the UN units. Such fanatical attacks often ended in hand-to-hand fighting. The war correspondents who reported on the raids of Chinese units described them as unimaginable hordes of savage soldiers attacking in a wild fighting frenzy, completely fearless of death and danger. In Korea, a typical Chinese unorthodox (or "asymmetrical" in today's parlance) approach to warfare took the form of attacking and pressing in an extremely bold way, without regard to casualties. This terrifying and ruthless Chinese way of fighting caused not only shock and embarrassment amongst the UN forces but also the intended horror. The Americans and Canadians commonly believed that no sane soldier would act like the Chinese. It was presumed that the only explanation for this fearless and totally irrational Chinese bravado was that it was drug induced.[23] So, within the allied forces a rumor was rife that the Chinese went into battle intoxicated with opium. Major Réal Liboiron, the commanding officer of Dog Company of the 2nd Battalion of the Canadian Royal 22nd Regiment, recalled that most of his men truly believed that

> the Chinese were doped before they were committed to battle because they were completely oblivious to danger. They stood up fully exposed when the heaviest of our mortar and artillery concentrations were coming down and apparently had absolutely no regard for their own personal safety.[24]

This utterly alien way of war, based on absolutely blind devotion and a contempt for life, frightened Western soldiers in Korea much as the equally fanatical Japanese way of fighting had earlier horrified the Americans during the Pacific War. The Chinese "human waves," which mounted attack after attack under heavy shelling without proper, if any, cover, greatly resembled the Japanese banzai attacks. Hence the Korean experience only reinforced the popular Western image of the "savage Asian hordes" going to battle high on opium. The rumor that the Chinese fought drugged has never been confirmed. Furthermore, Mao launched a decisive and victorious campaign to eradicate the opium habit amongst the military and civilian population. In February 1950 the communist authorities banned the cultivation of the poppy plant and prohibited the production, import, and sale of opium and other intoxicating drugs. Opium stocks were burned in public, and dope peddlers were sent to work camps. The use of opium was declared not only harmful to the individual's health but was also proclaimed an antisocial, antisocialist, and typically capitalist activity. Drugs, in a word, were equated with imperialist subversion. The antidrug policy proved so effective that by 1960 China's long-standing drug problem was successfully overcome.[25] Confronted with an alien strategic culture and unable to understand the enemy's mentality, Western soldiers explained the behavior of the Chinese troops through their supposed intoxication. In this context, too, we should consider the popular gossip that the drugged Chinese units were led by a woman in black, the so-called Dragon Lady.[26] Where did this story come from? The fact that much of the fighting took place in the dark facilitated a sense of surrealism and aggravated a deep fear of the unknown, ferocious, and elusive enemy, endowed with superhuman qualities. The enemy who appeared more like "a deadly shadow of a man, who stalked the overgrown rice paddies of no man's land with the cunning and skill of a professional hunter."[27] Paradoxically, however, it was not the Chinese but the American forces that were regularly and extensively popping pills for combat.

The Controversial Korean POW Episode

> We have not used germ warfare, CIA propaganda claimed, the Communists had used brainwashing.
> —Walter Bowart, *Operation Mind Control*

At the moment when the Korean War broke out none of the parties soon to be involved in the conflict was bound by the Third Geneva Convention of 1949 on the treatment of POWs. China and the Democratic People's Republic of Korea had not signed it, while the United States would ratify it in 1955. Despite this, the parties declared that they would observe the provisions of the Convention.[28] Such an informal application entailed risks and soon lengthy disputes erupted, particularly over Article 118, which provided that "prisoners of war shall be released and repatriated without delay after the cessation of active hostilities." During drafting of the Convention, the Americans strongly pushed for precisely such an uncompromising wording of the clause (i.e., "forcible repatriation"), seeing it as a useful propaganda tool against the Soviet Union, which still continued to hold large numbers of Axis POWs as forced labor. During the war in Korea, however, this provision was no longer desired by the United States.[29] Article 118 assumed that all POWs were willing to return to their home countries; by 1951, however, it became clear that significant numbers of North Korean and Chinese prisoners in the UN camps did not want to be repatriated. It was for this reason that the Americans began to advocate for "nonforcible repatriation," that is, giving the prisoners a fairly informed free choice between going back to their home country or staying in South Korea or Formosa. This option was, of course, unacceptable to China. Thus from the very beginning the belligerent parties saw the POW issue as a valuable tool of psychological warfare, and the topic inevitably became an important element in the early Cold War ideological struggle.

In order to indoctrinate the communist prisoners, the Americans used movies and lectures that were aimed at showing the true face of communism and telling a demythologized history of Korea, as well as presenting and instilling democratic values. The United States was interested in re-educating North Korean and Chinese POWs and sending them back home where they would form a focus of popular antiregime opposition. The goal was to turn them into a Cold War fifth column. The Chinese adopted a similar stance to the Americans over the POW issue. Enemy prisoners of war were so valuable a resource that one of China's war aims was to capture them in large numbers. In the spring of 1952 China admitted to holding 11,559 prisoners, including 3,198 Americans. In the course of the war, more than 7,000 American soldiers were interned in Chinese POW camps, while the UN forces held 137,000 North Koreans, Chinese, and South Koreans.[30]

Edward Hunter, a CIA propaganda operator working undercover as a journalist, was the first to use in print the term "brainwashing" in an article published in the *Miami News* in September 1950.[31] He popularized the concept in his book *Brainwashing in Red China* (1951) by describing the "thought reform" carried out by the Maoists after having seized and consolidated power in China.[32] "Brainwashing" went into widespread public use as the term to denote the methods for rectifying the mind employed by the communists in general. There is no question that the Chinese sought to take control of the minds of enemy POWs. The indoctrination began with the systematic destruction of group structures to undermine loyalty and authority. The ultimate goal was to lessen the sense of security and trust among inmates by weakening and eventually breaking solidarity, thereby impairing their group cohesion and brotherhood. The resulting conflict and social anomie were further fueled by camp authorities. All of this was thought to make prisoners more prone to manipulation.

Indoctrination was carried out in the form of compulsory daily lectures, movies, and reading of propaganda publications, as well as through total control of information. POWs were compelled to write their own autobiographies, emphasizing the errors, weaknesses, and evils of the capitalist world.[33] The Chinese developed a very close surveillance system over camp activities through informers in the POW ranks and intensive spying. Denunciatory activities eroded trust, hindered the development of closer relationships, and, above all, had a very demoralizing effect. The sense of alienation and loneliness was also deepened by strict control on correspondence with home since POWs were given only letters containing bad news. To sum up, brutal treatment, dire sanitary and nutrition conditions, and a very high mortality rate of 34 percent were the key factors that determined the behavior of prisoners. Cooperation and support were replaced by a fiercely egoistic struggle for survival.

The Chinese were extremely smart and effective in employing a complex system of rewards and punishments; thus they implemented what Joost Meerloo called "the negative and positive conditioning stimuli."[34] American POWs could gain better treatment in return for active propaganda activities, such as making radio broadcasts, organizing lectures for fellow inmates, signing statements supporting the North Korean case at the UN, and writing letters to their families condemning American imperialism and extolling the Chinese. Prisoners with a "progressive attitude" received higher food rations, cigarettes, warm clothes and blankets, more comfortable places to sleep, and easier access to mail.[35] Resistant and uncooperative prisoners were punished by being watertreated (waterboarded in today's parlance), exposed to cold and drenched with water, deprived of sleep, forced to remain in one painful position for many hours, and more.[36] Overall, the Chinese "re-education" methods proved so effective that many POWs broke down and agreed to far-reaching cooperation.

Information on the Chinese use of brainwashing techniques reached the American public while the war was still on. Confessions of American pilots who repeatedly confirmed that the United States used biological weapons in Korea deeply shocked U.S. society. Kenneth L. Enoch and John Quinn, two pilots shot down in January 1952 and taken as POWs, submitted a testimony that their mission was to deliver bombs containing anthrax, typhoid, and cholera spores. As the issue of germ warfare gained wide publicity in the communist countries, the Soviet bloc went on to accuse the United States of committing war crimes. Further, in February 1953, Colonel Frank H. Schwable, not just anybody but the chief of staff of the First Marine Air Wing, who was shot down over Korea in July the previous year, confirmed Enoch's and Quinn's allegations and provided the communists with an exhaustive account of the American biological weapons program. He was followed soon after by another thirty-five American pilots downed over Korea, who testified to the authenticity of the colonel's statements and confessed their involvement in the operation.[37] The whole story about germ warfare was, however, false. Pilots were forced to confess under the combination of psychological pressure (call it brainwashing) and calculated brutality (violence and threats).

The fact that 22,000 Chinese and North Korean POWs did not want to be repatriated was understandable to the Americans, but it was impossible to explain why twenty-one fellow citizens chose life in a backward and totalitarian country. Most of grief and accusations against the "pro-Red POWs" were expressed by journalists, Eugene Kinkead in particular. In his later book *In Every War but One* (1959) he presented biased, condemnatory, and pronounced opinions. As a result, in the popular view those American soldiers who were taken POW were morally frail and did not embody typical American traits.[38]

As the issue of the "procommunist POWs" became a frequent theme of Hollywood productions, movies reinforced perhaps not so much the image of a disgraced Korean POW but rather the Chinese methods of "thought reform," or "coercive persuasion," to use Albert Biderman's phrase.[39] In Andrew Marton's film *Prisoner of War* (1954) there is a memorable scene illustrating the use of violence to extort testimonies from POWs, in which Colonel Peter Reilly (John Lupton) confesses to fabricating the allegations concerning dropping biological bombs. Or take another example: Captain Edward Hall (played by Paul Newman), the protagonist of the 1956 movie *The Rack*, is accused of numerous violations of the military code of conduct during his captivity in Korea, such as giving propaganda lectures, distribution of leaflets, signing false testimonies, and ill-treatment of his fellow prisoners. The film suggests that it was not so much the American bodies that the communists racked but their minds.

The most famous film about the war in Korea and brainwashing is, however, John Frankenheimer's *The Manchurian Candidate* (1962), based on the 1959 novel by Richard Condon. It depicts the hypnotic science-fictionesque mind-control techniques through which the victims are totally deprived of their free will. Raymond Shaw (played by Laurence Harvey) is an American officer, captured by the Chinese, who undergoes a complete brainwashing in a secret location in Manchuria, hence the title. His brain is cleared of "those uniquely American symptoms—guilt and fear."[40] After being released from captivity, Shaw returns to the United States as a secret communist agent, secret even to himself. When his mental trigger is activated, he turns into a perfect assassin. Shaw's ultimate goal is to install a Kremlin stooge, the demagogic Senator Iselin, as the president of the United States. Condon did not make up Manchuria as the place where the communist performed their mind-control procedures but based his story on hearsay and the recollections of veterans. In May 1953, a Korean POW admitted to being drugged on the train returning him from Manchuria. A related CIA document reported, "The individuals who had come out of North Korea across the Soviet Union to freedom recently had apparently had a 'blank' period or period of disorientation while passing through a special zone in Manchuria."[41] Something dark was happening in this covert "special zone" somewhere in Manchuria. The CIA suspected that POWs were intoxicated there. Brainwashing—a powerful symbol of anticommunist hyperbole—proved to be a remarkably persistent and suggestive "cultural fantasy" and fodder for a variety of conspiracy theories.[42]

The "POW episode" sparked a wider discussion on a moral flaw in American character. Some disturbing questions were strongly raised, such as, "What was wrong with the new generation?" or "Were the young Americans wimps?" Fortunately, in the end some voices of reason were heard, maintaining that the entire issue should be approached with greater emotional detachment and objectivity. In 1962 a group of twenty-one academics who had researched the behavior of prisoners of war issued a statement in which they argued:

> The behavior of the Korean prisoners did not compare unfavorably with that of their countrymen or with the behavior of people of other nations who have faced similar trials in the past. Instances of moral weakness, collaboration with the enemy, and failure to take care of fellow soldiers in Korea did not occur more frequently than in other wars where comparable conditions of physical and psychological hardship were present. Indeed, such instances appear to have been less prevalent than historical experience would lead us to expect.[43]

So, how to understand the public discussion of the POW episode? Harold Wubben provided a simple but sensible answer: it was during the Korean War that the Americans had been confronted for the first time with an enemy who carried out a well-thought-out and calculated program of ideological indoctrination of enemy prisoners.[44] For the first time the adversary attempted, as Edward Hunter put it, to "murder minds" and "hijack the free will" of American POWs.[45] Would the American everyman have demonstrated moral strength and remained faithful to American values when faced with efficient and ruthless methods of mind control? Joost Meerloo was, indeed, acutely skeptical: "When, during the military inquiry into the Schwable case, I was called upon to testify as an expert on menticide, I told the court of my deep conviction that nearly anybody subjected to the treatment meted out to Colonel Schwable could be forced to write and sign a similar confession."[46]

The fact that communist indoctrination had proven remarkably effective paved the way for the common belief that the Chinese and the Soviets used not only behavioral scientific methods, such as Pavlov's conditioning, but also hypnosis, sex, and drugs. This was, however, a myth. There is no evidence that the Chinese had mastered the use of intoxicants as a means of "thought reform" or that they had administered any psychoactive substance to POWs, be it in Manchuria or anywhere else. Neither had they employed hypnotic methods, conditioned reflexes, or sex.[47]

In August 1955 two Princeton University academics, the psychiatrist Lawrence Hinkle and the neuroscientist Harold Wolff, prepared a CIA-commissioned report that debunked the claims that American POWs were put on drugs or hypnotized. The authors insisted that the confessions obtained by the communists were not the result of popping pills but rather of deliberate mental manipulation and psychological abuse, through methods and techniques such as sleep deprivation, isolation, threats, humiliation, forced

standing, induced disorientation, deprivation of the use of toilet facilities, and
the like. Prisoners would do anything to stop this cruel treatment.[48] In addition, a document published in 1956 by the Department of the Army read: "The
exhaustive efforts of several Government agencies failed to reveal even one
conclusively documented case of the actual 'brainwashing' of an American
prisoner of war in Korea."[49] Thus there was neither "Pavlov" nor drugged
prisoners. Furthermore, the interrogation of repatriated POWs revealed that
they had not necessarily been subject to a regimen of group indoctrination or
brainwashing. Quite the contrary; it appeared that on agreeing to cooperate
with the captors, they merely followed the army's instructions, known as the
"secret emergency code of conduct." They had been trained to cooperate with
the enemy if taken prisoner and not to give their captors any excuse to torture them. Soldiers had been strongly convinced not to feel remorse because
everybody at home would understand that they were acting under coercion.
Servicemen claimed to have performed in line with the army's recommendations. All this, of course, was denied by the armed forces.[50]

A similar situation occurred in May 1962, when an American U-2 spy plane
was shot down over the Soviet Union. During the public trial in Moscow, the
captured pilot, Francis Gary Powers, apologized to the Russian people for
doing them wrong. His behavior provoked shock and disbelief in the United
States, although a covert CIA instruction allowed him to admit anything if
taken prisoner. Powers was released in a trade for the Soviet spy Rudolf Abel.
Immediately upon crossing the border from East to West Berlin, blood samples
were taken from Powers which were, as he recalled in his memoir, "necessary
to determine whether I had been drugged. This seemed to be the first question of almost everyone to whom I talked: Had I been drugged? They seemed
almost disappointed when I told them I hadn't."[51] Is it possible, one must ask in
conclusion, that after Powers's release the CIA forgot about its own guidance
issued to the U-2 pilots? Or did it operate according to another rationale?

Myth often animates the real; fiction frequently impacts reality. Why have
I so extensively focused on the controversies surrounding Korean POWs? The
incident and the atmosphere surrounding the public debate on American soldiers' misbehavior, the suspicions over the Chinese techniques of mind control,
and the gossip about the communist use of pharmacology to foster ideological
re-education had pushed the authorities to establish one of the most futuristic,
controversial, and covert military and intelligence research projects. Studies
were carried out independently by the American armed forces and the CIA,
but at times the two institutions cooperated on some issues. Both the military and the CIA decided that large-scale experiments on humans with potent
psychoactive substances could be imperative for the United States' success
in the Cold War. In this regard, the aftereffects of the conflict in Korea were

experienced long after the ceasefire. In the next chapter I focus on army projects, leaving aside the CIA's MKULTRA program (1953–1973; its objective
was the search for novel pharmacologically assisted interrogation methods
and mind control techniques for covert intelligence operations; the program
involved ethically dubious experiments with drugs on uninformed citizens)
because this had to do with a secret intelligence war rather than the military
application of mind-altering agents.

9

In Search of Wonderful New Techniques and Weapons

So, first of all, let me assert my firm belief that the only thing we have to fear is fear itself—nameless, unreasoning, unjustified terror which paralyzes needed efforts to convert retreat into advance.
—Franklin Delano Roosevelt, "First Inaugural Address," 1933

The fear of communists intensified not only due to the Korean POW episode but also because of the threat of "brainwashing" and the vision of the enslaved human robot. It was also envenomed by the intelligence reports, from which it followed that the Americans were far behind in their works on psychochemical weapons. In 1951 intelligence sources informed that the Soviets were experimenting with a psychotropic drug known as "ketjubung."[1] It was also known that the Soviet Union was stockpiling large amounts of tabun and sarin gas, which it was producing with the significant support of German scientists taken to the Soviet Union after the collapse of the Third Reich. Sources in Europe also informed that the Soviets were bringing in vast amounts of ergot from the Balkan states. This parasitic fungus *Claviceps purpurea*, which attacks grains, rye in particular, contains numerous alkaloids, and lysergic acid diethylamide (LSD) can by synthesized from it. The *Report on LSD*, prepared by the CIA's Office of Scientific Intelligence and dated August 30, 1955, stated that ergot, abundant in nature, has a commercial value in Bulgaria, Czechoslovakia, the German Democratic Republic, Hungary, and Romania. The authors were convinced that the communists had begun to systematically collect large stocks of ergot. According to the report, radio stations in Poland and other countries of the Eastern Bloc were urging people to gather it and deliver to local purchasing centers.[2] The Americans had no doubts as to the purpose of these actions: the communists wanted to produce mass amounts of LSD for chemical warfare purposes. Soviet attempts to use pharmacological substances were also known.

In July 1951 the CIA captured two Soviet agents in West Germany, who were in possession of plastic cylinders containing a gray liquid and needles. The interrogated Russians confessed that the substance was a strong narcotic capable of depriving a person of free will and allowing one to take control of them. The drugged individual was to fulfill all orders given, regardless of the consequences. No laboratory in the United States was able to identify the contents of those vials.[3]

The real scare erupted in 1955 when an alleged English translation of a confidential speech given by KGB leader Lavrentiy Beria was disclosed to public knowledge. In a brochure entitled "Brainwashing: A Synthesis of the Communist Textbook on Psychopolitics," Beria discussed the plan for employing new weapons, specifically, drastic methods of interrogation using narcotics, hypnosis, and torture, thanks to which all the information that one wanted to obtain from someone would be possible. In Beria's opinion, "there will never be an atomic war, for Russia will have subjected all of her enemies."[4] The Americans had a large problem with this publication, as none of the intelligence community authorities was able to ascertain whether the document was falsified. One of the members of the National Security Agency commented: "If the booklet is a fake, the author or authors know so much about brainwashing techniques that I would consider them experts, superior to any that I have met to date."[5]

In 1959 the Soviet agents tried to poison the staff of Radio Free Europe in Munich, filling the salt shakers in the cafeteria with atropine.[6] The need for the immediate development of research on psychochemical agents was created both in military and intelligence agencies in the United States. In line with the Cold War arms race logic, the Americans could not remain behind the Soviets. The condition for making up for the alleged delay was the initiation and development of an extensive range of research, which would, however, require experiments to be carried out on human subjects.

Early American Military Experiments with Psychoactive Substances on Humans

[A]n experiment is never as uncertain as in the space of war, for here fate has a greater impact on life than anywhere else, resulting in each step having a decisive meaning which it is impossible to negate.
    —Ernst Jünger, "War and Technology"

Historically, experiments carried out on people, despite the fact that they are immeasurably controversial and in many cases at least ethically doubtful, were often necessary for the advancement of medicine, especially military medicine. During the First World War countries and their armies, for the first time on a large scale, had to deal with the problem of testing on humans substances that could prevent illnesses and injuries or treat them. The use of chemical weapons on the battlefield, albeit in contradiction to the Hague Conventions (1899, 1907), may have proven to be a way of taking the strategy from the impasse of trench warfare back to maneuver warfare. These hopes, however, did not come to fruition. The war gases not only did not become weapons allowing for victory to be achieved, but they also drastically contributed to the brutalization of war. Thus began the search for antidotes, which would allow the gassed soldiers to be saved. Gas masks and decontamination stations were insufficient, particularly after the Germans used mustard gas for the first time in July 1917, for it inflicted a much greater number of casualties than the "conventional" gases deployed earlier (such as hydrochloric acid and phosgene), causing severe skin and lung burs. Even a small dose of this poison produced oozing blisters and temporary blindness. Mustard gas stuck close to the ground for many days, sometimes even weeks. The scale of the use of chemical weapons increased along with the introduction of more lethal combat gases and new means for their delivery. From 1915 to 1916 the amount doubled, while from 1916 to 1918 it quadrupled.[7] As Martin van Creveld writes, "[O]nly 3 percent of all fatalities were caused by gas; yet the number of shells that were filled with it rose from just 1 percent in 1916 to as high as 30 percent in 1918."[8] The gases were useful for one main reason: when they settled near the ground, they "smoked" the soldiers from the trenches, thereby turning them into easy attack targets for conventional weapons. Chemical warfare, therefore, had but an indirect destruction capability. In total, over 1.14 million soldiers fell victim to chemical attacks, from which 90,000–100,000 were fatal casualties.[9]

The unsettling phenomenon of the growing use of poisonous gases on the battlefield made the U.S. Department of War seriously consider undertaking preparations for gas warfare. Thus in November 1917 a new military base was created in Aberdeen, Maryland, forty miles northeast of Baltimore: Edgewood Arsenal; its task was manufacturing shells filled with combat gases.[10] In the following year, the Chemical Warfare Service (CWS), which oversaw research on chemical weapons with the possibility of developing American offensive capabilities, was founded. Urgent action was badly needed, for if the war had lasted longer, the scale of the use of deadly gases would have significantly increased. This was, indeed, assumed by the British plan of action for 1919. Most probably also lewisite (dew of death)—a poisonous American-produced chemical weapon causing burning pain—would have been used. The initial experiments with the participation of soldiers, which were aimed to improve the defense methods against chemical weapons, were often accompanied by deadly accidents. One of the participants, an army electrician George Temple, perhaps did not make it up when recalling that "[m]ore men were killed by gas on the experimental side than in actual use" in the battlefield.[11] Following the end of the war, the CWS, being a temporary entity appointed for the needs of military operations in Europe, was restructured into a permanent bureau of the War Department.[12] It was, however, only in the aftermath of the Second World War when it was changed to the Army Chemical Corps and its true development began.

For decades venereal diseases were the real problem affecting combat efficiency. During the Second World War in North Africa more soldiers suffered from these than from injuries sustained on the battlefield. It was therefore no surprise that at the beginning of the 1940s, John Pershing, famed commander of the American Expeditionary Forces during the First World War, deemed that the fight against sexually transmitted diseases among American soldiers was of great significance, not just for health and moral reasons but, more importantly, for military reasons.[13] It was during the battle against venereal diseases conducted during the Second World War that the first effective method of treating syphilis via penicillin, the oldest antibiotic discovered in 1928 by Alexander Fleming, was developed in 1943.[14] The person who took an active part in the fight against sexually transmitted infections was Joseph Earle Moore, an outstanding venereologist from Johns Hopkins University who was granted the Medal of Merit for his services on this often forgotten and underappreciated front of the Second World War. In 1942, as the chairman of the Subcommittee for Venereal Diseases of the National Research Council, he received a letter from Charles Carpenter, a researcher from the University of Rochester, who in his study of "the chemical prophylaxis of gonorrhea" wanted to conduct experiments on humans. He asked Moore for his opinion, that is, whether this was recommended. Moore relayed Carpenter's doubts to the Committee on Medical Research (CMR). The committee, which was a body of the Office of Scientific Research and Development (appointed in 1941 for the duration of the war as an institution supporting medical research for military purposes), presented its stance on the matter relatively quickly:

> Human experimentation is not only desirable, but necessary in the study of many of the problems of war medicine which confront us. When any risks are involved, volunteers only should be utilized as subjects, and these only after the risks have been fully explained, and after signed statements have been obtained which shall prove that the volunteer offered his services with full knowledge and that claims

for damage will be waived. An accurate record should be kept of the
terms in which the risks involved were described.[15]

This opinion expressed the government's approach to medical tests conducted
on people: they were admissible under the condition that only well-informed
volunteers, who consciously expressed in writing their consent to participate,
would take part in them. In this manner the committee, and thus the administration, explicitly gave the green light for state experiments on humans.

In 1942, secretary of war Henry L. Stimson issued formal consent for
the recruitment of volunteers from among soldiers to participate in experiments with the use of chemical substances.[16] In the report published in 1993,
the National Academy of Sciences estimated that during the Second World
War experiments were conducted with the participation of 60,000 American
soldiers, from which mustard gas and lewisite were used on at least 4,000 of
them.[17]

Apart from research on combating sexually transmitted infections with the
help of penicillin and experiments with poisonous gases, an equally burning
issue, especially toward the end of the war, was efforts aimed at obtaining an
effective medication to treat malaria. Americans were aware that if they wanted
to force Japan into an unconditional surrender, then they would have to launch
a huge and costly invasion of the Japanese islands, during which they would
have to deal not only with a fanatical opponent but also with another unconditional and initially invisible enemy: a dangerous, chronic, tropical contagious
disease.[18] For this reason, the effectiveness of new antimalaria medications
was tested both on soldiers, civilian hospital patients, and prisoners.

Strong suspicions exist whether the American soldiers who participated
in the experiments during the Second World War were true volunteers or
they were rather merely executing orders or fulfilling their superiors' expectations. What were the consequences for refusing to participate in the experiments? Would this have been deemed insubordination? As it later turned
out, despite the recommendations expressed by the CMR, in many cases the
subjects were not adequately informed of the nature of the experiment or of
the substances' properties that were tested on them or of the risks to their
health and life. The authorities justified not disclosing full information on
the tests by citing requirements of national security. The research was subject to the "top-secret" clause, and the participants committed themselves to
remain silent and maintain confidentiality. After the end of the war, along
with the onset of the Cold War and in the face of the demonic, communist
enemy, the army felt badly in need of conducting more diversified experiments on humans.

Edgewood Arsenal: The Army's "Alchemical" Factory of Psychochemical Dreams

LSD can produce a temporary state of severe imbalance, hysteria, and insanity. It requires little imagination to realize what the consequences might be if a battleship's crew were so affected.
—Dr. H. K. Beecher quoted in Hank P. Albarelli Jr.,
*A Terrible Mistake: The Murder of Frank Olson
and the CIA's Secret Cold War Experiments*

Since the mid-1950s the Army Chemical Corps conducted experiments mainly at Edgewood Arsenal, testing mostly war gases, both aimed at offensive and defensive purposes. The scope changed and significantly expanded soon after a secret message was received in 1948 from Dr. John Clay, a high-ranking consultant in the chemical department of the U.S. European Command in Heidelberg, Germany. Clay informed on the existence of a new, very potent hallucinogenic substance called LSD-25, synthesized for the first time in 1938 by Albert Hofmann from Sandoz, a Swiss pharmaceutical company.[19] Sandoz was then testing a stimulant which would be helpful during childbirth, and Hofmann deemed that LSD was not what he was looking for, so he stopped working on it. He returned to the compound in 1943 and completely by accident discovered its potent hallucinogenic effects.[20] LSD has properties that are similar to mescaline (the alkaloid that is present, among others, in peyote), with the difference being that it is five to ten thousand times stronger. Thus it sparked a genuine interest in the armed forces, becoming one of the main substances tested at Edgewood.

Despite the fact that the army's experiments raised and continue to raise controversies, they were usually carried out in accordance with the accepted rules of safety, although, of course, there were exceptions to this rule. The basic problem concerned the army's violation of its internal procedures. In 1953 the army secretary issued guidance entitled *Use of Volunteers in Research* ("Army Chief of Staff Memorandum 385") that assumed the possibility of conducting experiments on volunteers upon obtaining the approval of the secretary of the army. The first program for testing LSD on volunteers was launched in 1955. Although it was presented to the secretary of the army on April 26, 1956, he did not issue any written approval for its implementation. Instead the scheme was based on the consent of the chief of army staff.[21]

The problem of the lack of volunteers on which the military medical experiments were to be conducted was solved in 1955 by deciding to use the soldiers stationed at the Edgewood Arsenal base. The Chemical Corps created a recruitment procedure for this purpose, in accordance with which the voluntary consent of all participants to undergo experiments was required. Each person was to be notified of the actions taken during the tests and the nature and effects of the substances to be used. This is, at least, how the procedures were to formally look, because in reality the manner of conducting experiments was at times quite different from the established model. As Dr. Gerald Klee, one of the psychiatrists working in the army's experimental programs, said about the volunteers, "Most of them were not highly educated, and even if they had been told exactly what they were to be given, they wouldn't have understood it."[22] It was most often assumed that the requirement of informing the persons participating in the experiment as to what substance they were to receive was not of great significance. Why disclose confidential information when the soldiers did not possess sufficient pharmacological knowledge?

In 2006 James Ketchum, a psychiatrist with an impressive career who played an important role in the research on psychoactive substances at Edgewood Arsenal, published his memoirs. Ketchum was recruited in 1955 at the age of twenty-nine. He was the first, and until 1963, the only psychiatrist who was appointed to the medical laboratories at Edgewood. Being a professional of the highest level, he always placed great emphasis on procedures and safety regulations. When reading Ketchum one needs, of course, to remember not only that he is fully aware of what he is writing about, as he was the creator and executor of the program, but also that he wrote his memoires over forty years after acceding to the project, and in such cases it is difficult to expect both full objectivity and stark self-criticism. Ketchum himself points out that he is presenting "a personal perspective on the clinical study of incapacitating agents investigated in the 1960s."[23]

According to his accounts, before selected volunteers were allowed to participate in the tests, they underwent a detailed interview. Most often, those who explained their willingness to participate in an experiment in terms of fulfilling their patriotic duty or the desire to try secret medications were rejected on the spot. The volunteers completed a psychological test (Minnesota Multiphase Personality Inventory) aimed at revealing any mental problems or unstable personalities. They then underwent medical screening. Persons who were qualified were divided into two categories: those who would be given small doses of the tested substances and those who would receive larger amounts. Before signing the consent, the doctors generally informed the soldiers about the effects of the substances they were to receive and the aims of the experiment.[24] Ketchum emphasizes that the volunteers could not learn everything as the doctors themselves were not fully aware of the scale and effects of the investigated agents—because the experiments were being conducted to learn precisely that. If all of this was already known, the testing would not have been needed. Ketchum responds convincingly to the charge that the volunteers were not informed in detail which substances would be tested on them. Most of the compounds simply did not have names, while the labels of the remaining ones meant nothing to the average person. Would informing soldiers that "1-methyl-4-piperidinyl" would be tested on them change anything apart from perhaps causing light terror through its mysterious name? The army designated a code for each of the intoxicating agents, for example LSD was "EA 1729," BZ (an extremely strong hallucinogen) was "EA 2277," and MDMA (now commonly known as ecstasy) was referred to as "EA 1475." There were also brand new drugs, introduced into the program, indicated solely by the use of a code, for example "EA 3443," having an almost identical time frame of duration as BZ but causing significantly stronger symptoms.[25] The volunteers were not fully informed, not only because of national security reasons but also because such knowledge would mean nothing whatsoever to them. After an almost two-month-long stay at the base, all the participants underwent additional medical testing, which was to provide certainty whether they returned to their normal psychophysical status. Taking all of this into consideration, Ketchum decidedly refutes the charges that those soldiers participating in the experiments were "guinea pigs." He argues, "If these were 'guinea pigs' or (as some writers have referred to them), 'unwitting guinea pigs,' one would have to assume that American soldiers in those days lacked basic intelligence."[26] What is more, many volunteers reported their participation in the studies several times, while after the first of them they had to be aware of what the experiments entailed.

Critics, however, cite examples that undermine the thesis that all the participants were well informed and conscious of the nature of the research in which they were participating. In February 1958, Army master sergeant James B. Stanley volunteered for the experiments on new agents aimed at combating the effects of the use of chemical weapons. As he claims, he knew nothing of the fact that he was given psychoactive substances, mainly LSD. At the end of the experiment he neither underwent any observation to identify possible long-term negative effects of the tested compounds nor provided with medical care. Meanwhile, Stanley was experiencing strong hallucinogenic states and serious emotional problems, which had a destructive impact on his private life, ultimately leading to his divorce in 1970.[27] Another example is Sergeant Wendell Queen, who participated in the experiments at Edgewood as a volunteer in 1964. When information on the topic of the research projects were publicized in the mid-1970s, Queen decided to find out what substances were tested on him. His surprise was huge when army representatives informed him that no documents confirming his participation in any experiments existed. Queen, however, all too well remembered how a secret intoxicant was administered to him: "They just took a small drop and put it on my arm, and my arm became inflamed and kinda itchy, something like a bad mosquito bite." Several hours after getting the drop, he felt intoxicated. "I had lost all my senses. I had no sense of balance or sense of the environment around me. . . . Later on that night I really got paranoid and if anybody would come close to me I would think that they were going to kill me."[28]

Overall, the truth lies somewhere in the middle—between the stark charges of the critics, deeming the army's experiments as being unethical tests on human "guinea pigs," and Ketchum's narrative, from which an image of professionally conducted research with the maintenance of rules, procedures, rights, and the dignity of the participants ensues. Thousands of soldiers encouraged by the vision of better service, free three-day weekends, symbolic financial compensation of one dollar and fifty cents a day, higher standard barracks, and comprehensive medical tests reported to participate.[29] For some, changing the location in which they were stationed was an opportunity to be housed closer to home. During the two decades of the program's functioning there was no lack of volunteers to participate in the experiments. On the contrary, more soldiers than were actually needed offered themselves since military experiments were moved to Edgewood in the mid-1950s. From the report of the army inspector general prepared in 1975, it follows that overall seven thousand soldiers took part in the experiments conducted in Edgewood Arsenal, most of them between 1961 and 1970. This was an entire army of volunteers, or as the critics say, "guinea pigs" whose "slight" sacrifice not on the battlefield but in the science field could have, it was believed, tipped the scales of the Cold War confrontation in the United States' favor.

The pharmacological substances were additionally tested in other army bases and on over a thousand civilians. The army contracted the research with universities, hospitals, and penitentiaries. An army inspector general reported: "In some of the tests and experiments, healthy adults, psychiatric patients, and prison inmates were used without their knowledge or consent or their full knowledge of the risks involved."[30] Within the course of twenty years the army signed forty-eight external agreements, twenty-nine of them were concluded with twelve universities, among others, in Indiana, Utah, and Washington; and also with Baylor University, the University of Pennsylvania, Tulane University, and Johns Hopkins University. The largest contract, the value of which was estimated at almost 327,000 dollars, was concluded by the University of Pennsylvania in March of 1964.[31] The university signed a total of six agreements, within the framework of which experiments were carried out on inmates held at the Holmesburg prison in Philadelphia for ten years. According to one of the reports, within twelve months from March 1965 experiments commissioned by the army were conducted there on 148 persons.[32] In fact, 75 percent of the medications marketed for sale in the United States were previously tested in penitentiaries until 1974.[33] At Holmesburg, various types of allergological and dermatological experiments were conducted on humans. These tests were initiated and executed by Albert Kligman, dean of the faculty of dermatology at the University of Pennsylvania, who discovered the famous Retin-A anti-acne medication. The fame and money that the discovery brought him would not have existed had it not been for the experiments performed on the prisoners. Kligman's actions raised a lot of controversy, and years later he was charged with unprofessional conduct, lack of ensuring specialized scientific and medical supervision, transgressions in regard to safety during the experiments, abuses, lack of full medication records, and even their falsifications. This resulted in Kligman being deleted from the list of investigators approved by the Food and Drug Administration. The Chemical Corps, specifically James Ketchum, repeatedly but to no avail asked Kligman to hire a psychopharmacist to assist with the research work on the psychoactive substances. Despite this, the army continued its subcontracted experiments.

At Holmesburg there was never a lack of volunteers willing to risk their physical and mental health, ready to have the strongest chemical substances, which were in the possession of the American armed forces (including, for example, dioxin, one of the most toxic synthetic compounds) injected into them. This was, in fact, not a bad form of income for the inmates. They received between thirty and fifty dollars for allergy tests and biopsies, while the rates for experiments commissioned by the army reached as much as seven to eight hundred dollars. Prisoners participating in such research wore special plates which read: "Please excuse this inmate's behavior. He can't think or act in a coherent manner and is part of the U.S. Army testing program."[34] EA 3167 was among the substances that the army was specifically interested in and that was researched at Holmesburg. In a confidential report Ketchum affirmed that "EA 3167 is a highly potent, extremely long-lasting" agent.[35] It left people delirious for even up to two weeks. Participation in the tests did not remain without an impact on one's health. Many years after the experiments their effects were, among others, tumors and lung diseases. In 1984 a group of former prisoners sued the University of Pennsylvania and the city of Philadelphia. By virtue of the final agreement, they were paid a sum of between 20,000 to 40,000 dollars compensation. The prison in Holmesburg was shut down in 1995.[36]

What were all of these secret, often morally doubtful experiments aimed to serve? One can observe two of the army's basic motives. First, they were searching for an agent that could be used as a nonlethal weapon. Second, they were dreaming of discovering a compound that would facilitate obtaining information from an interrogatee despite their will to resist. The substance could also be helpful in testing the effectiveness of training soldiers in the event of being held captive and thwarting attempts at extracting confidential information from them under the influence of torture or sophisticated interrogation techniques, including the use of narcotic drugs. In this way, the military was trying to avoid a repeat of the disgraceful Korean POW episode. Both of the aims were of a clear "offensive" nature, each of them, however, also had its "defensive" extent, for finding antidotes to adverse chemical substances could significantly strengthen American defense capabilities. During the Cold War the threat of chemical warfare was not only real but also relatively high, given the steady development of the Soviet chemical weapons arsenal. Americans were also very apprehensive, as we know, of the use of psychotropic substances by the communists for the purpose of "breeding" an army composed of "Manchurian candidates." So, let us now take a closer look at these two aims.

The Hallucinogenic Arsenal of the "Anchor of Democracy": In Search of Nonlethal Psychochemical Weapons

> Generally in war the best policy is to take a state intact; to ruin it is inferior to this. To capture the enemy's army is better than to destroy it; to take intact a battalion, a company or a five-man squad is better than to destroy them.
>
> —Sun Tzu, *The Art of War*

Despite the fact that the Geneva Protocol of 1925 prohibited the use of chemical weapons in armed conflict, during the Cold War both the United States and the Soviet Union were developing their arsenals with fervor. The United States collected over 30,000 metric tons of various military chemical substances and the Soviet Union some 40,000 tons.[37] At the same time the goal of the American armed forces was to find such agents that would not kill or result in permanent physical injury but incapacitate. In other words, they were working on obtaining a means of temporarily paralyzing the enemy's soldiers. After the end of the Second World War, the Americans relatively quickly began their search of substances, which dispersed on the adversary's forces, added to their food, dissolved in water, or delivered in any other effective form, would transform them into a group of undisciplined units devoid of their elementary fighting abilities and unable to offer resistance. The enemy would thereby be more easily defeated without the need to use traditional, lethal means of combat. Thus the army unwittingly tried to carry out a prediction made by the American writer Don DeLillo in his novel *End Zone* (1972), in which one of the characters says: "I think what'll happen in the not-too-distant future is that we will have humane wars," because "Nagasaki was an embarrassment to the art of war."[38] Along with the onset of nuclear weapons, as Alvin and Heidi Toffler noted at the beginning of the 1990s, "the maximization of lethality has reached its outer limits"; military history has got to "the point of dialectical negation."[39] Hence it began to reverse itself and started going in the direction of minimizing the deadliness of war.

The search for chemical substances, which would not kill but would weaken the combat abilities of the opponent and help tip the scales of victory, was not, by any means, an original creation of the nuclear era. It was said that 2,500 years ago, the Chaldeans were to have set high heaps of Indian cannabis and a huge, thick smoke cloud was formed, which aimed to strip the opponents of their spirits and fighting power. The effectiveness of such a method was most probably limited, as the smoke would have also weakened the Chaldeans' defensive capabilities.[40] The Americans wanted to obtain much more powerful, efficient, and reliable means to immobilize the enemy's units with the use of hallucinogenic compounds. Ephraim Goodman from Edgewood Arsenal conducted literary research on the history of using atropine and its derivatives. He summed up his results in a report from 1962, describing documented accounts of the inadvertent consumption of fruits and vegetables containing atropine, which in each case caused stupefaction, disorientation, and delirium. This happened to the colonial units in Virginia in 1667, and it took the soldiers over a week to recover.[41] Atropine was, however, also used purposefully and consciously as a weapon that was to help defeat the enemy without combat. Around 200 BC Maharbal, Carthaginian military commander and one of Hannibal's lieutenants, knowing that an African tribe, which revolted against the Carthaginians, loved to drink wine, mixed it with mandrake (a perennial containing atropine) and left in the abandoned camp. The Africans, not suspecting anything, drank all the poisoned wine. When Maharbal returned, he found the enemies totally unable to show any resistance as they were felled with strong intoxication and hallucinogenic psychosis. He took some of them as prisoners and killed the rest.[42] In 36 BC, during the campaign against the Parthians in Asia Minor, the Roman soldiers under Mark Anthony were severely affected after eating "one plant that killed them after driving them mad."[43] On the basis of the described symptoms, the toxicologists assumed that this may have been the atropine-containing Jimson weed (devil's snare or *Datura inoxia*). Moving to more contemporary times, in 1881 a French unit traveling through the desert from Sudan to Algeria was poisoned with atropine by warriors from the Touareg people, with the soldiers becoming overpowered by hallucinogenic delirium.[44] The conclusion that followed from Goodman's report was that some psychoactive substances could be used to undermine the enemy's fighting power by causing disorientation, panic, irrational actions, and, first and foremost, an inability to show resistance.

For some time, the Americans did not only test atropine but also the so-called red oil (EA 1476), that is, a highly concentrated cannabis extract. Its effects, however, were too weak for military purposes.[45] Paradoxically, while marijuana had been one of the main controlled substances in the United States under the Marijuana Tax Act of 1937, synthetic "weed" was tested as a potential instrument of war in the government's laboratory. Parallel to combating marijuana at home, the United States also considered its use on the battlefield as an intoxicating, nonlethal weapon. The history of drugs and warfare often abounded in such ironic cases.

In 1947 in his letter to the Chemical Corps Technical Command Dr. Alsoph H. Corwin, a professor of chemistry at Johns Hopkins University, argued that it was worth considering the use of psychochemical substances for the purpose of causing "mass hallucinations and uncontrolled hysteria by intoxication."[46] He therefore recommended searching for and testing suitable agents. The letter reached a very receptive audience as it found its way to the desk of L. Wilson Greene, the technical director of the Chemical and Radiological Laboratories at Edgewood Arsenal. In just several weeks Greene took action. After examining a vast amount of Nazi files and documents he prepared a list of close to 1,000 chemical substances that were known to cause mental disturbances in people.[47] Inspired by the idea of a "bloodless war," in 1949 Greene drafted a report entitled *Psychochemical Warfare: A New Concept of War*, in which he urged the United States to elaborate and develop a doctrine for a new kind of warfare. He speculated that if the soldiers or civilians of the enemy were exposed to the effects of incapacitating means, to which he included sixty-one substances, then they would inevitably suffer from attacks of hysteria, hallucinations, and panic. As a result, Greene concluded, "There can be no doubt that their will to resist would be weakened greatly, if not entirely destroyed."[48] Victory would become possible without unnecessary casualties and material damage. War would revolutionarily change its face. Waged on a hallucinogenic battlefield, it would become much "more humane."

The vision of creating such an incapacitating psychochemical weapon also fascinated the head of the Army Chemical Corps, Major General William Creasy, an unusually eccentric and determined man. With the fervor of a great visionary, he tried to convince his superiors and politicians to build weapons that would not kill but would still be uniquely effective. These arms were to enable the conducting of bloodless wars; in other words, they would allow for winning with no or minimal causalities on both sides. What Creasy sought was to downplay the reputation of chemicals as cruel and odious weapons of mass destruction. As perverse as this may sound, in certain situations their use would be the more humane option. It was not without reason that some of the observers during the First World War proclaimed chemical weapons as much more humane than conventional ones. Whereas the mortality rate from war gases remained at an unusually low level and amounted to 3 percent of the total number of casualties, in the case of conventional weapons it reached 25 percent.[49] In the context of the Second World War, Creasy referred to a different argument, citing the example of the battle of Iwo Jima. The Americans seized the island, defended by 21,000 Japanese troops, at the cost of unusually large casualties. At that time the army already had chemical weapons at its disposal. Should they be used, the fight would prove less bloody for the Americans. Such actions were, however, deemed as overly inhumane and very un-American. Despite the fact that the United States did not ratify the Geneva Protocol, President Franklin Delano Roosevelt accepted the policy of possessing "abject" chemical weapons in the arsenal but refrained from being the first to use them. Meanwhile, Creasy argued, moving away from the no-first-use doctrine and the deployment of chemical weapons in the war in the Pacific would save the lives of many combatants. But the American authorities had objections of a moral nature, as they did not want to treat the Japanese in the same manner in which they treated their enemies: cruelly and ruthlessly. Creasy then further developed his argument:

> Let's observe what the result of the entire humanitarian fervor was: 7,000 dead marines, 18,000 injured. And what happened to the 21,000 Japanese soldiers? Most of them died anyway due to the white phosphorus [material used in incendiary bullets] as well as from flammenwerfers [flame throwers].[50]

Paradoxically, however, when President Harry Truman finally justified the decision to use the atomic bomb on Japan, he made references to the "humanitarian" argument, notably quickly ending the war, limiting the number of its further casualties, and avoiding the need to invade the Japanese islands, which would have resulted in hundreds of thousands American deaths. According to an exaggerated prediction by the secretary of war, Henry L. Stimson, the bombs on Hiroshima and Nagasaki would save the lives of 500,000 Americans.[51] In the Cold War era, the use of chemical weapons, even on a mass scale, would certainly bring less tragic effects than the use of nuclear weapons, even on a limited scale, whatever that was supposed to mean. Would psychochemical weapons therefore not be a less bloody alternative? In light of atomic annihilation, would this not be a humanitarian weapon, bringing barely minimal and reversible immobilization and incapacitation of the enemy?

In June 1955, the Chemical Corps commissioned its Technical Advisory Panel on Biological and Chemical Warfare to prepare a report on potential military applications of psychoactive substances. A six-person working group supervised by Harold Wolff, a neurologist from Cornell University, was appointed. Wolff's committee decisively recommended conducting research on a hundred of these types of compounds, and particularly the testing of the combat capabilities of trained soldier and volunteer units in the field before and after receiving 150 micrograms of LSD. As a result of these suggestions, in February 1965 a program under the leadership of Van Sim was initiated. Three months later, following the decision of Secretary of Defense Erwin Wilson, the Chemical Corps obtained approval for running experiments with hallucinogens on volunteer soldiers.[52]

In May 1955, hence before the Wolff Committee was appointed, Creasy decided to reach a wider circle with his vision of "war without casualties" and was quite willing to grant interviews to the media. While traveling the country, he also gave a series of open lectures. In a conversation with *This Week* magazine, for example, he confessed:

> I do not contend that driving people crazy—even for a few hours—is a pleasant prospect. But warfare is never pleasant. And to those who feel that any kind of chemical weapon is more horrible than conventional weapons, I put this question: Would you rather be temporarily deranged, blinded, or paralyzed by a chemical agent, or burned alive by a conventional fire bomb?[53]

Was this not a rhetorical question? The vision of a cloud of incapacitating agents, specifically LSD, which dispersed over the enemy's forces would paralyze even the best trained and disciplined units without killing or injuring them, seemed very attractive. Creasy tried to popularize his ideas. In September 1959 he published an article in *Reader's Digest* entitled "Can We Have War without Death?"[54] Apart from firmness, determination, and faith, he had a great talent for convincing people, which he used to his advantage when he sought to sell his vision to the politicians. His contribution was that the congressmen unanimously agreed to the proposal of tripling the Chemical Corps' budget, which was to allow testing of incapacitating substances and running experiments on volunteers. When asked whether he was going to incapacitate congressmen as he did soldiers, he wittingly responded that he had not seen a need to do so thus far.[55]

Ultimately, however, Creasy became very disappointed. When he wanted to expand the research testing on psychedelics by going beyond the army bases, he was met with strong opposition. His argument on the need to move to a new stage in the process that was to give the United States the ability to wage a "war without casualties" was not accepted. Creasy proposed the implementation of tests with hallucinogenic gases in the subway systems of America's largest cities. Such experiments, he argued, would allow the possibilities of conducting a real psychochemical war to be verified. Highly dissatisfied, he complained with bitterness: "It was denied on reasons that always seemed a little absurd to me."[56] But it was Creasy's ideas that were too absurd and risky for his supervisors.

In 1961, chief of the Army Chemical Corps, Major General Marshall Stubbs, in his speech before the Subcommittee on Science and Astronautics of the House of Representatives spoke directly and rather convincingly, although somehow futurologically, on humanizing war through the use of compelling, psychochemical weapons:

> We are attempting to completely separate the incapacitating agents from the lethal agents so that any castigation normally given to toxic agents will not be associated with them, since they do not maim or kill. As a result we hope to have a weapon which will give the commander much freer rein in its use as compared to the toxic agents. It is my hope that through the use of incapacitating agents, the free world will have a relatively clear and rapid means of both fighting and deterring limited war, which has come to the forefront in the international political scene in the last several years. It is one means by which we can maintain some degree of equality in the face of overwhelming manpower superiority of the Communist-dominated nations.[57]

The use of deadly weapons, specifically weapons of mass destruction, in a limited war would automatically mean there would be a serious threat of escalating violence to a higher level. This was not in the interest of the parties in the Cold War, who had to calculate their operational, tactical, and strategic plans in the shadow of the threat of nuclear armageddon. After 1945 the superpowers appreciated security, and their very survival required the "renouncing" of a total war. This did not mean the end of conventional wars, however. On the contrary, in the shadow of the threat of nuclear annihilation relatively "safe" limited proxy wars were conducted, during which the politicians of both blocs did not allow their militaries to use all available means to achieve their strategic objectives. This refusal has been a fundamental condition for the survival of humankind. In many cases, this became the reason for either a tactical "tie," not achieving a full strategic victory or suffering a defeat; a good example of which were the wars in Korea and Vietnam. Limited wars, therefore, use limited military means, although this certainly is not their only fundamental trait. Since the deployment of the full spectrum of weapons (of mass destruction) was excluded in principle (or forbidden), the armed forces began searching for new methods of conducting limited wars, and psychochemical arms seemed to be an unusually attractive option to be explored and developed.

In his report of 1970 on combat tactics in the urban area entitled *Nonlethal and Nondestructive Combat in Cities Overseas,* Joseph Coates from the Institute for Defense Analyses in Washington presented the first all-encompassing methodological and explanatory approach to the issue of nonlethal weapons.[58] He noticed the overwhelming need to minimize damages and casualties during combat in urban areas, in which the United States, as he accurately argued, was to be more and more inevitably involved. In the course of fighting in the city, a large number of civilians are present, and their lives and health are threatened by the use of conventional armaments. Thus, "As the number of noncombatants increases, both relatively and absolutely, the requirements for less deadly techniques go up."[59] Coates discussed different types of nonlethal weapons due to their operating mechanisms and the possibility of using them during various types of missions. From among all the analyzed categories of less lethal measures, the chemical agents had, according to him, the greatest value, especially during operations carried out in populated and built-on areas. For intoxicants'

> mental effects such as disorientation, confusion, and hallucinations by no means exhaust the range of potentially militarily interesting mental derangements. Other effects of some potential value would be induced susceptibility to fear, amnesia, dyschiria (confusion of touch), indecisiveness, heightened suggestibility, or dyskinesia.[60]

Hence, what does the essence of nonlethal chemical weapons entail, and what would its use look like? Let us imagine the following scenario. A saboteur on the enemy's territory facilitates the contamination of its water and food. At the same time, the army disperses gas into the air, which permeates into the body through the respiratory system and skin. The army assumed that if an operation of this type was to succeed in a city, the enemy would have to be totally paralyzed and thus conquered without the need of intense fighting involving heavy bombings and gunfire. What is interesting is that the ideas of Greene, Creasy, Stubbs, Coates, and other military leaders forcing the concept of a psychochemical warfare brought Americans remarkably close to Sun Tzu's unorthodox thinking on war and his famous maxim that "to win one hundred victories in one hundred battles is not the acme of skill. To subdue the enemy without fighting is the acme of skill."[61] So, thanks to the "hallucinogenic water" and the "deranging gas," one could avoid a siege, which would undoubtedly bring numerous casualties. The armies would simply enter the cities with minimal resistance. The following day, or after several days, when the residents returned to their normal psychophysical state, they would already be under occupation.[62] The local economy would also not suffer, as no significant material damages would occur. Such a war would be a peculiar "economic blessing." Let us further assume that great museums and galleries, gathering valuable collections of world famous pieces of art were located in the city. The use of traditional methods of conquering urban areas would mean the threat of cultural barbarism, a kind of "artiscide." Nonlethal weapons would allow this to be avoided. This was the notable humanitarian thinking: the art of war needed to be transformed to protect true works of art. What Europe experienced during the Second World War—as for example, when 434 outstanding works of art including paintings by Caravaggio, Titian, and Veronese were destroyed as a result of a single air strike on Berlin—seemed no longer acceptable.[63] Thanks to the new psychochemical weapons, the great cultural inheritance of humanity could therefore be saved. What was surrealistic in this form of argumentation was the fact that it was being developed in the nuclear age, in which the use of atomic weapons would mean the threat of total annihilation of not only works of art but also of their creators. Such a threat was most clear, particularly a year after Stubbs's address to the House of Representatives, during the Cuban Missile Crisis in October of 1962.

Of course, all these were fantastic scenarios along the lines of "science fiction," perhaps even "warfare fiction," more the dreams of the army rather than real tactical plans. Conducting such a campaign even in modern times would have been unusually difficult, if at all possible, due to logistical reasons. If such an operation were to bring the desired effect, then the psychoactive agent should attack and affect the largest number of residents. The contaminated water would require a large concentration, which would be beyond reach in the case of a developed municipal water works system. James Ketchum, someone who knows exactly what he is talking about, does not leave any illusions:

> The assertion that one could affect a city with "an easily portable" quantity of LSD dumped into its water supply is outrageously inaccurate. Powerful as it is, tons of LSD would be required to create an effective concentration in the huge volume of a major city's reservoir. In the presence of sunlight and chlorination, it is doubtful that residual LSD would have any perceptible effect by the time it reached consumer faucets. The amount of chlorine in a glass of ordinary tap water is sufficient to rapidly deactivate a full dose of LSD.[64]

Some people did not give up. For example, Henry K. Beecher, an anesthesiologist and CIA and army consultant, strongly suggested taking seriously the possibility of contaminating municipal water reservoirs or at least the reservoirs located on the enemy's army bases or water supplies on warships.[65] Until 1963 experiments with LSD were carried out by administering it orally, but the army was interested, first and foremost, in preparing effective methods of its dispersal, so as to throw the "acid rain" down on the enemy's units, its cities, and civilian population. Yet it quickly turned out that LSD in gaseous form was three times weaker than when administered orally, which hampered even more the precise indication of the minimum incapacitating dosage. Dispersal could have a limited effect also due to the fact that residents of cities spend most of their time in closed premises. Finally, the difference in the concentration of hallucinogens can have various effects on individual people, often causing serious mental disorders. What is more, it is known that the nature of hallucinations and illusions caused, for example, by LSD largely depends on the current emotional status of the person subject to the effects of the drug. To simplify, LSD may strengthen the feeling of either euphoria or depression. It would therefore be difficult to precisely foresee people's reactions and behaviors. An additional problem was how to secure one's own soldiers against exposure to the effects of nonlethal chemical attack. Let us imagine a situation in which a city paralyzed by psychochemical arms could not be taken over by the American unit because it also was incapacitated by a random gust of hallucinogenic wind. Such a threat, which was precisely one of the fundamental reasons for the low effectiveness of war gases during the First World War, is attested to by the incident that took place in 1968 during the experiment at Dugway Proving Grounds in Utah. When VX, a nerve agent and one of the strongest war gases, was sprayed from an airplane, an unexpected gust of wind caused the toxic cloud to drift in a different direction than the one planned. This did not, albeit, cause any casualties among humans, nevertheless many sheep that were grazing in the neighboring fields were killed.[66] The problem of the "boomerang effect" was not solved until 1975, when an effective antidote for LSD was discovered. Equally important though, the army failed to create the means to deliver hallucinogenic weapons.

In 1965 the technological capabilities of achieving what military writers referred to euphemistically as "nonlethal violence" were starting to be considered. In a short article published in 1968 in the pages of *Air University Review*, Lieutenant Colonel Arnold J. Celick proposed, in a utopian manner for that time, the use of nonlethal weapons, especially chemical ones, during peacekeeping operations. He argued: "A capability already exists for mankind to wage an unusual kind of warfare, one which can be accomplished with relatively little, if any, killing."[67] Despite these visionary, optimistic, and humanitarian assumptions, the materialization of the concept of nonlethal violence did not become realistic until the development of science and technology made it possible by the end of the 1990s. Still, psychochemical weapons have not dominated today's nonlethal inventory.

Yet in the 1960s the research on this type of armament not only had a large scope but was also treated as being the most serious. Albert Hofmann admitted that the American army on a fairly regular basis, say every two years, contacted him, asking the Sandoz pharmaceutical company to actively participate in its military programs, but the Swiss firm always rejected these requests.[68] In many cases the experiments entailed administering an appropriate dose of LSD to the servicemen without their knowledge (for example, by dissolving it in coffee) and sending them on their routine training. Toward the end of the 1950s, the staff of the Edgewood Arsenal conducted these types of tests outside its home base, at locations such as Fort Bragg (North Carolina, 1958), Fort Benning (Georgia, 1960), Fort McClellan (Alabama, 1959–1960), and Aberdeen Proving Ground (Utah, 1959).[69] Many of the experiments were filmed with a hidden camera, and later the army presented fragments of the recordings to members of Congress to show the potential destructive impact of the psychochemical weapons on the combat readiness and efficiency of the enemy, to prove the legitimacy of developing these types of projects and hopefully increase their funding.[70] So how did the soldiers behave "on acid"? They could not, in any way, carry out basic and routine tasks and orders. Most of them giggled, cackled, and were very happy for the rest of the day.[71] If this happened to the enemy troops, they would be literally defeated by laughter. Such would be an extremely humanitarian way of waging a war, an interesting but strange American Cold War idea of "humane warfare."

In 1964 the British Army conducted experiments with LSD, which it also filmed.[72] The task of the units was simply to protect their positions against attacks by enemy forces. On the first day the servicemen were given a placebo, and the unit proved its outstanding training by defeating the enemy easily. On the second day, they were unknowingly given "acid" dissolved in water (150 micrograms). Its first effects were felt after twenty-five minutes. The soldiers became more and more relaxed and amused. The radio operator was unable to use his equipment, the shooters were not able to hit their targets, and the commanding officer was not able to locate his position in the field and needed help reading the map. Persons with the strongest reactions to acid had to be evacuated from the training site. Fifty minutes after ingesting LSD, radio communication with the unit became impossible, and the soldiers were laughing, staggering, and in no way were they able to concentrate on carrying out even the simplest of tasks. In other words, they were overcome with a state of mindless amusement, for practically everyone was giggling. Soldiers with the highest feeling of responsibility tried to act constructively, attempting to control the strange psychophysical symptoms. Seventy minutes after taking the drug, the commanding officer finally surrendered. He confessed that after one of his men started climbing a tree to "feed the hungry birds" he was no longer able to control himself, let alone his own people. Hence, LSD could potentially conquer even the best trained and armed units. On the third day, after administering the placebo, the soldiers once again functioned as an expert unit. These scenes from the British experiment proved the potential usefulness of LSD as a weapon that could incapacitate the enemy, paralyzing him with mindlessness and bliss.

In the 1970s the Czechoslovak army also conducted tests with LSD.[73] The drug was given to selected commanding officers, who behaved totally irrationally under its influence and were unable to perform their assigned tasks properly. Several days after the experiment, the commanding officer was given a list of decisions made that day for review and with great horror realized that he sent his soldiers to sure death. Luckily, these were only exercises in experimental conditions, but they proved the potential of LSD for asymmetrical use during wartime. Perhaps it would suffice to intoxicate just the enemy's commanding officer? Regardless, the basic problems were not solved: How to attack the enemy with the use of LSD? In other words, what means of delivery could be employed?

In searching for a substance with which one could poison the enemy water supply system or spray from the air, the Americans tested the usefulness of not only LSD but also BZ, colloquially known as "Agent Buzz." The Army Chemical Corps regularly received samples of "rejects" from pharmaceutical companies, that is, substances unfit to be marketed and used by patients due to some serious adverse effects that they caused. And what the army was interested in was precisely the side effects of pharmaceuticals. The Army Chemical Corps received samples of 3-quinuclidinyl benzilate, a substance referred to by the abbreviation BZ (from benzilate), which it gave the code EA 2277, from Hoffmann-La Roche based in New Jersey. In 1951, in searching for a medication for ulcers, the company created a substance much more effective in causing hallucinations than in the treatment of stomach conditions. Acting similarly to atropine, however exceptionally stronger, BZ seriously disrupts the normal mechanisms of perception, so the person under its influence loses full contact with reality and is unable to function at all. Consider the following two examples. One of the soldiers on BZ took a shower in full uniform while smoking a cigarette.[74] Another serviceman, who in the course of one of the field experiments was given an order to deliver information to the commander, saluted, went off but half way there made a ninety degree turn and started running right into the forest. When stopped by the paramedic, he explained that the order was to run in the other direction. Later in the course of the experiment, the same participant suddenly got up and ran straight ahead.[75] Under the influence of BZ many of the soldiers held two- or three-day conversations with imaginary people. In short, subjects affected by benzilate behaved in an awkward and unexpected manner.

The "incapacitating" influence of BZ lasts for around eighty hours, in comparison to up to twelve hours in the case of LSD. The culmination of the effects takes place after eight hours, then the strange behavior alternately intensifies and weakens. A person moves around chaotically, fully disoriented, and incapable of doing anything reasonable. Around forty-eight hours after ingestion, one can observe somewhat more normal behavior; however, returning to the preadministration state takes another one to two days.[76] Hence the effects of BZ last for at least three days, although the adverse symptoms, such as headaches, disorientation, hallucinations, amnesia, and manic behavior, may last for some weeks. Although LSD incapacitates with much smaller doses (150 micrograms) than BZ (one-half milligram), in comparison to "acid," BZ proved to be a "superhallucinogen"—ten times stronger and longer lasting. One should not be surprised then by the memoirs of Dr. Solomon Snyder, professor of psychiatry and pharmacology at Johns Hopkins University School of Medicine, previously working at Edgewood, who admitted: "The Army's testing of LSD was just a sideshow compared to its use of BZ."[77] In fact, about 90 percent of the testing on LSD was carried out before 1961, and around 1966 the army lost interest in it, becoming more attracted to BZ.[78]

When Doctor Van Sim, chief of the Clinical Research Division at Edgewood (whom James Ketchum uniquely described as "brave and dedicated" because he had the habit of testing all the substances on himself before giving them to the subjects) tried BZ, he described his experience in the following manner: "It zonked me for three days. I kept falling down and the people at the lab assigned someone to follow me around with a mattress. I woke up from it after three days without a bruise."[79]

BZ, which causes delirium and could knock down a person, was an ideal substance for literally defeating the enemy's army without combat. Between 1959 and 1975 it was tested in clinical trials on 2,800 soldiers at Edgewood Arsenal.[80] In addition, field experiments were conducted. For example, in the autumn of 1964 Operation Dork was carried out on a desert range in Utah which entailed the spraying of BZ from a distance of 500 and 1,000 yards from the volunteer soldiers. What was the aim of this experiment? It resulted from the request of a four-star general who wanted to check the possibility of using a cloud of sprayed BZ on the crews of Soviet trawlers, which lurked off the coast of Alaska making the Department of Defense extremely nervous. Operation Dork cost over one million dollars, and its results did not clearly ascertain whether the United States would be technically able to neutralize the Soviet trawlers by releasing an incapacitating chemical cloud on their crews.[81]

The tests and experiments with BZ continued, since the army correctly deemed that it was a much more suitable for a nonlethal weapon than LSD. It also proved to be less expensive and easier to disperse. In 1964 BZ became the "standard incapacitating agent" adopted for tactical use and available for delivery via grenades, mortars, cluster bombs, and rocket warheads. Thus the army filled its experimental weapon with the initial ulcer medication, and BZ became the combat agent of the Chemical Corps. According to unconfirmed rumors, the Americans considered using it against the communist guerrillas in Vietnam.[82]

While in 1961 the effects of BZ were already well known, what remained undiscovered was how to stop them and all the more so, how to reverse its massive effects. If the military wanted to use psychochemical agents as weapons, it would have to find antidotes that would protect its own military personnel in the event of their being exposed to the effects of the incapacitating substances. Hence, as Ketchum recalls, "finding antidotes was a top priority."[83] The most effective countermeasure proved to be physostigmine (an alkaloid obtained from the African Calabar bean plant). What is interesting, atropine, which from the beginning was tested as a potential combat substance due to its hallucinogenic properties (although it was abandoned relatively quickly as much stronger agents appeared), is also an effective antidote to BZ. But the case is similar with paralyzing agents such as sarin or VX, one of the most dangerous war gases.[84] Quite often one poison neutralizes another or, as Paracelsus famously put it, all substances are poisonous, and only the dosage makes one either a poison or a remedy.

The Hallucinogenic Arsenal of the "Empire of Freedom": In Search of a Truth Serum

Therefore I say: Know the enemy and know yourself; in a hundred battles you will never be in peril.

—Sun Tzu, *The Art of War*

The "discovery" of the truth serum is traced to the beginning of the twentieth century and the use of a mixture of morphine and scopolamine by German obstetricians for alleviating labor pains. The doctors observed that under the influence of these substances women under light anesthesia often spontaneously began disclosing intimate details of their private lives and were also willing to answer any questions. In 1922 Robert House, an obstetrician from Dallas, came to the conclusion that a similar technique could be used while interrogating suspects about their alleged crimes. Thus he conducted an experiment on two prisoners who after receiving scopolamine denied per-petrating the acts they were charged with. He believed that proof of the effec-tiveness of this method was that they were cleared of all charges during the court proceedings. House announced the results of his study and later went on researching the application of other medications. The term "truth serum" was first used by a *Los Angeles Record* journalist in a report on House's first experiment. Because the use of scopolamine as a "truth" drug was disqualified in the 1930s due to its numerous side effects, the police began adopting barbi-turates while interrogating witnesses and suspects. It is known, for example, that in 1935 Clarence Muehlberger, director of the Michigan Crime Detection Laboratory in East Dansing, employed barbiturates while examining highly resistant suspects. However, with the exception of several cases, the courts did not, as a rule, admit testimony obtained under the influence of drugs as evidence.[85]

During the Second World War barbiturate thiopental (sodium pentothal), commonly used in general anesthesia, was employed in the treatment of sol-diers suffering from combat stress injury. The medication was effective as a means supporting the release of suppressed fears and traumas, since when in a state of semiconsciousness, the mind is not capable of controlling hidden and painful secrets.[86] It also turned out that thiopental helped unmask the soldiers who feigned illness to tried to dodge military service. It bore, in a word, the traits of a truth serum.[87] The Office of Strategic Services, the American intel-ligence agency appointed by President Roosevelt in 1942, created a commit-tee chaired by Winfred Overholser, superintendent of St. Elizabeths Hospital in Washington, DC, the aim of which was to carry out research on a "truth serum." Thus the possibilities of using mescaline, several barbiturates, and scopolamine were analyzed and tested. They were, however, rejected as inef-fective. In the spring of 1943, the committee concluded that marijuana seemed an unusually promising substance. So experiments were commenced; it was tested on the staff working on the Manhattan Project.[88] Why such a choice? The safety and confidentiality aspects were most likely the decisive factors. No military program in the United States was as top secret and protected as the atomic bomb project. Hence, its employees were to contribute to the United States' attainment of not only nuclear but also psychochemical weapons. Initially, concentrated marijuana was administered in liquid form; however, because oral ingestion caused vomiting, in May 1943 the Manhattan Project staff was given marijuana cigarettes, as this intake method was already known to jazz musicians and hipsters in general.[89] In working on the atomic bomb program, the essence of which was to harness the atomic fission of uranium, they received joints from the authorities, who expected that, in leading to a "fission" of the brain cells, marijuana would prove an effective truth serum.

Was this not also a perfect opportunity to uncover any would-be spies among the staff?

Despite this episode, it was not until the end of the war that the American armed forces began intensive research aimed at discovering a truth serum for the purposes of the Cold War. In the autumn of 1947, the navy initiated the CHATTER program, developed under the supervision of Charles Savage from the Naval Medical Research Institute in Bethesda, Maryland. In 1951 command was taken over by Samuel Thompson, a psychiatrist, physiologist, pharmacologist, and navy commander who headed psychiatric research at the Naval Medical Research Institute.[90] The goal of CHATTER was to identify and then test chemical substances that could help obtain information against the will of the interrogated party. The knowledge of experiments that were run during the war by Nazi doctors provided additional inspiration. In 1942, thanks to breaking the Enigma code, the Allies learned of tests conducted on German pilots using mescaline and scopolamine.[91] The Nazis then carried out experiments on concentration camp prisoners, among others, in Dachau, where Kurt Plotner was searching for mind-controlling substances, which could weaken the combat abilities of the opponent's army. The Jewish and Russian inmates were given large doses of mescaline, and their schizophrenic behavior was carefully observed. They started to speak directly, without any inhibitions and fears, about how much they hated their oppressors, thus acting irrationally against the instinct for self-preservation.[92]

The motive for the navy's commencement of the research was rumors that the Soviets had achieved excellent results with tablets, known only to them, given to subjects undergoing interrogation. Thus a truth serum, which could secretly be used on the enemy's prisoners of war or secret agents, or also during the recruitment procedure for intelligence service, was being intensively searched for in the United States.[93] The following substances were tested, among others: scopolamine (with a weaker reaction on the nervous system compared to atropine, causing sedation, sleepiness, and stupefaction when given in small amounts, and delirium when issued in large doses), mescaline (a semisynthetic peyote extract causing similar hallucinations to those associated with LSD), and anabasine (an alkaloid occurring in tobacco, used as an insecticide). One of the main investigators of the CHATTER project was Professor Richard Wendt, chairman of the Psychology Department at the University of Rochester, who for a long time had been testing medications to be used by the air force. Up until this time, he had always tried the substances out on his assistants and students before moving to the stage of experiments on volunteers. Within the framework of CHATTER, however, Thompson decided to not only speed up the procedure but also to carry out the tests on people who were neither volunteers nor informed of the medical experiments performed on them. Although aware that such actions were unethical, Thompson confessed: "We felt we had to do it for the good of country."[94] Reasons of national security and raison d'état were employed to justify illegal actions, which broke not only the memorable CMR recommendations of 1942 but also the general standards for the conduct of medical trials. Wendt's breakthrough experiment, which was to bring the navy closer to the truth serum, entailed the testing of a miraculous medication, the content of which was not revealed until the very end. The shock of the officials observing its course was great when it turned out that the secret drug was a cocktail of commonly known and already widely tested substances: secobarbital, dextroamphetamine, and THC. What Wendt probably hoped to achieve was a powerful effect resulting from the interaction of these compounds. But the entire experiment turned out to be a fiasco because contrary to expectations no desired effects were observed in subjects, and project CHATTER was terminated shortly after the end of the Korean War in 1953.[95] Thus the navy's search for a truth serum had so far come to nothing.[96]

Yet it was not the navy that was running the most extensive research in this matter but the army. Experiments on humans were carried out in various military bases and mostly at Edgewood Arsenal as the Chemical Corps was the main executor of experiments. The following were among the 254 most commonly tested substances: poisonous gases, incapacitating agents (mainly BZ), anticholinergics (smooth muscle relaxants), sedatives, atropine and its derivatives, amphetamines, LSD, marijuana, mescaline, and morphine. The army was specifically interested in psychoactive compounds with unique, strong psychedelic properties. From 1950 to 1975, around 6,700 persons were the subjects of experiments using LSD and phencyclidine (PCP, colloquially known as angel dust).[97] What was searched for were substances that would affect human behavior, thereby helping obtain reliable information.

Tests on LSD as a potential truth serum, being a joint experiment of the Medical Laboratories of the Army Chemical Corps at Edgewood and the Army Intelligence Center, were run in three stages. In the first one, between 1955 and 1958, the hallucinogen was given to over 1,000 military personnel and their combat abilities were then carefully observed to see whether and how subjects were able to function as soldiers. In the second stage in 1958, LSD was tested on ninety-five volunteers in laboratory experiment conditions. Finally, in the third stage, under the consent granted in 1960 by the deputy army assistant chief of staff for intelligence, trials were conducted on unknowing soldiers and civilians, who were given LSD and then questioned. The procedures of the Department of Defense and particularly the Department of the Army were violated, as experiments with the participation of volunteers required the written consent of the secretary of defense. More important, tests carried out on persons who were not volunteers remained in contradiction with standards accepted long ago. Still, the Department of the Army for Special Tasks went on to launch two projects: the THIRD CHANCE run in Europe from May to August 1961, and the DERBY HAT run in Hawaii from August to November 1962.[98]

James R. Thornwell, a black private stationed in France, was one of the participants of the series of tests under the THIRD CHANCE project. He was arrested in the course of a military investigation on the theft of confidential documents. Thornwell was treated in a drastic, torture-like manner; he was detained in isolation; not allowed to sleep; not given water, food, and access to a toilet; physically abused; hurled with racial slurs; and threatened with death on many occasions. Finally, after six weeks of humiliation and such treatment designed to "break" him, he was given LSD during a lengthy interrogation; thus the drug was being tested on him as a truth serum. Thornwell was told that if he did not talk, then his unpleasant and horrifying mental state would not only be prolonged into eternity but would also ultimately turn into paranoia. Only in 1978 he learned that back in the 1960s he was an involuntary experiment participant—his own country treated him like a guinea pig. Thus he confessed: "I had no life after they gave me LSD. I had nothing. I lived in a twilight world where nothing was real or important."[99] He made attempts at pursing compensatory claims in court and demanded the sum of ten million dollars. But he lost in circuit court, which dismissed his claims on the basis of the so-called Feres doctrine: a Supreme Court ruling of 1950 (*Feres v. United States*) stating that neither a soldier nor his family could sue the federal government for injuries or damages incurred during, or death resulting from, military service. Yet in 1980 the House of Representatives granted him a compromised compensation in the amount of 625,000 dollars, thereby recognizing not only the legitimacy of his demands but also the illegal nature of the actions of the government's bodies.[100] Four years later Thornwell was found dead in his outdoor swimming pool.

Under the second project, DERBY HAT, seven foreigners involved in drug trafficking or intelligence activities were experimented on. They were given LSD while being interrogated. Each time, the investigators managed to obtain information that they were not able to acquire earlier when using traditional techniques. Some of the interrogees pleaded not to be kept in a continuous terrifying psychedelic state, saying it was torture; others threatened to commit suicide; many decided to cooperate fully in exchange for regaining control over their own thoughts and bodies.[101] Eventually, in April 1963 the deputy army assistant chief of staff for intelligence decided to abandon further field experiments with LSD "based on a lack of data, inconclusiveness of the testing and the legal, political and moral problems inherent in the use of EA 1729."[102]

Although the army's experiments with LSD did not directly lead to the death of any of the participants, the same could not be said for experiments with psychedelic substances in general. The death of Harold Blauer was a tragic accident, which saw the light of day after many years. In 1952, at the age of forty-two, this professional tennis player leading a comfortable and generally happy life began suffering from what doctors would today refer to as a typical case of the andropause, the male version of the menopause.[103] Things were no longer working out for him, he decided to get a divorce and, in the end, fell into deep depression. Searching for psychiatric help, he made his way to Bellevue Hospital in New York. He was diagnosed with clinical depression and referred to the New York State Psychiatric Institute, a renowned institution founded in 1896, which employed many outstanding specialists. Blauer was admitted on December 5, 1952, started psychotherapy and reacted relatively well to it. From December 11 to January 8, he underwent experimental therapy with the use of EA 1298. It was a psychoactive substance synthesized for the first time in 1910 and known as MDA (3,4-methylenedioxyamphetamine), the effects of which are similar to those of MDMA (ecstasy). As it turned out later, the Institute was one of the civilian institutions secretly cooperating with the Chemical Corps. The army provided psychochemical means, and then selected doctors tested them on patients without their informed consent. The team was led by Paul Hoch who was not only under contract with Edgewood Arsenal but also worked as a consultant for the CIA.[104] Although Blauer was aware that he was being subjected to some type of experiment, he was convinced that it was part of his therapy: in fact, he was participating in the search for a "magic" Cold War weapon.

Blauer received a total of five injections. Just before the third one, in simulating a cold, he unsuccessfully asked the nurse to help him avoid participation in the subsequent tests. When, after receiving the third injection, he declared that he no longer wished to receive any more, the psychotherapist threatened that he would be sent away to other, less specialized hospitals for treatment; it was commonly known that the conditions for caring for mentally ill patients in these institutions were much worse. Despite his firm protests, Blauer received two subsequent injections. The final dose proved lethal. At 9:53 a.m. on January 8, 1953, the day before his planned release from the hospital, he received 500 milligrams of MDA, which was sixteen times greater than the first dose. At 11:45 a.m. he fell into a deep coma and was pronounced dead half an hour later.[105] The army and the CIA made sure to cover up the entire case. His former wife learned that her husband died due to an "atypical" reaction to a medication. Doctor Hoch asked the army to consent to conducting an autopsy of his brain to better learn the effects of EA 1298 on human tissues. He received approval under the condition of keeping the whole matter confidential; however, the army changed its mind at the very last minute—to the doctor's great dissatisfaction.[106]

Blauer can in fact be recognized as a victim of the Cold War, as an innocent scapegoat offered by the state to the ritual altar of secret experiments performed on the human body and mind. He is just one of the many unaware
citizens who were incidental victims of the national security state. Along with
him, several other patients received mescaline injections at the New York State
Psychiatric Institute, but they had more luck then he did. One woman, while
being administered mescaline, became so aggressive that the experiment
had to be halted. That perhaps saved her life. After some years she wondered:
"I've been in hell. Why did they put me in hell?"[107] This was yet a totally different hell than the one described by Dante, for his *Inferno* can be deemed as
more "natural," that is, in accordance with the traditional historical vision and
Christian theology. It constituted a "normal" place, where condemned souls
went. Dante's *Inferno* was divided into circles, in which sinners were kept,
depending on the wrongs they committed. This was not the hell on earth
to which the state threw its citizens, even though they did not deserve to be
condemned. Despite that, the motto visible on the gates to the *Inferno* could
have well been found on the gates to the hell of the national security state:
"Abandon every hope, ye who enter here." The state decided to send some of its
own citizens to the "hell" of psychedelic experiments because the stakes in the
Cold War were believed to be "hellishly absolute": victory or defeat, salvation
or damnation. Although the United States fought in the name of democracy,
all too often security became more important than the fundamental values of
liberal democracy that it was supposed to secure. The secret state experiments
on humans with psychoactive substances, motivated by the alleged fact of the
narcotic-assisted brainwashing techniques mastered by the communists, were
to bring the authorities the capability of not only controlling the human body
but also the mind. All efforts, however, proved futile.

10

Vietnam

The First True Pharmacological War

Instead of taking away marijuana from the soldiers—we ought to be
giving it to the negotiators in Paris.
—Bob Hope, comedian, 1970 quoted in Jeremy Kuzmarov,
*The Myth of the Addicted Arm: Vietnam
and the Modern War on Drugs*

The Vietnam War was unquestionably one of the most landmark and tragic
events in modern American history. In *A Rumor of War*, one of the finest war
memoirs ever, Philip Caputo explained that Vietnam was a watershed event
because it

> has severely called into question American myth. Americans entered
> Vietnam with certain expectations that a story, a distinctly American
> story, would unfold. When the story of America in Vietnam turned
> into something unexpected, the true nature of the larger story of
> America itself became the subject of intense cultural dispute.[1]

What rendered the Vietnam War a truly harrowing experience was notably
its unusually irregular character, which makes it probably one of the best
examples of asymmetrical war in the twentieth century. Vietnam was not a
conventional war with the frontlines, rears, enemy mobilizing its forces for
an attack, or a territory to be conquered and occupied. Instead, it was a formless conflict in which former strategic and tactical principles did not apply.
The Vietcong were fighting in an unexpected, surprising, and deceptive way
to negate Americans' strengths and exploit their weaknesses. All this made
Vietnam the "last modern war" as some claim, or the "first postmodern war"
as others suggest. The American response to the Vietcong's asymmetry was
the heavy deployment of modern military technology. The more asymmetry
the Vietcong generated, the more technology the Americans deployed. Thus

the war turned out to be a tragic example of a "techno-war." Still, the conflict also came to be referred to as the first "pharmacological war" because
both the prescribed and self-prescribed consumption of psychoactive substances by military personnel assumed alarming proportions, unprecedented
in American history. The British philosopher Nick Land aptly described the
Vietnam War as "a decisive point of intersection between pharmacology and
the technology of violence."[2]

At times the Americans fought the enemy in Southeast Asia nearly as resolutely and brutally as they did some sixty years earlier in the Philippines, which
they acquired control over in 1898 after the war with Spain. Then they ruthlessly
suppressed a popular anti-American rebellion under the foregoing ally Emilio
Aguinaldo. During the colonial war that dragged on for four years, American
soldiers adopted the local habit of smoking opium, which soon grew to be so
common in the ranks that in 1903 the American Pharmaceutical Association
felt compelled to address this alarming problem.[3] Later, such drugs as cocaine,
marijuana, and heroin gained in popularity among the troops, with the latter
being particularly attractive due to rumors about its amazing power to boost
male potency. Officers usually followed a relatively restrictive policy, so that
soldiers who got caught taking cocaine or heroin were punished, often even
discharged. What the authorities feared most was the domino effect of one
abuser infecting the entire unit.[4] And it was precisely this problem, yet on a
massive scale, that the command of the American forces in Indochina had to
tackle in the 1960s and 1970s.

 According to the Department of Defense, in 1968 as much as half of
American men deployed in Vietnam took some kind of drugs. In 1970 this
rate increased to 60 percent and in 1973, the year of the United States' withdrawal, some 70 percent of soldiers used intoxicants. In 1971 nearly 51 percent
smoked marijuana, 28 percent took hard drugs (mostly heroin), and almost
31 percent used psychedelic substances.[5] These were but estimates that obviously worried many and seemed to justify the claim that most American soldiers serving in Southeast Asia did drugs regularly and on a massive scale.
The Tet Offensive launched by the Vietcong on January 31, 1968, served as a
catalyst for the further "pharmacologization" of the war, since the consumption of substances increased considerably in its immediate aftermath.[6] On
his return from the trip to Vietnam, Egil Krogh, President Richard Nixon's
liaison to the Bureau of Narcotics and Dangerous Drugs, reported: "Mr.
President, you don't have a drug problem in Vietnam; you have a condition.
Problems are things we can get right on and solve. Conditions we have to
ameliorate as best we can. I don't think we can solve this short of bringing
everybody home."[7]

Drugs "Prescribed" by the Military

Although since the Second World War no cutting-edge research proving that amphetamine had a highly positive impact on soldiers' performance had been carried out, the American military continued to supply its troops in Vietnam with speed. Pep pills were usually distributed to men leaving for long-range reconnaissance missions and ambushes. The opening lines of *Dispatches* (1977), the acclaimed book by Michael Herr, a war correspondent for *Esquire*, bring this out superbly: "Going out at night the medics gave you pills. Dexedrine breath like dead snakes kept too long in a jar."[8] The standard army instruction (twenty milligrams of dextroamphetamine for forty-eight hours of combat readiness) was rarely followed; and amphetamine was issued, as one veteran put it, "like candies" with no attention given to recommended dose or frequency of administration; hence the American troops consumed a massive amount of speed.

In 1971 a report by the House Select Committee on Crime revealed that from 1966 to 1969 armed forces used 225 million tablets of stimulants, mostly Dexedrine (dextroamphetamine), an amphetamine derivative that is nearly twice as strong as the Benzedrine used in the Second World War.[9] The annual consumption of Dexedrine per person per military branch was 21.1 pills in the navy, 17.5 in the air force, and 13.8 in the army. Statistically, it was thirty or forty five-milligram Dexedrine tablets per fighting man per year.[10] Elton Manzione, a member of a long-range reconnaissance platoon (or Lurp), revealed: "We had the best amphetamines available and they were supplied by the U.S. government." He also quoted a navy commando saying: "When I was a SEAL team member in Vietnam, the drugs were routinely consumed. They gave you a sense of bravado as well as keeping you awake. Every sight and sound was heightened. You were wired into it all and at times you felt really invulnerable."[11] Soldiers in units infiltrating Laos for a four-day mission received a medical kit which contained, among other items, twelve tablets of Darvon (a mild painkiller), twenty-four tablets of codeine (an opioid analgesic), and six pills of Dexedrine. Before leaving for a long and demanding expedition, members of special units were also administered steroid injections.[12]

A study revealed that 3.2 percent of soldiers arriving in Vietnam were heavy amphetamine users; however, after one year of deployment this rate rose to 5.2 percent.[13] Further studies revealed that 7 percent of servicemen were heavy amphetamine abusers. In short, the administration of stimulants by the military contributed to the spread of drug habits that sometimes had tragic consequences, because, as many veterans claimed, next to alertness, amphetamine increased aggression.[14] Some remembered that when the effect of speed faded away, they were so irritated that they felt like shooting "children in the streets."[15] For example, a member of the elite Green Berets nicknamed "Bill," who was so heavily addicted to amphetamine that he needed to take as much as one hundred milligrams per day, during one nighttime river patrol "was so jumpy after twenty-six sleepless, drugged hours on duty that, when startled by a noise, he machine-gunned an accompanying boat, killing and maiming a number of his colleagues."[16] Hence amphetamine was to blame for some incidents of friendly fire and unjustified violence against the civilian population.

Psychoactive substances were issued not only for boosting the war fighters but also to reduce the harmful impact of combat on their psyche. In order to prevent soldiers' mental breakdowns and their suffering from combat stress, the Department of Defense employed sedatives and neuroleptics. By and large, writes David Grossman, Vietnam was "the first war in which the forces of modern pharmacology were directed to empower the battlefield soldier."[17] For the first time in military history, the prescription of potent antipsychotic drugs, such as chlorpromazine, manufactured by GlaxoSmithKline under the brand name Thorazine, became routine. The massive use of psychopharmacology and the deployment of a large number of military psychiatrists to the frontline explain the unprecedentedly low rate of combat trauma recorded in wartime.[18] Whereas during the Second World War the rate of mental breakdowns among American soldiers was 10 percent (101 cases per 1,000 troops) and 4 percent in the Korean War (37 cases per 1,000 troops), in Vietnam it fell to 1 percent only (12 cases per 1,000 troops).[19] What was achieved, however, was a short-sighted outcome, because by merely alleviating the symptoms, antipsychotic medicines and narcotics brought immediate but short-lasting effects. Drugs taken without proper psychotherapy only assuage, suppress, or freeze the problems that remain deeply embedded in the psyche and which later, sometimes even years afterward, can explode unexpectedly with multiplied force.

Intoxicants do not eliminate the causes of stress but, observes Grossman, do "what insulin does for a diabetic: they treat the symptoms, but the disease is still there."[20] That is precisely why, when compared with previous wars, in Vietnam very few soldiers required medical evacuation because of combat stress breakdowns. By the same token, however, the armed forces contributed to the outbreak of a major PTSD epidemic in the aftermath of the conflict, as the number of veterans suffering from posttraumatic stress disorder was unprecedentedly high. This resulted, to a large extent, from reckless use of pharmaceuticals and drugs. In her book with the telling title Flashback, Penny Coleman tells the stories of wives whose Vietnam veteran husbands committed suicide, and she quotes a military psychologist who astutely says that

> if drugs are given while the stressor is still being experienced, then they will arrest or supercede the development of effective coping mechanisms, resulting in an increase in the long-term trauma from the stress. What happened in Vietnam is the moral equivalent of giving a soldier a local anesthetic for a gunshot wound and then sending him back into combat.[21]

The essence of war trauma and PTSD can be captured in many ways. Philip Caputo does it particularly well in his novel *Indian Country* (1987): "[W]ars don't end when the shooting stops and the treaties are signed. They go on and on in the wounded minds of those who did the fighting."[22] This is also what Tim O'Brien, perhaps one of the greatest authors ever to write about the Vietnam War, talks about time after time: "[Y]ou go into war 'clean' and you get 'dirty,' and afterwards you are never the same."[23] The precise number of Vietnam veterans who suffered from PTSD remains unknown. Estimates vary widely and range from 400,000 to 1.5 million.[24] According to the *National Vietnam Veterans Readjustment Study* published in 1990, as many as 15.2 percent of soldiers who experienced combat in Southeast Asia suffered from PTSD.[25]

Drugs "Self-Prescribed" by Soldiers

What made Vietnam the first true "pharmacological war" was not only the official administration of psychoactive substances but most of all their self-prescription by soldiers. The unauthorized use of drugs is often described in the Vietnam War literature. Take, for example, Tim O'Brien's story *The Lives of the Dead* (1989): "Ted Lavender had a habit of popping four or five tranquilizers every morning. It was his way of coping, just dealing with the realities, and the drugs helped to ease him through the days."[26] Also Michael Herr tells the story of a Lurp member "who took his pills by the fistful, downs from the left pocket of his tiger suit and ups from the right, one to cut the trail for him and the other to send him down it."[27] Such a pharmacological cocktail of downers and uppers calmed him down and at the same time sharpened his senses so that he could unerringly find his way in the jungle at night. He was, according to Herr, one of the best killers around.

In fact, anything that would help mitigate the consequences of being in Vietnam could be taken for self-medication (see table 10.1). Apart from

Table 10.1 **The most common intoxicants used by the American servicemen in Vietnam**[*]

	Percentage reporting use
Alcohol	92
Marijuana	69[**]
Opium	38
Heroin	34
Amphetamines	25
Barbiturates	23

[*] Based on interviews, general sample of 451 Vietnam veterans
[**] Estimated

Source: Lee N. Robins, *The Vietnam Drug User Returns: Final Report* (Washington, DC: Special Action Office for Drug Abuse Prevention, 1974), p. 29.

alcohol popular self-prescribed intoxicants were above all: marijuana; heroin, morphine (popular especially among medics); opium; sedatives and hallucinogens (mostly LSD); (meth)amphetamine (soldiers who wanted to supplement the amphetamines issued by the military could easily obtain on the black market French-made ampuls of one-hundred-milligram dextroamphetamine liquid for injection called Maxitone Forte); and amphetamine-like uppers, mostly Ritalin (methylphenidate), a psychostimulant in use since the early 1960s in the treatment of attention deficit hyperactivity disorder, or ADHD.[28]

Marijuana was the most common nonalcoholic drug. Soldiers called it by various names depending on the region or province where it came from—Pleiku Pink, Bleu de Hue, Cambodian Red, and so forth. The concentration of THC in the local cannabis plant was high, about 5 percent compared with 1 percent in the marijuana available in the United States.[29] It was easily accessible and as a military psychiatrist cited by the *U.S News & World Report* affirmed: "The drug is everywhere. All a person has to do to get the drug in any village hamlet or town is say the word Khan Sa."[30] Thomas Boettcher in *Vietnam, The Valor and the Sorrow* (1985) quotes a Marine Corps colonel saying: "When a man is in Vietnam he can be sure that . . . there are probably drugs within twenty-five feet of him."[31] Marijuana was ridiculously cheap—a carton of ready-made cannabis cigarettes could be purchased for five dollars or exchanged for a package of American cigarettes. A veteran recalls:

Pot was a funny thing there. Not everybody smoked it. I've heard all sorts of reports of the time I was there . . . 20 percent, 80 percent. . . . I would say in my area, maybe 40 percent of the people were smoking pot, another 40 percent were getting drunk. There were 20 percent who just wrote letters home. And listened to Barbara Streisand. Most people smoked their pot in a pipe, because cigarette papers were always getting sticky and soggy.[32]

At first, the army ignored the marijuana habit; in 1968, however, under the heavy pressure of alarming media reports, which presented marijuana as a plague debilitating American troops in Vietnam, action had to be taken. Education programs on the harmful and habit-forming effects of cannabis were introduced (compulsory lectures, radio broadcasts, pamphlets, warnings issued by the chaplains and doctors, etc.). When all these attempts proved ineffective, the army undertook more penitentiary actions. It was apparently, though probably unwittingly, assumed that the results of research carried out by the army in the Panama Canal Zone nearly half a century earlier were not reliable. The American troops deployed in the Canal area took from the local people the habit of smoking cannabis as a mild mood enhancer. Farmers who grew it for their own use began to sell the surplus to soldiers. The first military report on the scope of marijuana smoking in the American ranks comes from 1916.[33] In 1925 and 1931 the army carried out research which proved that cannabis does not affect the combat efficiency and fighting spirit of the individual soldier nor does it undermine military discipline.[34] In Vietnam, the army adopted a totally different stance toward smoking marijuana. Apparently, the command considered wrong or outdated the view of Colonel James Phalen, editor of the *Military Surgeon*, expressed in his 1943 editorial entitled "The Marijuana Bugaboo." He wrote: "The smoking of the leaves, flowers, and seeds of Cannabis sativa is no more harmful than the smoking of tobacco. . . . It is hoped that no witch hunt will be institutionalized in the military service over a problem that does not exist."[35] During the Second World War, however, the use, possession, and introduction of marijuana were prosecuted as drug offenses by American military courts. It was believed that marijuana produced a deleterious effect upon human conduct and behavior inconsistent with the "requirements of military efficiency and discipline."[36] In line with this logic, the amendment to the *Army Regulation 600-50* introduced in January 1968 widened the category of harmful substances and prohibited the use, sale, transfer, or introduction of depressants, stimulants, and hallucinogens except for authorized medical purposes. All servicemen taking medicines were obliged to keep prescribed drugs in the original container.[37] It was precisely on this legal basis that the armed forces in Vietnam began to scout the barracks for marijuana, arresting roughly a thousand GIs per week.

Compared to the U.S. Army, the Marine Corps in Vietnam did not face the problem of drug use, because it placed much greater emphasis on maintaining rigid discipline and high morale. Also, the possession or use of even the smallest amount of marijuana was a court-martial drug offense, while the army brought to trial only the heavy drug abusers and dealers.[38] But still the army's court system did not work very efficiently, in part, because until 1968 there was no crime laboratory in Vietnam. So, urine samples had to be sent to Japan for testing, and it took about forty-five days for the procedure to be completed. This was a major obstacle to the army's attempts to punish marijuana users. When the judicial system could not punish the drug offenders, administrative discharges were used to expel them from service.[39] In 1970 as many as 11,000 soldiers were prosecuted for the use of hard drugs, but the overall detection rate was still low, as it is estimated that only one in five soldiers doing drugs was identified.[40] Anyhow, by 1972 the military judicial system in Vietnam became almost paralyzed by drug offenses, which, as one counsel of the defendant soldiers put it, became for the military courts what car accidents were for the civilian courts in the United States.

In order to reduce the availability of marijuana, aircrafts were used to seek out cannabis fields, which were then destroyed by South Vietnamese troops.[41] All these efforts, as might have been expected, did not produce impressive results. In 1969 it was estimated that while some 30 percent of soldiers had smoked marijuana prior to their departure to Indochina, when deployed in Vietnam, 60 percent of them would smoke a joint.[42] A survey commissioned by the Department of Defense revealed that in 1971 almost 51 percent of army personnel in Vietnam used marijuana.[43]

The army's more restrictive policy on marijuana had a serious unintended consequence: heroin quickly gained ground in popular use. Indeed, as much as 79 percent of all soldiers who tried any drug in Vietnam used heroin.[44] By 1970 heavy increases in heroin use were frequently reported, and when it became commonplace, it was realized that marijuana, which would nevertheless remain the most popular drug of choice, was not a problem at all. One army commanding officer captured the essence of this change: "If it would get them to give up the hard stuff, I would buy all the marijuana and hashish in the Delta as a present."[45] But it was too late.

By the end of spring of 1970, with the opening of drug trafficking routes from the Golden Triangle through Cambodia, pure and cheap heroin became even more easily obtainable. By 1971 as many as twenty-nine laboratories operated in Vietnam that produced cheap and powerful heroin (94–98 percent pure and smokable "white snow") flooding the country with the "white junk" to meet the rising demands of the American troops.[46] The remarkable purity of heroin, which enabled its oral ingestion instead of intravenous application, made it an extremely attractive drug of choice. So, American servicemen smoked it like cigarettes, mixed with tobacco or marijuana, inhaled its heated fumes, or snorted it like cocaine. It was, by the way, Thai soldiers who introduced these nonintravenous heroin-intake methods to Vietnam.[47] Heroin was, therefore, extremely attractive, especially for those who were reluctant to inject (only 9 percent of soldiers doing drugs took it intravenously), as there was no risk of infection, and one did not have to remember about keeping synergies or needles—what was needed was only a joint, a pipe, or sometimes just a paper bag.[48] Although the risk of fatal overdose was relatively low, between April 1970 and January 1973 half of 112 GIs' drug-related deaths resulted from heroin overdose.[49] The assumption that the intoxicant was less harmful and less addictive when inhaled compared with taken intravenously was dangerously deceptive, because heroin in Southeast Asia had, in fact, a higher addictive potential than the weaker and less purified injectable narcotic available in the United States.

Unlike marijuana, odorless heroin was hard to detect without urine or blood sample tests, nonetheless soldiers did not hide their habit, which was often almost as common and ordinary as puffing a cigarette. Drugging became so overt an activity that GIs engraved their Zippo lighters with drug-rhymes such as "Say Hi! If you're high" or

> Always ripped
> Or always stoned
> I made it a year
> I'm going home.[50]

In the spring of 1971 military doctors estimated that 25,000 to 37,000 soldiers, or 10 to 15 percent of troops, were addicted to heroin, but in some units it was almost 20 percent. Surveys and studies showed that 85 percent of all American servicemen in Vietnam were offered heroin, of which 35 percent tried and 19 percent became habitual users.[51] In 1973 the Pentagon confirmed that about one-third of soldiers used heroin and 20 percent of them became habitual users.[52] Late in the war, drug taking was so excessive that, as one veteran said, "Near the end of my tour, when everybody was doing heroin, I remember there was a pool of vomit outside our hootch that never dried up completely. Like for days on end. Because heroin makes you vomit."[53] In the final stage of the war, drug use was omnipresent and in some bases the problem was so severe that commanders would allow prostitutes to the barracks with the goal of deterring soldiers from going to downtown brothels where they usually got supplied with drugs.[54]

use to talk about
why they used drugs for rec usage

Why?

Why is it, in fact, that so many soldiers reached for psychoactive substances and medications? There are no simple answers to this question, and one needs to take a chain of various factors into consideration.

Firstly, the nature of the conflict and the conditions in which the American soldiers had to stay in and fight were extreme, physically exhausting, and— most importantly—psychologically devastating. When entering a euphoric mood and by numbing the psyche, intoxication allows one to view one's, even uniquely difficult, situation with more optimism. Drugs are "consolers" that help one get through a difficult time, and it is for this reason that they are so easily addictive. They are a means to escape from the hopelessness, tragedy, nonsense, and brutality of the surroundings. According to the research conducted by John Helmer, 43 percent of American soldiers in Vietnam indicated "escaping" from the depressing reality as the main reason for taking drugs.[55] In one of the key stories from Tim O'Brien, *The Thing They Carried*, the titular "thing" embodies, among others, the difficult conditions of the war and the problems that the soldiers had to face.

> They carried infections.... They carried diseases, among them malaria and dysentery. They carried lice and ringworm and leeches and paddy algae and various rots and molds. They carried the land itself—Vietnam, the place, the soil—a powdery orange-red dust that covered their boots and fatigues and faces. They carried the sky. The whole atmosphere, they carried it, the humidity, the monsoons, the stink of fungus and decay, all of it, they carried gravity. They moved like mules.[56]

"They carried their own lives" in a very unfriendly environment, which was, apart from the Vietcong, their most serious enemy. This is what Vietnam was—foreign, unfriendly, horrifying, and, above all, unusually uncomfortable. In *A Rumor of War* Philip Caputo writes: "We fought the climate, the snipers, and monotony, of which the climate was the worst," and the heat was terrible; it could kill a man, "bake his brains, or wring the sweat out of him until he dropped from exhaustion."[57] Relief did not come until nighttime. Then the insects, specifically the malaria-carrying mosquitoes, tropical ants, and leeches, which were unimaginably severe, took their toll. The dark jungle was not very hospitable, and despite what the army manuals wrote—"The jungle can be your friend as well as your enemy"—in Vietnam it turned out to be only the enemy. And the soldiers had no understanding of it whatsoever. The unusually naturalistic and moving description of the extreme conditions, in which the divisions had to stay for longer periods of time, was given by James Webb:

> You spend a month in the bush and you're not a Marine anymore. Hell. You're not even a goddamn person. . . . You're an animal. It gets so that it's natural to squat when you take a shit. You get ringworm and hookworm and gooksores. You roll around in your own filth. You forget how bad you smell. Dead people, guts in the goddamn dirt, miserable civilians, it all gets sort of boring.[58]

Drugs allowed the soldiers to lessen the burden of feeling what they were "carrying"; they fulfilled the function of a kind of pharmacological exoskeleton. Intoxicants, in a word, facilitated the easier endurance of an unusually difficult stay in Indochina. They numbed the psyche, allowing the body to bear the huge inconvenience of this "Indian country," as the soldiers often described Vietnam, and as Caputo titled one of his books.

Secondly, intoxication was an effective way for survival given the increasing disillusionment with the war, its purpose, and one's efforts and sacrifice. Tim O'Brien (echoing Clausewitz) remarks on Vietnam: "It was my view then, and still is, that you don't make war without knowing why."[59] The United States, however, ignored this fundamental principle. The Americans fought because a defeat would mean a catastrophe in the Cold War confrontation with the Soviet Union. It would mean that the superpower would not be able to beat the determined guerrillas. Still worse, in essence the United States did not have a strategy for trying to win over an enemy who was highly unconventional and difficult to grasp, had wide support among the population, and fought on its own uniquely inaccessible territory.

The said lack of a strategic objective, evident on the highest levels of the military, destroyed the morale of the American troops. One of the officers recalled: "I'm not sure that anyone in the higher up levels knew what we were supposed to be doing. Like my troops, I just wondered, . . . if we do all this, what's going to happen, what are we doing, what's the goal of the whole thing?"[60] In a bold and well-known article, "The Collapse of the Armed Forces," published in 1971, Colonel Robert D. Heinl Jr. presented the image of the American armed forces in Vietnam. They were, in his opinion, in a state of decline: "By every conceivable indicator, our army that now remains in Vietnam is in a state approaching collapse, with individual units avoiding or having refused combat, murdering their officers and non-commissioned officers, drug-ridden, and dispirited where not near mutinous."[61] Samuel Hynes offers a very accurate perception in this context by claiming that if the army was subject to degeneration, it was not because the soldiers were decomposed from the very beginning, but because it was the war itself that degenerated them.[62]

The lack of strategy compensated by the "search and destroy" tactics plunged Americans into sheer brutality, as the goal was to "find, fix, and finish" the enemy. The aim of the search and destroy operations was simply to maximize the kill ratio, as it was believed that the huge and unacceptable level of losses would ultimately force the enemy into negotiations. Philip Caputo writes: "Our mission was not to win terrain or seize positions, but simply to kill: to kill Communists and to kill as many of them as possible.... Victory was a high body-count, defeat a low kill-ratio, war a matter of arithmetic."[63] As a result, many innocent civilians lost their lives, and this was not only due to the difficulties in differentiating the Vietcong from the ordinary peasants but also due to the huge pressure of the commanders expecting measurable effects, that is, a great number of communists killed. This intensified an unhealthy and morbid competition between the divisions and their commanders. In such a political climate, extreme situations occurred because of the solution commonly accepted by the commanders and described by Caputo. For each killed member of the Vietcong, confirmed through a trophy, such as a cut off ear or penis among others, a soldier could receive an additional ration of beer. Thus morality sunk into a dark jungle; the American army found itself in a deplorable condition: "We were going to kill people," Caputo observed, "for a few cans of beer and the time to drink them."[64] It is, in fact, difficult to find a more moving comment on the emptiness in which the GIs found themselves.

Given the lack of clear political and strategic objectives, and the doubtfulness on the part of the politicians and society of the legitimacy of the American involvement in Vietnam, the basic aim of each soldier was simply to survive. The questions that the combatants asked themselves reflect the soldier's psychological state. The troops were overcome by helplessness toward the senselessness of the war in which they were forced to fight, despite no one really knowing for what purpose. Caputo captured these doubts particularly well: "How to find meaning in such a meaningless conflict? How to make sense out of a succession of random fire-fights that achieved nothing? How to explain our failings? And what heroes could be found in a war so murky and savage?"[65] In his outstanding memoirs *Born on the Fourth of July* (1976), on the basis of which Oliver Stone made a well-known film with the same title, Ron Kovic noted in one sentence, which pointedly reflects the tragic situation of the American men in Vietnam: "All I could feel was the worthlessness of dying right here in this place and in this moment for nothing."[66] A very similar confession, attesting to the commonness of such a stance, is found in O'Brien's work: "I did not want to die. Not ever. But certainly not then, not there, not in a wrong war."[67]

And here we arrive to the clue. Intoxication became the manner for survival and keeping psychological balance in the wake of the need to participate in the mission, in the sensibleness of which no one believed. Psychopharmacological self-medication gave the soldiers a feeling of control, even if just over themselves in the conditions, in the wake of which they were usually helpless. The possibility of using drugs was a sign of individualism, the freedom to impact one's own life, in other words, the symbol of power over oneself. In short, drugs became the substitute for everything that was lacking in this war. They restored balance, gave a feeling of solace and temporary peace, they brought back faith and a sense that things are not all that bad. They fulfilled the void emanating with senselessness and pointlessness, hopelessness and helplessness. Drug taking may thus be considered as an existential activity. A truly human thing in a war that was increasingly dehumanizing combatants.

Thirdly, the war in Vietnam was a war of young men, even more important, it was the "youngest" war which the United States fought in its history. Insofar as the average age of the fallen soldiers in the Second World War was twenty-six years, the average in Vietnam was barely nineteen. Kurt Vonnegut marked his story on the Second World War, *Slaughterhouse-Five*, with the telling subtitle *The Children's Crusade*, as the main characters and the victims were mostly young people. "But the average age of the American corpse in my war," Vonnegut wrote in another place, "was an unchildlike twenty-six. In the Vietnam War your average American corpse was six years younger."[68] This was the first American "teenager's war," and youthfulness follows its own course. It is, in short, a time of rebellion, fun, and experimenting with tobacco, alcohol, drugs, and sex. The state called upon young people who were slowly entering adulthood and sent them to the Asian "heart of darkness." It should therefore come as no surprise that most of them reached for intoxicants. This is what their peers who stayed back in the United Sates were doing overtly without having to go through the extreme experiences of combat. Thus, as George Herring noted, "the drug culture that attracted growing numbers of young Americans at home was easily transported to Vietnam."[69]

The hippies took advantage of life, enjoying sex, drugs, and rock 'n' roll. And drugs became, to put it reductively, one of the key elements differentiating the hippie lifestyle. The cultural revolution of the 1960s was taking place under the banner of total liberation, and intoxicants, next to sexual liberation, were the main ways of achieving this individual freedom.[70] Additionally, the use of drugs became a form of political activism, a symbolic gesture of opposition against the war in Vietnam. Thus marijuana and the antiwar movement came to be joined at the hip.[71] Research conducted in 1971 by the National Institute on Drug Abuse revealed that 7 percent of the young people between the ages of twelve to seventeen smoked marijuana on a regular basis, and in 1974 this percentage increased to 12.[72] Among college students, however, the rate of marijuana smokers skyrocketed from 5 percent in 1967 to as much as 51 percent in 1971.[73] Since the young people in the United States were using drugs routinely, why should the situation be any different in Vietnam? Why should the young soldiers differ from the behavior patterns of their peers who remained in the United States? In fact, in the 1960s the consumption of intoxicants among private soldiers increased similarly as in the entire population.[74] The recruits were coming from a society that was much more tolerant of recreational drug use than the previous generations. Additionally, social factors and standards, specifically bans and castigation on the part of the family, that could prevent reaching for intoxicants, did not function in Vietnam. The fact that it was young people who were sent to Southeast Asia resulted in the war introducing, in a dramatic manner, both the present tense and "drug culture" into the discourse. The boys, therefore, took their lifestyles, needs, and desires typical of youth with them to Vietnam. And it is precisely for the huge consumption of drugs, alcohol and the common use of prostitutes, that the war was deemed as the "big rock 'n' roll-war." In the Second World War soldiers placed slogans like "Big Mama" or "Lazy Harriet" on the hoods of cars and jeeps; in Vietnam one found vehicles with the phrases "Purple Haze" or "Window-Pane," which were common names for LSD. Life in Vietnam was passing, in the words of one of the veterans, "in a haze of highs and heat and Jimi Hendrix."[75] Ultimately, the drugs not only strengthened and relaxed the servicemen but also accompanied them at parties.

Overall, the soldiers and veterans regarded society's attitude as greatly unjust. Why was something seen domestically as fashionable and liberating a misdemeanor in Vietnam? Why was taking drugs by soldiers perceived as a pathological phenomenon, while in hippie culture it was viewed as a desirable search for different states of consciousness? One of the veterans accurately expressed his distaste toward this double standard:

> They turned us into murderers and addicts. It wasn't important if this really had to do with you. Were you in Vietnam? Then you had to kill and dope. Simple. I just couldn't fathom how much emotion our drug-taking actually sparked. Hold on, hold on! Just a moment there daddy-o! Before casting the first stone, why don't you visit your son at the campus . . . Go and see how the drugged "promising future of America," who couldn't even move their ass to do something for their country, parties.[76]

Fourthly, the GIs' feeling of alienation and loneliness was drastically increased by the rotation policy. Introduced for the first time during the Korean War, it was aimed at minimizing the negative impact of the war on the soldier's psyche. Since the statistical data stemming from the period of the Second World War rather explicitly showed that psychological breakdowns increase sharply after one year in combat, the infantry service in Vietnam lasted for twelve months and one month longer for Marines.[77] However, as is commonly recognized, the greatest mistake was taking on the principle of the individual commencement of service. Each soldier, when leaving for Vietnam, knew his DEROS (Date Eligible for Return from Overseas), that is, the precise time of his return. Entire divisions were not withdrawn, but individual soldiers were taken out and replaced with new incoming ones, known pejoratively by the old troopers as the FNGs (fucking new guys). Since they were inexperienced, they constituted a threat to the units in which they were stationed. When one was successful at creating a well-integrated team, in which everyone was able to count on each other, some sort of rotation took place. This broke unit cohesion and the feeling of security. The unfledged newbie, who would have to be met and tested to know if he could be trusted, arrived. Until a newbie was accepted, he was treated very impersonally. New soldiers often felt alienated, rejected, and mistrusted by their colleagues. Moreover, adaptation required an adjustment and assimilation to the life of the unit, its customs, and the rules of its operations. The socialization process was taking place, one of the elements of which was the drug use. Smoking marijuana was more of a group rather than of an individual nature. It took on the form of a ritual, more of a public scope than a private and hidden one. Group rituals in the army are of great significance; they facilitate the individual soldiers in dealing with fear and stress in a brotherly atmosphere. Smoking joints also became an important element of initiation for the newcomers. In Oliver Stone's film *Platoon* (1986), drugs appear to play such a role: the transformation of an inexperienced recruit Chris Taylor (played by Charlie Sheen) into a true and hard warrior, who passed his combat christening. Hence intoxicants were of key socializing and ritual value. Even without the peer pressure, the new soldiers did seek help in order to survive this psychologically difficult period. Chris writes letters "from hell" to his grandmother, in which he complains about the anonymity. No one has even asked for his name yet. Most of the FNGs felt the same way as Chris— exchangeable and exchanged elements of the system, not very important gear wheels in the superpower's war machine.

Fifthly, Vietnam was an "intoxicating paradise," where drugs were common and accessible, dirt cheap, and of very good quality. The availability of psychoactive substances is presented in table 10.2. One can say that the soldiers took drugs because they were more easily available than alcohol, which could legally be purchased at the age of twenty-one. And although most of the recruits were between the ages of eighteen to twenty, the armed forces placed even further limitations on its consumption. An interesting correlation was observed: those who numbed themselves with alcohol did not use opiates, while those who took drugs did not abuse alcohol. This was a tendency other than the phenomena observed in civilian life, where alcoholics much more

Table 10.2 **Availability of drugs in Vietnam (in percent)**[*]

Marijuana:		
Always available	70	
Usually or always	92	
Half of unit (or more) used it regularly	71	
Heroin:		
Available in own unit	76	
Within an hour	98	

	Most common[**]	Available in own unit[***]
Marijuana	81	91
Heroin	78	92
Amphetamine	14	45
Opium	15	40
Barbiturates	7	31
Hallucinogens	3	28
Cocaine	4	15

[*] A general sample of 451 Vietnam veterans

[**] In answer to "What were the drugs most commonly used in your unit?"

[***] In answer to both "What were the drugs most commonly used in your unit?" and "What other drugs did you see or hear about being used in your unit?"

Source: Lee N. Robins, *The Vietnam Drug User Returns: Final Report* (Washington, DC: Special Action Office for Drug Abuse Prevention, 1974), p. 26.

 willingly also reach for drugs compared with abstainers. In Vietnam, drugs were so common that they were treated like cigarettes.[78] A gram of pure heroin could be purchased for two dollars, meaning that it was at least fifty times less expensive than it was in the United States.[79] In 1967 opium cost one dollar per vile, while morphine was five dollars. Binoctal, an addictive French medication, containing amobarbital and secobarbital sodium, used medically as a headache reliever, could be easily purchased from Vietnamese children and at local pharmacies: twenty tablets for one dollar.[80]

Egil Krogh reminisced when, while visiting one of the American bases in Vietnam, he said to those gathered:

Post war

"Gentlemen, I'm here from the White House to find out about the drug problem." The soldier looks up at me, and he takes a deep toke and says, "And I'm from Mars, man." I never forget that. But I said,

"No, really, I'm from the White House. What's available?" And he said, "You want pot? You want shit? Whatever you want, just go down there." I went to thirteen firebases ... and the experience was replicated.[81]

In his book *The Tarnished Shield*, Colonel George Walton cites Senior Master Sergeant Ernest R. Davis, who reported on the horrid drug situation: "The further north you go in Vietnam, the more drugs there are. Some of the forward fire bases are among the worst."[82] The stuff could be scored at stands along the road to Saigon. On the way to the main American base in Long Binh, they could be purchased in restaurants, brothels, newspaper stands, ice cream sellers, in a word—everywhere.[83] Since Vietnam was a drug paradise, it was naive to expect that the soldiers would not want to try them.

Sixthly, the soldiers also reached for intoxicants and experimented with medications because they simply had not much else to do. They did drugs to kill the utter boredom and monotony. One of the American war correspondents, who in January of 1971 visited the divisions in Vietnam, noticed:

> The most persistent enemy a U.S. soldier faces in South Vietnam these days is not the Communists—it seems to be boredom. . . . In this strange state of listlessness, commanders face new problems: a sharp drop in troop morale, increased use of drugs, and alcohol, touchy relations between black soldiers and white.[84]

Boredom, in fact, became one of the characteristics of modern war in general, and it accompanied the combatants during the earlier conflicts to almost the same extent as it did the soldiers in Vietnam. In writing about the First World War, Ernst Jünger noted: "Worse still was the boredom, which is still more enervating for the soldier than the proximity of death."[85] The topic of severe and unbearable monotony appeared in many of the veterans' accounts. Caputo did not hide his surprise caused by a confrontation with the reality of war. He thought that, of all things, in Vietnam he would not have time to read books, while it turned out that "nine-tenths of war is waiting around for the remaining one-tenth to happen."[86] Sheer boredom drove servicemen mad; one veteran confessed, "It was so terrible there, so boring. That was the worst part—every day was just like the one before. The only difference was maybe today would be wetter than yesterday."[87] O'Brien describes the fury caused by boredom in a very moving manner:

> I remember the monotony. . . . Even in the deep bush, where you could die any number of ways, the war was nakedly and aggressively boring.

But it was a strange boredom. It was boredom with a twist, the kind of
boredom that caused stomach disorders. . . . You'd try to relax. You'd
uncurl your fists, and let your thoughts go. Well, you'd think, this isn't
so bad. And right then you'd hear gunfire behind you and your nuts
would fly up into your throat and you'd be squealing pig squeals. That
kind of boredom.[88]

Every third veteran surveyed by Lee Robins confirmed that he did not have
much to do at all, and his tasks were deathly boring.[89] In order to kill the monotony of life in the camp, the soldiers thought up the most diverse games: contests
involving drinking, smoking, or experimenting with medications. Boredom
had a very negative impact on servicemen, as not being occupied by anything
serious, they had too much time to think and brood. They contemplated the
nonsense of the war and their role in a conflict with no clear purpose. It led to
greater depression and weakened the will to fight. It undermined the morale of
the troops. Boredom favored reflection, which could also produce a feeling of
guilt over the death of friends or civilians. Already during the "dirty war," the
French soldiers suffered from a spiritual disease that they called *la cafard* and
which the Americans later became victims too. It manifested, Caputo recalls,
as "occasional fits of depression combined with an unconquerable fatigue that
made the simplest tasks, like shaving or cleaning a rifle, seem enormous. Its
causes were obscure, but they had something to do with the unremitting heat,
the lack of action, and the long days of staring at that alien landscape."[90]

It is known that in periods of lesser activity on the battlefield, the number
of soldiers experiencing psychological difficulties rises. This phenomenon was
also noted in Vietnam. In the years 1965–1970, the number of patients with
neuropsychiatric symptoms doubled. In 1970 twenty-four cases were noted
for 1,000 soldiers, in comparison with the previous ratio for the American
army which was 15.4.[91] The situation would be much more grim had it not been
for the soothing means that the soldiers "treated" themselves with. Intoxicants
allowed the negative thoughts to be muffled, the damaged psyche to be bri-
dled. Drugs were, to a certain extent, a response to *la cafard*. They killed time
in expectancy of the return to the "world," as soldiers described the United
States, a home, or in a wider sense, to everything that was not the damned
Vietnam.

Seventhly then, drugs and pharmaceuticals limited the negative impact of
the conflict on the psyche of young soldiers, many of whom got high to numb
the severe experiences and memories of the atrocities of war. And there was
quite a lot to suppress. The Americans were unscrupulous in achieving their
undefined strategic objective: they deployed carpet bombing carried out by
B-52 bombers, napalm, and search and destroy tactics. Since the character of

the war was uniquely asymmetric, so that it was extremely difficult to differentiate the Vietcong guerrillas from the population, civilians were killed on a mass scale. And as David Grossman tells us, the killing is always traumatic, but "when you have to do it not from twenty thousand feet but up close where you can watch them die, the horror appears to transcend description or understanding."[92] According to the previously cited research by John Helmer, 37 percent of the soldiers took drugs "to forget the killing and relieve the pressure."[93]

On the other hand, the opponent was just as ruthless. Guerrilla warfare tactics, booby traps, tunnel warfare, and a sudden sniper firing gathered a bloody crop among Americans. During the Second World War and the Korean War, traps resulted in 3 to 4 percent of American casualties, while in Vietnam booby traps and land mines, massacring the human body in an especially cruel and repulsive manner, were responsible for 11 percent of the casualties and 17 percent of the injured soldiers.[94] The infamous booby traps not only brought death and severe injuries but were also a tremendous fear factor. A soldier on patrol would suddenly sink into the ground, getting wounded or killed by the hidden blades; he could step on a mine or hook the cable that activated explosives hidden in the treetops. In short, he could vanish in a moment. Very often the sight of what remained of their killed colleagues was the most traumatic life experience. One had to become indifferent, not to go crazy. A common way of dealing with the all-embracing death and destruction was the saying, "It don't mean nothin," yet the gruesome images remained in the memory and kept coming back in a pestering way. O'Brien describes one such distressing story:

> This one wakes me up. In the mountains that day, I watched Lemon turn sideways. He laughed and said something to Rat Kiley. Then he took a peculiar half step, moving from shade into bright sunlight, and the booby-trapped 105 round blew him into a tree. The parts were just hanging there, so Dave Jensen and I were ordered to shinny up and peel him off. I remember the white bone of an arm. I remember pieces of skin and something wet and yellow that must've been the intestines. The gore was horrible, and stays with me. But what wakes me up twenty years later is David Jensen singing "Lemon Tree" as we threw down the parts.[95]

Given such horrific scenes, intoxication was a common attempt to erase haunting and traumatic images. Drugs, in a word, played, as Sigmund Freud would put it, a typical function of drowning soldiers' sorrows.[96]

Additionally, the war was a forced and accelerated lesson in growing up for the young soldiers. During a war a man "ages" much faster than as a civilian. "Most of all," writes Caputo, "we learned about death at an age when it is common to think of oneself as immortal. Everyone loses that illusion eventually, but in civilian life it is lost in installments over the years. We lost it all at once and, in the span of months, passed from boyhood through manhood to a premature middle age."[97] Herr shares a similar thought with readers, by writing about his experience from the Tet Offensive period: "I realized later that, however childish I might remain, actual youth had been pressed out of me in just the three days that it took me to cross the sixty miles between Can Tho and Saigon."[98] Can one be surprised that such an unnatural and dramatically accelerated growing up was a serious problem, which the soldiers tried to bridle with the help of alcohol and drugs? Can one be surprised that they sought to slow down the process, that they wished to remain boys as their peers back in their home country? Of course, the fact that they could succeed in doing so was a great illusion, but they had to try, and this is something that needs to be understood. Intoxicants were an intrinsic part of this attempt.

Eighthly, pharmacology was a way of dealing with the soldiers' ever-present and biggest enemies: stress, fear, and anxiety. Many soldiers reached for drugs as a means to calm their frayed nerves, especially after difficult skirmishes. During a battle adrenaline and tension keep the fighting men at the highest stages of alertness, so that the negative impact of stress is usually not visible until afterward. One of the infantry soldiers recalled: "We only used [drugs] after we got back from a mission, particularly if it was a hard one. Sometimes we'd just sit under a tree, smoke dope and cry. It was a good way to unwind; a wonderful anesthetic and escape."[99]

One veteran, Yoshia Chee, remembered that it was in Vietnam that for the first time in his life he felt real, unique anxiety, totally different than just average fear. He was not afraid that he could be killed or maimed, but, he recalls, "I had fear of something. I can't describe it. It's like some people get in elevators. It was like a phobia. A phobia for the whole thing, the whole country."[100] How did Chee deal with this overwhelming, previously unknown severe fear? "What I decided to do was completely obliterate my brain the best way I knew how, which was opium. When I wanted to put away the war, opium was the best thing in the world."[101]

Many young men, who in the early stages of the war enlisted to Vietnam, were "intoxicated" with the Hollywood images and myths along the lines of John Wayne and Audie Murphy, who in their movies idealized, and even sanctified, war as the most noble attempt at American patriotism. Soldiers were apprehensive whether they would disappoint. Thus, "[t]hey carried their reputations. They carried the soldier's greatest fear, which was the fear of blushing."[102] In a situation of threat, the hormones secreted by the adrenal cortex cause an entire range of unforeseen reactions which is called the "fight-or-flight response." In fact, the universal topic, which has for centuries been entwined in the memoirs and the accounts of war veterans, is not so much the fear of death, pain, disability, or killing, as the fear of weakness, not performing according to expectations, the fear that one can chicken out, or be incapable giving one's all. Ultimately, fear can be brought down to a test of manhood or, to a wider extent, of humanity. Caputo captured this timeless thought in soldiers' literature concisely and accurately: "I felt the worst fear of all: the fear of fear."[103] In the context of Vietnam, it was inconceivably difficult to meet the idealist models of heroism created by the earlier generation, for they sounded like platitudes. Drugs were the ideal way to regain control over one's nerves, to combat fear and anxiety, and to maintain a psychological balance. In a word, they were medicine for the shaken soldier's soul. In many cases they helped dispel the fear and take on the fight, rather than opting for flight.

Ninthly, the soldiers took drugs for the same reason the army gave them amphetamine stimulants, namely, in order to strengthen their body and increase efficiency during the mission. What was interesting, smoking a joint to relax can be also perceived in these categories of performance enhancement, as Jeremy Kuzmarov, quoting Dr. Morris Stanton, writes, "Marihuana and some other illicit drugs may help certain individuals function on the job by assisting them in maintaining an adequate psychological adjustment while under the stresses of a combat environment and separation from home."[104] Other doctors in the 1970s were of the same opinion, arguing for the beneficial impact of marijuana on the psyches of soldiers, which translated into their combat capabilities. What is more, at times smoking a joint between patrols allowed soldiers to continue their task altogether.

Finally, some of the servicemen using and abusing drugs in Vietnam did so before they even made it to the war. From Lee Robins's research it follows that before leaving for Southeast Asia, 47 percent of the soldiers had contact with drugs, mainly with marijuana; however, only 1 percent used them on a regular basis.[105] War did not change much if they were already addicted at home. One might assume that going to war and participating in battles would disrupt the use of intoxicants; however, Vietnam was different. As we know, Americans had much easier access to less expensive and very good quality drugs in Indochina than they did at home. Therefore, almost everyone who had some sort of contact with intoxicants before leaving also used them in Vietnam.[106] Table 10.3 lists the factors that Robins's respondents indicated when answering the question on the purpose of taking drugs in Vietnam.

In summarizing this analysis of the reasons that induced the combatants to use and abuse intoxicating substances, one can cite Sigmund Freud's general diagnosis. Hence soldiers could have explained that during the Vietnam War: "The life imposed on us is too hard for us to bear: it brings too much pain,

Table 10.3 **Reasons for using drugs among American servicemen in Vietnam (in percent)**[*]

	Spontaneous	*Agreed when asked*	*Total agreed*
To get a high	41	47	88
More tolerant of army rules and regulations	13	61	74
Less homesick and lonely	12	**	–
Less bored	10	72	82
Less depressed	9	64	73
To sleep better	9	**	–
Made time seem to pass quickly	7	66	73
Improved social skills: patience, sensitivity, communication	7	**	–
Less fearful	6	40	46
Fitted in better with other soldiers	3	43	46

[*] A general sample of 196 of Vietnam veterans
** Not asked specifically

Source: Lee N. Robins, *The Vietnam Drug User Returns. Final Report* (Washington, DC: Special Action Office for Drug Abuse Prevention, 1974), p. 32.

too many disappointments, too many insoluble problems. If we are to endure it, we cannot do without palliative measures. As Theodor Fontane told us, it is impossible without additional help."[107]

The Government Steps In

On May 27, 1971, two Republican congressmen, Morgan F. Murphy and Robert H. Steele presented an influential report "The World Heroin Problem" to the House Committee on Foreign Affairs. Although their estimates, which assumed that 25,000–37,000 soldiers serving in Vietnam were addicted to heroin, resembled the aforementioned statistics gathered earlier by military doctors, the public exposure of these figures caused a media frenzy and an atmosphere of moral panic. In a memorandum to Secretary of Defense Melvin R. Laird, President Nixon called for the urgent need to establish a program identifying soldiers who had a problem with drugs. The goal was "to maintain military readiness by removing incapacitated servicemen from the field, if necessary, in order to provide rehabilitation. Veterans who are identified as addicted to opiates should undergo treatment and not simply be released into our cities."[108] Because the media coverage created general anxiety in society, President Nixon felt obliged to take a firm response. In his famous special message to Congress on June 17, 1971, he asserted that the "public enemy number one in the United States is drug abuse" and announced measures for "a full-scale attack on the problem."[109] Thus the president declared the "war on drugs." Nixon acknowledged, "While by no means a major part of the American narcotics problem, an especially disheartening aspect of that problem involves those of our men in Vietnam who have used drugs."[110] However, apart from domestic policing and treatment programs, the core initial measures of the antidrug abuse efforts were the screening of all servicemen returning from Indochina, and if necessary, their detoxification and adequate drug and psychological treatment programs. This action was thought essential to prevent the epidemic of addiction spreading across the United States. With the Vietnamization of the war and the gradual withdrawal of the American troops, nearly 1,000 soldiers returned home every day. Assuming that up to 25 percent of them were heroin addicts, there was a serious threat to American society. Preventive measures were therefore needed because it was feared that veterans would commit crimes to get heroin and to bring about a similar intoxicating effect experienced in Vietnam, since the drug available in the United States was not only much more expensive than in Indochina but also much weaker and much less pure. Thus Nixon warned that "a habit which costs five dollars a day to maintain in Vietnam can cost one hundred dollars a day to maintain in the United States, and those who continue to use heroin slip into the twilight world of crime, bad drugs, and all too often a premature death."[111] This was not only a gross exaggeration but also a harmful one as the president frightened the society not with a threat (a real danger) but with a risk (a probable danger). He presented the risk as if it was a threat. Thus, in the public mind, the fear of an addicted veteran returning home and endangering an orderly civilian world was created. A new "other" was born.

To thwart this risk, preventive actions were required to create a sort of *cordon sanitaire*. Nixon demanded from the Secretary of Defense Laird swift action for the identification and detoxification of drug-using servicemen departing from Vietnam.[112] The military responded promptly, and in mid-July 1971 the program, under the grotesque name "Operation Golden Flow," was launched. It required compulsory urine tests for the presence of heroin of all American servicemen before leaving Vietnam. Only those who tested negative could fly back home. Those found positive had to undergo a compulsory five- or seven-day methadone detoxification.

As new technologies allowed for assembly-line-like testing, in late 1971 army laboratories in Vietnam could analyze up to 7,500 urine samples a day. According to a report by Jerome Jaffe, the director of the newly established Special Action Office for Drug Abuse Prevention (SAODAP), by September 1971 as many as 92,096 soldiers were examined and 4,788 (5.2 percent) tested positive for heroin. The idea which guided Jaffe was that the threats of a delayed return home, dishonorable discharge, and court-martial were highly effective measures of deterrence.[113] In March 1972 the number of servicemen testing positive fell to less than 2 percent. The urinalysis, however, was not a credible indicator of heroin abuse. Firstly, it only showed whether soldiers had taken it in the five days prior to analysis. Because servicemen knew the exact date of their testing, they could stop taking the drug and get negative results. Therefore, almost 93 percent of soldiers who would normally be classified as addicts were able to temporarily give up taking heroin during their final days in Vietnam. Secondly, the research carried out by Lee N. Robins of Washington University in St. Louis on a sample group of veterans showed that 3 percent of soldiers who tested positive claimed that they had not taken heroin and 3 percent of those who tested negative admitted using the drug. One method of distorting results was to get heavily drunk before the urinalysis; another was submitting a sample of pure urine bought on a "black market for clean urine," which developed among soldiers. Overall, it seems that the idea behind Golden Flow was less to help addicted soldiers and more to clear the consciences of politicians and the military, and solve an imagined and exaggerated national emergency.

Soldiers who passed the second test could return to the United States, but those who tested positive twice in a row (1,000–2,000 cases a month) were processed for dishonorable discharge and then sent back home.[114] Such a discharge often worsened their drug problem, especially because only 5 percent of those vets who needed professional assistance were given any medical treatment. For many, a true readjustment to civilian life proved impossible, which only further deepened their drug habit. The hell of Vietnam was often replaced by a hell of rejection, lack of understanding, condemnation, stress disorders, in a phrase—by the misery of the inability to get back to "normal" life in a society that did not, and did not want to, understand their experience and condition.

The Myth of the Addicted Army

The Vietnam War called the American myth into question, yet it also created a new one. The drug problem gave rise to the myth of a weak and degenerated, addicted American army. According to the widespread opinion, drugs made most soldiers unfit for combat, hampered units' fighting power, broke down the military discipline, destroyed the troops' morale, and resulted in the collapse of the entire war effort. A popular view of the "junkie army," which was persistently reinforced by gloomy press reports and politicians' public appearances, implied that drugs and addiction were among the main reasons to be blamed for the American inability to win the war.

Myriad hyperbole and false stories emerged about the use of intoxicants in Vietnam. Jeremy Kuzmarov traced their spuriousness and deconstructed "the myth of the addicted army"—the army that allegedly lacked a fighting spirit and combat effectiveness. The myth was invented by John Steinbeck IV, the son of the famous writer, who upon his return from Vietnam, where he served as a war correspondent, published an article entitled "The Importance of Being Stoned in Vietnam" in the January 1968 issue of the *Washingtonian* magazine. Kuzmarov notes that "by his own admission, Steinbeck overdramatized the nature of drug abuse in Vietnam for political purposes," claiming, for example, that 75 percent of soldiers got high regularly.[115]

The media quickly struck this hysteric tone and fostered the claim so much that it reached its absurd and apocalyptic peak. For example, a headline in the *U.S. News and World Report* read: "Marijuana—The Other Enemy in Vietnam." On May 24, 1971, *Newsweek* published a photo of a syringe hitting a soldier's helmet.[116] In the same issue of *Newsweek*, Stewart Alsop presented emotional and populist arguments, reporting that "the drug epidemic" was "horrifying . . . worse even than My Lai."[117] And *Newsweek*'s cover of July 5, 1971 featured an image of a civilian junkie shooting up heroin and the blazing headline: "The Heroin Plague: What Can Be Done?" The lead story described the spread of addiction from "the back alleys of Long Binh and Saigon" to "Middle-American towns and neighborhoods."[118] The authors exaggeratedly demonstrated that

> heroin has exploded on us like an atom bomb. Ten years ago, even three years ago, heroin was a loser's drug, an aberration afflicting the blacks and long-haired minorities. Now all this has changed. Nice Jewish boys are coming out of the woodwork as well as Mormon kids, Japanese Americans and all other exemplars of hard-working middle-class ideals.[119]

The parallel was as inappropriate as that sometimes drawn by antiwar activists between the My Lai massacre and the Nazi atrocities.[120] Without common-sense limits, the media expanded the "drug epidemic" in the military so much that it was matched up to the worse "medieval plagues." These hyperbolic analogies were accompanied by unreliable statistics equating substance "use" with "abuse." Thus the category of "addict soldiers" usually encompassed those who merely tried drugs and never turned into habitual users.

The media and politicians resorted to the rhetoric that closely resembled the language of the cocaine panic in Britain during the First World War, when cocaine was perceived as a weapon used by the Germans to undermine British combat performance. Half a century later, heroin was seen as the vile weapon used by the communists to disintegrate American units in Vietnam. In November 1967 Walter Cronkite, the editor and host of the *CBS Evening News*, introduced the report by correspondent John Laurence with a comment that the "Communists are battling American troops not only with fire power, but with drugs."[121]

The myth of the addicted army, as Kuzmarov aptly remarks, turned "attention away from the escalation of American atrocities and the ravaging of the Vietnamese countryside."[122] Long before Kuzmarov, however, a prominent psychiatrist Thomas Szasz, fought against the myth of the addicted army by attempting to refute the ridiculous accusations that junkie veterans returning home posed a vital threat to public safety and national security. In his pursuit to unlock the truth, Szasz claimed that soldiers who abused drugs were made scapegoats for the total fiasco of the American strategy in Vietnam and were turned into national antiheroes of the "pharmacological Gulf of Tonkin." He noted:

> Like the Germans after World War I who claimed that their troops were stabbed in the back by pacifists and other "unpatriotic elements" at home, we claim that our troops are being stabbed in the back by heroin and the pushers responsible for supplying it to them. As we deescalate against the "Vietcong," we will escalate against heroin. No doubt we shall find it easier to control Americans who shoot heroin than Vietnamese who shoot Americans.[123]

As Szasz saw it, Nixon's war on drugs was a curveball to distract public attention from the United States' strategic failure in Vietnam.

He was right; the truth was far more different from the popular view. As an army-commissioned survey revealed, even soldiers who were addicted to heroin could conduct their normal duties. Drug taking was not an obstacle to fighting efficiency, and intoxication did not render troops inoperable.[124] Michael Herr described the siege of Khe Sanh of January–July 1968, during which GIs would voluntarily quit smoking marijuana because they did not want to risk their lives.[125] There is plenty of evidence for such self-disciplining behavior. Soldiers usually reached for drugs in situations where it was not too risky to get intoxicated: in the rear, after the completion of a mission, or in between patrols. They did not carelessly go into action on drugs; that would go against the natural instinct of self-preservation. As the noted social psychologist Lieutenant Colonel Larry H. Ingrahm observed:

> Soldiers are not fools. They know the dangers of working around heavy equipment or going into combat unable to function. Individuals who threaten the lives of others are oftentimes violently excluded from the combat group. In Vietnam, during 1970–1971, there were performance problems which resulted from heroin *withdrawal*, but not from heroin addiction per se.[126]

Less effective soldiering might indeed be induced not so much by drug usage, but by drug withdrawal and its poignant psychophysical symptoms. To sum up, contrary to the popular view, drug use did not, overall, seriously interfere with combat performance.

A Painful Homecoming and "Othering" of Veterans

Following David Campbell's postmodern analysis of foreign policy, the myth of the addicted army can be perceived in the context of the formulation and implementation of American foreign policy. In his renowned book *Writing Security*, Campbell demonstrated how national identity is continuously constructed by the perception of threat.[127] Foreign policy becomes a grand nonobjective discourse on the dangers posed by "aliens" or "others." As the title of his book implies, security is "written," meaning it is continuously constructed and created, rather than resulting from objective, fixed, and unchangeable factors. The politicians and influence groups who shape public opinion choose some aspects of reality and describe them as dangerous threats to the state and society's security. For Campbell, the aim of national security strategy is first and foremost to define and uphold the identity of a state and its nation. And identity is always relational—it is created through establishing borders between "us" and "them" (i.e., other or stranger). The perception and interpretation of specific factors, groups, and phenomena in terms of threat help highlight the hallmarks of a society and reinforce the feeling of belonging, identification, attachment, and solidarity.

Post

Interpreted from Campbell's perspective, American soldiers returning from Vietnam were "othered" by politicians and society. Because the popular image presented them as excessive drug abusers, they were unjustly labeled as potential disturbers of the social order. The veterans were portrayed as a threat to American identity and to society's safety. The media and politicians exposed this atmosphere of fear with President Nixon at the forefront. The comparison of drug addiction to a plague, to a fatal contagious disease that develops like a cancer, debilitates armed forces, and then "invades homes and threatens our children" was useful for constructing the image of the hostile other and heightened the sense of insecurity. The use of metaphors of poison or disease has always been a common means of differentiating between us and them. Thus the border was drawn between normal, healthy Americans and unhealthy, filthy drug users.[128] A similar demarcation was also made between the forces of modernity and nonmodernity.

Post

By its nature addiction can be seen as nonmodern, in the sense that addicts are cut off from their society and alienated from the mainstream of community activities.[129] Strong addiction is the very negation of modernity as it turns users into economically unproductive and socially dysfunctional individuals. Substance abuse is nonmodern also because it is irrational in a sense that by providing artificial and inauthentic pleasures, it detaches the person from reality. Pleasures derived from drugs go beyond the category of delight allowed by law and society. By depriving people of free will, addiction undermines the essence of individual freedom that is one of the pillars of American identity. While modernity frees people from the old social, economic, customary, and mental limitations, drugs enslave them in a novel and toxic way. Heavy addiction degrades, consumes, and can turn life into a painful experience, all of which conflicts with the American credo that praises pragmatism, productivity, in-group solidarity, and individual freedom.

Looking on the Vietnam veteran as the other, as a potential threat to American identity, significantly contributed to the development of the "post-Vietnam syndrome," because those men who had risked their lives for the defense of American values, on their return home were considered a severe challenge to Americanness. Young boys, who had been called for service in a hostile Southeast Asia and who turned to drugs to stay sane and to deal with the reality of a truly terrible war, were portrayed as frightening addicts. They were stigmatized and victimized by politicians, the media, and society. In his book *The Drugged Nation* (1973), John Finlator, a former agent of Federal Bureau of Narcotics, expressed a popular sentiment of the day—the fear of the highly destructive drug plague that would flood America. He warned in an utterly hysterical tone: "The junkman has descended on us like the Vandals upon Rome . . . assaulting an unsuspecting and unprepared people." Soldiers returning from Vietnam were perceived as the Vandals who endangered the very spirit of America—in effect, another Rome.[130] It was feared, as President Nixon expressed directly in June 1971, that junkie veterans would turn to "Vandal violence," exacerbating domestic crime rates and disorder.

Of course, the apocalyptic visions were not fulfilled. However, unlike the myth of the addicted army, the problem of drug abuse among veterans was not a fabrication, although it was vastly overstated. The image of a maladjusted addicted veteran lived through the 1990s largely due to pop culture and movies in particular, for example the Oliver Stone film *Born on the Fourth of July* (1989), which exaggerated the scale of addiction by showing vets doing drugs in the back of the veterans' center. The American withdrawal from Vietnam did not mark the end of the drug problem as heroin arrived in America along with the returning soldiers. Many brought a stash of drugs with them, and many had sent some home in advance. For example, one veteran confessed that a year before his date of return he smuggled opiates in a stereo set sent to his father in the United States. Soldiers arranged special transfers of heroin from Vietnam, which they shared after homecoming.[131] New York City Mayor's Office for Veterans Action estimated that in 1971 between 30,000 and 45,000 Vietnam veteran heroin addicts lived in the city.[132]

A survey on soldiers who returned from Indochina in September 1971, which was commissioned by SAODAP and conducted by a team led by Lee Robins, revealed, however, that the majority of interviewees were not habitual users. The results of Robins's survey, presented here in table 10.4, were startling: 43 percent of servicemen reported having consumed drugs in Vietnam but only 10 percent after their return. This meant that the level of drug use dropped to its pre-Vietnam level. Many soldiers had quit by the time they left for home: 75 percent of those who had used drugs before departing for Vietnam and continued using them, and 80 percent of those who used drugs for the first time in Vietnam. "More than 60 percent of detected addicts stopped all narcotic use as they left Vietnam and did not resume after their return to the United States."[133] These findings were so astonishing and so severely undermined the prevalent view that some commentators ridiculously assumed that they had been counterfeited at the request of the authorities. The truth, however, is that drug use in Vietnam was contextual—it resulted from the extreme conditions and the nature of the combat, and when the factors that forced servicemen to take drugs ceased to operate, most of them gave up their habit. An additional reason for a high rate of remission was that soldiers were generally averse to the intravenous application of heroin, so if they wanted to stick with "hitting the stuff," they would have to forget about smoking heroin doobs and inject instead. Operation Golden Flow also contributed to this effect of unexpected remission because the threats of a delayed return home, dishonorable

Table 10.4 **Drug consumption by the American soldiers in three time periods (in percent)**[*]

	Since Return	*In Vietnam*	*Before Vietnam*
Any drug use	10	43	11
Any heroin use	7	34	2
Drugs more than weekly for a month or more	4	27	1
Addicted to drugs at any period	1	20	<0.5
Urine positive for drugs	1	10.5	–

[*] General interview sample of 451 Vietnam veterans

Source: Lee N. Robins, Darlene H. Davis, and David N. Nurco, "How Permanent Was Vietnam Drug Addiction?," *American Journal of Public Health*, vol. 64, Supplement (1974), p. 39.

discharge, and court-martial seemed to be effective deterrent measures for some soldiers.

Commenting on this paradoxical tendency in drug use, Richard Davenport-Hines wrote that "the fact that U.S. servicemen had experimented with heroin as a result of alcohol and marijuana prohibition, voluntarily renounced its use and did not relapse undermined most assumptions of U.S. drug policy."[134] It also punctured the myth of the veteran as a dangerous other. The most important conclusion of Robins's findings, I think, is that there was nothing exceptionally distressing about the homecoming "junkie soldiers" that the Americans should fear.

Nonetheless, intoxication by alcohol and drugs, such as heroin and marijuana, became inherent in the lives of some veterans, particularly those who suffered from PTSD. Although they managed to survive combat, they were still the victims of war. And this is precisely how Ron Kovic perceived himself and his fellow men—war did not kill them in Vietnam but was slowly consuming them back in America. Jonathan Shay tells a moving story of a military medic nicknamed "Doc." He enlisted in 1964, arrived in Vietnam in July 1967, and was assigned to the Military Assistance Command as a medical advisor based in Hue City. During the Tet Offensive, Doc lost his close friends and despite great commitment did not manage to save the lives of many wounded soldiers. It was then that he witnessed a horrific event that caused his trauma. A Vietcong sniper hit him and the captain he was standing next to. Doc's face was splashed with blood squirting from the captain's severed neck arteries. Despite being wounded himself, he refused to be evacuated and continued to dress the heavily injured men. Since then Doc suffered from nightmares full of mutilated bodies. The Tet Offensive was a turning point not only in the war but also in his life. Before leaving for Vietnam, he did not drink or use drugs. After the Tet Offensive, to escape painful and tormenting memories, he started abusing alcohol, marijuana, and heroin. At the moment of his honorable discharge in June 1969, he was an alcoholic and a regular heroin user. The army enlisted a healthy young man and discharged a sick addict suffering from PTSD who would hold and lose over fifty menial jobs in twenty years and get married three times. PTSD and self-medication with alcohol, heroin, and cocaine ruined Doc's life. Similar was the experience of many other Vietnam vets who at all costs tried to forget the hell they went through in Indochina. In the pursuit of oblivion, 45.6 percent used alcohol while 8.5 percent took drugs. If a veteran had PTSD, these rates were, however, higher—73.8 percent and 11.3 percent respectively.[135] For Doc, detox and withdrawal of intoxicants always meant a resurgence of PTSD symptoms. Eventually, he entered a specialized outpatient combat PTSD program, managed to overcome his addictions, and ultimately started regaining control over his mental disorder. Everything seemed to be on the right track until an ill-fated day in the early 1990s. After the Department of Veterans Affairs (VA) rejected his claim for a disability pension for combat PTSD, he fatally overdosed on heroin. The coroner ruled the death accidental, but Jonathan Shay, Doc's doctor and therapist, believes that he killed himself by intentionally overdosing on heroin "in despair, anger, and humiliation after the value of his service was—in his eyes—'officially' rejected by the VA."[136] His understanding of "what's right" was ruthlessly abused.

11

The Red Army in Afghanistan and the Problem of Drug Addiction

> Before they went to Afghanistan, they were just normal guys. They
> drank, like everybody else, but that was all. They learned that in
> Afghanistan, life was impossible without drugs. They needed them
> there because of the heat and because they had to carry 40 kilos up
> and down the hills. Then there was the fear—drugs helped with that.
> —Edi, heroin-addicted Afghan veteran quoted in
> Mark Galeotti, *Afghanistan: The Soviet Union's Last War*

Soviet Vietnam

Not only Americans in Indochina but also Russians in Central Asia learned what a tragic experience, both in individual and collective terms, it is to engage in combat with an asymmetric adversary waging a people's war in an extremely difficult terrain. The Soviet intervention in Afghanistan (1979–1989) became the "Soviet Vietnam." It was also the most pharmacological war in Russian military history to date, as soldiers used drugs on a rampant scale.

Both the United States in Vietnam and the Soviet Union in Afghanistan hoped for a speedy and final victory. Meanwhile, despite passing years, mounting costs, and growing numbers of casualties, the victory still remained elusive. The mujahideen, like Vietcong militants, adopted the tactics of prolonged conflict, using time against the invaders. Fighting on their own territory, they employed asymmetrical methods, characteristic of guerrilla operations. They would carry out hit-and-run attacks: avoiding direct confrontation with regular Soviet troops and operating from ambush in small groups.[1] Just like in the case of Vietnam, the techno-war, that is, escalating operations with the use of ever increasing numbers of weapons systems, proved not only ineffective but also resulted in huge damages and losses among civilians.

Insofar as Americans permitted for great openness in reporting on their operations in Indochina, Russians completely censored the conflict in Afghanistan. The control of information extended further than just the media to encompass also soldiers and veterans, who were not allowed to describe what they had experienced and seen. For many years the society was kept in the dark as to the number of Soviet servicemen killed in Afghanistan. Eventually, by the time the Soviet Union pulled all its troops out of Afghanistan, Soviet casualties had risen to 13,833 dead.[2] Approximately 50,000 soldiers suffered injuries while 11,600 were invalided.[3]

Becoming mired in an unpopular war, withdrawing from which would be equivalent to a damaging blow to prestige and reputation, the elusive adversary difficult to tell apart from the civilian population, the lack of clear distinction between the front line and the hinterland, huge problems related to reconnaissance and scouting in harsh terrain, difficult combat conditions, ruined esprit de corps, high economic costs, society's undermined confidence in authorities, and disgraceful treatment of veterans by the state and society alike are only some of the most prominent common characteristics of American Vietnam and Soviet Afghanistan.

American army privates and officers alike kept asking both the politicians and the society: "Why did you order us to fight in Vietnam?" Soviet soldiers, although most often they were careful not to voice their doubts, also wondered: "Why did you send us to Afghanistan?" After the war, a private from a grenadier regiment spoke out: "Apparently my friend died for nothing, and I might have died for nothing too."[4] Veterans of wars in Vietnam and Afghanistan were in fact soul mates; they could also count on greater mutual understanding than on understanding on the part of their own families, society, and politicians. Some of them had an opportunity to meet when a small group of Afghan war veterans took part in therapeutic programs and conferences in the United States, organized in the frames of a project financed by American authorities.[5] In 1989 the *New York Times* published Peter Mahoney's account of meetings and conversations with veterans of the Afghan war:

> Each time, after an initial denial, Sergei responded to a Vietnam story of mine with a parallel story of his own: about drugs, about wanting revenge on the enemy, about not being able to tell the enemy from the local population and beginning to regard everyone as the enemy. It is as we expected. Their war was our war, their experience our experience.[6]

Yuri Khlusov, who served in Afghanistan from May 1980 until November 1981, confessed:

> It seems to me that there are many similarities between the Afghan and the Vietnamese wars. During both wars people in the home country were living in a time of peace, but soldiers were dying. I believe that I could find a lot to talk about with an American veteran of Vietnam, and I think he would too.[7]

Seeking consolation in drugs would undoubtedly be one shared topics. In this context, Lieutenant Colonel Yuri Shvedov admitted openly, having the drug problem in mind: "It was very sad. We realized what you Americans went through in Southeast Asia."[8] Considering multiple similarities between the conflicts in Vietnam and Afghanistan, especially the character of those wars and individual experience of the combatants, to answer the question of why the consumption of intoxicants was pervasive among Soviet soldiers, one might, in principle, reply by referring to the earlier attempts at explaining the reasons driving American boys in Southeast Asia toward drugs.

The 40th Army Heavy on Drugs

What made Soviet combatants seek oblivion in mind-altering substances was, first and foremost, the debilitating and grinding conditions in which they had to live and fight. Sixty-five percent of all soldiers who served in Afghanistan suffered from a variety of diseases.[9] The most common afflictions included dysentery, typhoid, hepatitis, pneumonia, and a host of skin problems. More than often, 50 percent of servicemen in individual units were ailing.[10] The situation was not helped by the difficult living and combat environment, stress, insufficient medical care, poor sanitary conditions, increasing sense of meaninglessness of their tasks, homesickness (they were seldom given leaves during their two-year long tours), ethnic animosities, and conflicts between conscripts from various regions of the Soviet Union.[11] Yet it was boredom and cruelty of superiors and soldiers of higher ranks that had a particularly negative effect on the psyche. Similar to Vietnam, boredom weakened motivation and the psychological status of soldiers, at the same time encouraging them to deal with ennui using mind-altering substances. Many servicemen were assigned to monotonous and routine activities: they stood guard, protected outposts, watched the area, guaranteed supplies, and so forth. Frequently, nothing would happen day after day. Divisions controlled up to 500 outposts scattered over an area of several hundred kilometers. Regiments commanded more than 100 positions deployed along the length of approximately 130 kilo-meters.[12] Soldiers serving on those numerous outposts were afflicted by lone-liness, isolation, and intense boredom, all of which substantially contributed to undermining their morale. One of the veterans admitted: "Most soldiers smoke hashish or opium because they are bored. There is nothing to do over there, nothing to entertain yourself with . . . it's just torture, nothing else."[13] Another one confirmed, "In Afghanistan drugs were our only amusement."[14]

Young boys aged seventeen to nineteen, arriving in Afghanistan for the first time, were afforded extremely brutal and humiliating treatment by "old troops," that is, soldiers with at least one year of experience. Not only were the so-called old men entitled to better food rations, but they also usurped the right to physically humiliate (by beating, breaking in, and intimidating) and inflict psychological torment on young conscripts.[15] *Dedovshchina*, that is, this organized and ritualized system practiced in the Soviet army since the aftermath of the First World War in which soldiers with longer service history take advantage of new recruits, was one of the significant causes of desertion. Moreover, combat missions that resulted in civilian casualties, destroying vil-lages, slaughtering livestock, and forced relocation added to the psychological strain experienced by the younger ones. Before arriving in Afghanistan, they had been subjected to indoctrination aimed to persuade them that they would be bringing Afghans happiness, yet soon they were to learn that more often their adversaries were civilians whose better lot they were supposedly fighting for. These were frequently traumatic experiences, and intoxicants, which pro-vided detachment and oblivion, were a proven method for soothing the psyche torn apart by tragic dilemmas. As one of the veterans confessed: "War is miser-able without anasha [marijuana] . . . anasha helps me understand Asia."[16]

Motivation was not the only thing that the soldiers were short of. As finally admitted by government agencies, they also lacked military training. The 40th Army deployed in Afghanistan was, in essence, neither well prepared in psy-chological terms nor motivated to fight. Young conscripts frequently showed little commitment in combat; they were not aggressive or confident enough.[17] The issue of insufficient qualifications was also present among the officer corps. Summarily put, in Afghanistan the army was corroding, and its morale was seriously weak from the very beginning.

Conditions of service and the character of the war in Afghanistan forced soldiers to adapt to them in order to survive, thus driving them to become ruthless and brutal. A veteran, Yuri Tinkov who served in Afghanistan from May 1979 to May 1981, admitted: "We were savage. The circumstances made us like that."[18] Suffice it to say, this is a recurring theme in recollections from the war. Under such extreme and difficult-to-bear circumstances, Russians in Afghanistan, just like Americans in Vietnam, came into contact with readily available drugs of high quality. However, unlike the case of the United States, it is difficult to obtain any reliable data on the scale of consumption of intoxicants. If the authorities kept the number of fatalities and wounded soldiers secret, all the more so no statistics on drug use and the problem of addiction among soldiers were kept. The Cold War was, first and foremost, a psychological and propaganda war, and such transparency in terms of the issue of drug abuse in the military could be a serious challenge for the communist regime. After all, stoned and high American soldiers in Vietnam represented the degenerated imperialist West. The allegedly "dry" Red Army had no such problems. Hence only on the basis of accounts, recollections, and confessions of veterans is it possible to state that intoxication was a very common phenomenon among Soviet troops in Afghanistan, affecting at least 50 percent of servicemen, although in some units the number of substance addicts could be as high as 80 percent.[19] Intoxicants became an inseparable part of everyday life for a majority of soldiers. Vladimir Rudoi, who served in Afghanistan from 1983 to 1985, confirmed that "[a] great many of us used drugs and took them in large doses."[20] And another veteran declared: "There wasn't a single person among us who did not try drugs in Afghanistan. You needed relaxation there, or you went out of your brain."[21]

The publication of a book by the leading journalist of the young generation, Artyom Borovik, was a watershed event for the discourse on the Afghan war. Borovik had accompanied the troops in Afghanistan and put his observations to paper without any embellishments. It was General Secretary Mikhail Gorbachev himself who permitted the book's publication.[22] On one hand, it was a result of a transparency policy (glasnost) that Gorbachev the Reformer set out to implement. On the other hand, Gorbachev wanted to prepare society for the withdrawal from Afghanistan. In the era when perestroika was gathering momentum, open criticism of war and decay of the Red Army became not only possible but, amazingly, also fashionable in a sense. Antiwar sentiments were revealed by public opinion polls commissioned by authorities: in January 1987 almost 17 percent of Muscovites overtly expressed their criticism of war, blaming it for the spread of drug addiction in society and an increase of criminality among minors.[23] Now, authorities, who at the beginning of the intervention implemented restrictive censorship, allowed citizens to express such brutally frank opinions as those Borovik took the liberty to present: "With each passing day, the war more and more resembled the sexual performance of an impotent."[24] Finally, Russians could read and hear opinions that Philip Caputo may well have offered on American involvement in Vietnam:

> In Afghanistan we bombed not only the detachments of rebels and their caravans, but our own ideals as well. With the war came the

re-evaluation of our moral and ethical values. In Afghanistan, the policies of the government became utterly incompatible with the inherent morality of our nation.[25]

Borovik graphically and naturalistically showed the horrors of war, in particular bloody ambushes sprung by the mujahideen, nighttime skirmishes with an invisible enemy, and the stench of charred bodies of crews in destroyed helicopters or vehicles. Above all else, however, he baldly described the demoralization of the Red Army, to which massive consumption of drugs had greatly contributed.

A very substantial factor pushing private soldiers toward drugs was the fact that the traditional consolation of the Russian soldier, that is, alcohol, was very difficult to obtain in Afghanistan and, on top of that, it was extremely expensive. For these reasons, it was mainly officers who could afford alcohol, and they did drink often and a lot.[26] Obviously, soldiers would smuggle alcohol from home: "Customs regulations permitted two bottles of vodka, four of wine, but unlimited beer, so we'd pour out the beer and fill the bottles with vodka. Or else you might open a bottle of mineral water and find it was 40° proof!"[27] Privates supplemented alcohol deficits not only with hooch, cologne, and such inventions as brake fluid, toothpaste, or shoe polish, but also mainly with drugs that were easier to obtain, cheaper, and had stronger effects.[28] In some respect, smoking cannabis was even more beneficial than drinking alcohol, for, as emphatically expressed by one of the servicemen, it "affected you much in the same manner as vodka except that by the next morning you would be okay."[29] The most popular intoxicants were hashish (*plant*), marijuana (*anasha*), and opium (*khan/chars*), but also heroin and cocaine.[30] Opium poppy has always been a traditional crop in the region of the so-called Golden Crescent spanning Afghanistan, Pakistan, and Iran. Afghans were accustomed to using opium paste both for medicinal purposes and as a stimulant smoked or chewed mixed with tobacco. And so, soldiers also sampled the local delicacies, such as partly refined opium (a substance further processed to make heroin and, therefore, with effects stronger than opium but weaker than heroin), *koknar* (infusion obtained by boiling poppy heads), or *cheffir* (very strong tea).[31]

Many mujahideen used hashish or opium to unwind and boost energy and pluck before engaging in combat against Russian soldiers, many of whom were drugged as well. During one of his missions with the mujahideen in eastern Afghanistan at the initial phase of the conflict, Tom Carew, a British special forces (SAS) soldier, wanted to leave the camp. When he began to look for his Afghan brothers-in-arms, he "found them all, sitting round getting stoned out of their brains on opium."[32] In turn, Afghan soldiers who collaborated with Soviet troops and fought against the mujahideen also received hashish in their food rations since "[w]hen you get high on hashish, you become completely revolutionary and attack the enemy—fear simply disappears."[33]

Russians most often obtained intoxicants during patrol missions and usually got high to relax upon return. At times, they would get drugged before fighting, seeking to boost their energy and courage. Borovik quoted one veteran, Igor Koval'chuk, saying:

> It's best to go into an operation stoned—you turn into an animal. If you drink vodka or dry alcohol that's diluted in water, you can still feel your whole body. But taking a drug is like anesthetizing your soul; you stop feeling altogether. Later, when you come back, you just collapse, like a watch spring that needs to be rewound. And all your muscles ache. As long as you're in combat, however, you just get high and run around like a maniac. Hashish stifles emotions, smoothes over nervous fits. And there are lots of those, especially in the beginning.[34]

Intoxication alleviated the sense of fatigue, boosting uncommon energy, self-confidence, and bravado. One of the servicemen put it this way: "It is no longer so frightening to die. You become sort of indifferent."[35] At times, stoned soldiers tended to be exceptionally aggressive, brutal, and ruthless. Ruslan Kust, a veteran who served in Afghanistan from 1987 to 1988, recalled:

> The pressures of army life were usually vented in senseless cruelty— not only toward Afghans, but also toward our own men—especially when the soldiers were high from smoking drugs. First you could be hugging someone, and the next minute you'd find yourself beating the same guy on the head with a boot. People began gradually to turn into animals. The continual bitterness and hate all the time sought an outlet. The Afghans were the ones who had to suffer the most.[36]

At times, the consequences of intoxication proved tragic for soldiers since narcotics, which lowered their combat capacity and alertness, brought death upon them. Cases of fatal overdoses were also recorded. It was common for many army drivers to be drugged while driving, which adversely impacted their spatial orientation and ability to assess distance. This, in turn, led to frequent accidents.[37] Furthermore, intoxication caused risky and reckless behavior. One artillery captain reminisced: "We smoked hash. One friend of mine got so high in battle he was sure every bullet had his name on it, wherever it was really headed."[38] Sometimes, narcotic visions posed a threat to life. An army major reported, "Some got high on it, others got into the state we called *shubnyak*, where a bush turned into a tree, or a rock became a hill, so that when they marched they had to lift their feet twice as high as the rest of us. That made the world even more frightening for them."[39]

Soviet soldiers quickly became addicted. Yet, just like in the case of Americans in Vietnam, the consumption of drugs frequently was a collective ritual, which strengthened community bonds and increased mutual trust. Mark Urban thus recalls tales of veterans who admitted that "for the most part they smoke hashish and cocaine. There are also those who inject. There are not many of them of course, but there are some. The soldiers get hold of drugs by means of sale and exchange."[40] A dose of drugs could be obtained in exchange for as little as a bar of soap.[41] The soldiers' pay did not allow them to purchase greater amounts of intoxicants since it was a mere ten rubles monthly, which they mostly spent on food, since the food rations were unfit to eat and insufficient. Hence drugs also helped stave off hunger. Yuri Tinkov recalled, "On a combat mission we didn't eat all day. In the morning we were given just tea, and only at 11:00 at night did we get food for the first time. The food was awful, but when you haven't eaten all day, you'll eat anything."[42] And another veteran Yuri Yurchenko added:

> During the whole time I was in Afghanistan, I got proper food only
> for a month and a half.... When I went into the army, I weighed 80
> kilos. I wasn't fat; I practiced wrestling. Later, when I had to go to the
> military hospital and I was weighed, I weighed only 61 kilos.[43]

To get hold of drugs, soldiers "sold literally everything possible; fat, butter, canned goods, soap, hardware, but also arms and ammunition."[44] The real problem was that to obtain goods for barter, not only did they ransack Afghan households, but above all else they also stole Soviet state property: they took apart the equipment, and they moved spare parts for cars, fuel, and clothes. Those serving in construction battalions stole and sold construction machinery and materials. One of the former soldiers confessed: "In my unit, which was guarding the *komendatura* in Kabul, we had a lot of vehicles, so we sold gasoline mostly, but also boots and uniforms. I smoked hashish so I needed the money."[45] Not merely paradoxical but rather tragicomic seems the fact that weapons were also used for barter: machine guns, grenade launchers, and ammunition. Afterward, in the hands of the mujahideen, these weapons brought death to Soviet soldiers. Trade in stolen military goods became so widespread that in order to facilitate exchange a special market, called the Russian bazaar, was set up in Kabul. Russian soldiers selling goods and buying hashish met there on regular basis.[46]

The problem of drug use and abuse had become so serious that in the mid-1980s the army command decided to intensify the rotation and shorten the term of service of certain units and personnel in Afghanistan from twenty-four to nine months. It did not, however, prevent the wave of addiction spreading in the ranks of the Red Army.[47] Moreover, the higher number of soldier-addicts returning home meant an increased risk of the drug problem developing in the Soviet society. Servicemen would come back home, bringing a stash of hashish, heroin, or opium to sustain their habit for some time. The return of veterans resulted also in intensified smuggling of drugs from Afghanistan and Pakistan to the Soviet Union.[48]

Insofar as the United States had its Vietnam syndrome, the Soviet Union had its Afghan syndrome. The Soviet society turned its back to the returning soldiers—the so-called Afghantsi—affording them the same dishonorable treatment that had been the share of Vietnam veterans in America. Forty-six percent of Russians considered Afghanistan to have been a national disgrace, whereas a mere 6 percent admitted they were proud of their servicemen who had fulfilled their patriotic duty.[49] This attitude was largely due to the fact that the authorities officially underestimated and passed over in silence both merits and sacrifices of Soviet soldiers of the 40th Army in Afghanistan. And so, veterans began to organize, this time to peacefully fight on the home front for the social recognition of their fallen and invalided comrades. Many Afghantsi returned with severely damaged psyches. Colonel General Boris Gromov, who supervised the withdrawal of the Soviet troops from Afghanistan in 1989, admitted the truth that was obvious but concealed, namely: "Psychologically, some *Afghantsi* 'can't take it and go to pieces.'"[50] Many former soldiers who suffered from the combat stress reaction were institutionalized in psychiatric wards. In 1990 in Moscow itself, approximately 44 percent of Afghantsi (between 30,000 and 40,000 veterans and their families) required specialized psychological assistance, although in fact no such support was available. Thus, inevitably, "those who needed it were being drawn to alcohol, toxic substance abuse, substance addiction and even suicide."[51] Afghantsi were too often treated as freaks, and they felt this way. They were rejected, scorned, condemned, and forgotten, as one of them remarked:

> The young people ignore us. There's absolutely no mutual under-
> standing. Officially we have the same status as the World War II vets.
> The only difference is, they were defenders of the Fatherland, whereas
> we're seen as the Germans—one young lad actually said that to me!
> We hate the younger generation.[52]

For most of them the war did not end when they returned home; it was to persist in their psyche often until the end of their lives. Others had to fight yet another war—the war to adapt to life in society, and to overcome poverty, disability, and addiction.

Although the communist propaganda, very much like the Nazi propaganda in the past, held that drugs and addiction were afflictions only of degenerated Western societies, along with the perestroika, authorities and media began to admit that the problem also affected citizens of the Soviet Union. Indeed, substance use did not appear in the Red Army only with the advent of the Afghan war. In 1988 officials from the Ministry of Internal Affairs confirmed that military doctors, psychiatrists in particular, had identified the problem a quarter of a century earlier. It was estimated that in the 1960s and 1970s, almost 20 percent of drug addicts in the Soviet Union first used intoxicants while in the army.[53] In January 1987 the government admitted that 175,000 inhabitants of the Soviet Union regularly reached for psychoactive substances, of which number some 49,000 used "hard" drugs, such as heroin and cocaine. Obviously, it is impossible to verify the data, all the more so that in September 1990 General Nikolai Khromov, the head of the Soviet criminal investigation service, estimated that 500,000 citizens of the Soviet Union took drugs regularly.[54] Therefore, a sharp increase in the number of addicts could not be linked directly to the aftermath of the Afghan conflict as the problem of drugs in society developed independently. Moreover, just like was often the case with American Vietnam War veterans, many soldiers managed to kick the habit after demobilization.[55] When the communist authorities first began to disclose alarmist statistics on high rates of drug consumption in the Soviet Union, the problem was automatically associated with the destructive influence of returning veterans. Meanwhile, as Mark Galeotti noted, "The impact of the war on substance use in Soviet youth culture was more subtle than many would suggest."[56] The connection between the spread of substance addiction in the ranks of the 40th Army in Afghanistan and deliberate activities of the mujahideen, Americans, and Pakistanis was, however, much more evident.

Drugs as a Weapon and Source of Funding for Military Activities

Vladimir Rudoi, who served in Afghanistan in the years 1983–1985, noted, "It seemed to me that the Afghans had the intention of making us addicted to drugs. Almost all the Afghans used drugs. Primarily they smoked grass; as far as I could see, they didn't use heroin. Our men, on the other hand, mostly used just heroin."[57] Rudoi was right; drugs became a weapon that both mujahideen and the United States decided to use against the Red Army.

In January 1981, soon after President Ronald Reagan had assumed the office, he met with Count Alexandre de Marenches, the head of the French External Documentation and Counter-Espionage Service (Service de Documentation Extérieure et de Contre-espionnage, SDECE). Marenches suggested Reagan preparing and carrying out a joint French-American Operation code-named "Mosquito." It was to consist of sabotage activities targeted at the Red Army in Afghanistan: a disinformation campaign (among others, distribution of fake Soviet newspapers), but first and foremost supplying Russian troops with drugs previously confiscated in the United States by the Drug Enforcement Administration, FBI, and customs authorities.[58] The SDECE would establish a network of drug dealers composed of Pakistani agents and Afghans. Systematic drugging of Soviet servicemen was to undermine their morale and operational capacity. Moreover, upon their return home, soldier-addicts would spread the epidemic in society. Reagan found Marenches's proposal excellent, but the French withdrew from the project while William J. Casey, the new director of the CIA, was not entirely convinced whether the operation could be kept undercover. The idea was, therefore, officially abandoned. Yet the CIA might have undertaken some activities of this kind, since fake copies of a Soviet military magazine *The Red Star* appeared in Kabul, as did substantial quantities not only of hashish, opium, and heroin but also cocaine, which, at the time, was not produced in South Asia.[59] Accounts also indicate that Soviet troops would frequently find abandoned drugs that Afghans would throw, for example, on passing armored vehicles or plant in the barracks.[60] So, did the CIA implement the plan of spreading drug abuse among Soviet soldiers, even if on a limited scale only? It seems very probable.[61] Finally, by providing the mujahideen with financial and technological support (for example with land-to-air Stinger missiles), the United States could have easily inspired such activities.[62] For as one mujahideen put it, "We try to poison the Russians with it . . . they sell opium and hashish but now also heroin to the Russian soldiers in exchange for guns and to poison their spirit."[63]

Americans could now repay the Soviets for the support they had given to the North Vietnamese and Vietcong combatants. It was a perfect opportunity to let the Soviets taste their own medicine—the atmosphere of Vietnam— by "making the occupation of Afghanistan politically and economically as expensive as possible."[64] While in the years 1980–1986 the total American aid for Afghan insurgents was estimated at 625 million dollars, in 1989 alone the Americans and Saudis transferred the total of 1.3 billion dollars to the mujahideen.[65] The Inter-Services Intelligence (ISI), the Pakistani secret service, served as the channel to distribute this aid and support for the "anti-Soviet jihad." The ISI, similar to the Pakistani military, was also involved in massive drug smuggling.[66]

Pakistanis sent transports of weapons and equipment for the mujahideen in Afghanistan, bringing drugs on return.[67] Revenues from smuggling were used to finance the ISI's secret operations abroad.[68] Until the fall of the Shah in Iran, most opiates reaching the West came from Iran or Turkey. When, in the aftermath of the 1979 Islamic revolution, Iran had ceased to be a significant transit channel and production center for the international drug trade, its place was taken by Pakistan and Afghanistan, which until then exported only insignificant amounts of heroin to the West. This resulted in a huge opium and heroin boom, the increase in the poppy cultivation area, and the creation of laboratories and smuggling networks. By 1981 the production of opium had increased so significantly that its price fell by more than 20 percent. In short, a huge illegal drug economy had been established in the region, and its development substantially intensified as a result of the Soviet invasion of Afghanistan. In the early 1980s, heroin from northern Afghanistan and northwestern Pakistan constituted almost 85 percent of all heroin intercepted by British customs.[69] In turn, American government estimates in 1984 indicated that as much as 51 percent of all heroin available in the United States came from the border areas of Afghanistan and Pakistan.[70]

Yet it was mainly the mujahideen who financed their forces and their struggle against the Red Army through the revenues from cultivating poppy and trafficking in opiates.[71] All this took place with the connivance of the United States that, yet again, preferred subversive anti-Soviet activities over the war on drugs. As graphically put by Artyom Borovik,

> The "migration" of poppies from Afghanistan to other countries lines the pockets of the rebels and permits them to buy modern weapons. The drug-addict's vein is merely the last stop on this charming but deadly flower's itinerary. Deadly indeed. What other flower can shoot down a Mi-8 hanging in the sky overhead?[72]

The Soviet Union, too, tried to compensate for the huge costs of the continued Afghan operation (each day cost the Soviet budget approximately fifteen million dollars) by partaking in the international trafficking of opium, heroin, and hashish.[73] Soviet bombers were destroying Afghan corn fields, yet they mysteriously left poppy fields nearly untouched. It is worth considering the following examples. In June 1986 Dutch police intercepted 220 kilograms of heroin, the black market value of which was thirteen to twenty million dollars, hidden in a cargo of Afghan raisins dispatched from Kabul and transported across territory of the Soviet Union. The cargo arrived in Rotterdam on board a Soviet ship with a fetching name of *Kapitan Tonson*.[74] In turn, in 1988 some 3.5 tons of hashish was intercepted in London. This time the cargo had first traveled from Afghanistan to the Soviet Union, to be then dispatched from Leningrad to Great Britain by sea.[75] Incidents of this type were more than frequent. Obviously, soldiers and officers resorted to drug smuggling for their own needs, yet it is difficult to imagine that contraband operations on this scale could take place without the consent of the communist authorities.[76]

Thus all the parties involved in the conflict engaged in the local game played on the opium board: the mujahideen, Pakistan, the United States, Afghanistan, and the Soviet Union. As a result, the region has been transformed into the world's main opium-and-heroin center, which it remains until today. According to the UN estimates, in 1991 the annual opium production in Afghanistan exceeded 4.6 thousand tons.[77] Currently, heroin obtained from opium produced in Afghanistan accounts for more than 90 percent of the world's demand for this drug.[78] Regular production and export of opiates increased significantly after the Soviet withdrawal, followed by the abandonment of American financial aid for the mujahideen. For many Afghan refugees returning to their completely obliterated farms and villages, poppy cultivation was the only relatively quick way to obtain funds for reconstruction and to start their lives anew. In 1996 Afghanistan supplanted Myanmar as the world's largest producer of opium.[79] Operation Enduring Freedom (OEF) only further contributed to the country's status as "a virtual monopoly producer of the world's opium and heroin supplies."[80] The consequences of which were captured remarkably well by the 2009 report by the United Nations Office on Drugs and Crime:

> Every year, more people die from Afghan opium than any other drug in the world: perhaps 100,000 globally. The number of people who die of heroin overdoses in NATO countries per year (above 10,000) is five times higher than the total number of NATO troops killed in Afghanistan in the past 8 years, namely since the beginning of military operations there in 2001.[81]

PART THREE

TOWARD THE PRESENT

Contemporary Irregular Armies
Empowered by Drugs

The use of drugged combatants by non-state groups lends itself to
asymmetric approaches to counter the superior technical firepower
and skills of Western militaries.
                    —Paul Rexton Kan, *Drugs and Contemporary Warfare*

Postmodern terrorists motivated by religion are in a way close to the premodern archetype originating from the legend of the Assassins. How this archetype
of an intoxicated "monster" is materialized nowadays and the way it self-repli-
cates are interestingly presented in a seminal book by Paul Rexton Kan. Iraqi
insurgents; Taliban fighters; Al Qaeda terrorists; rebel groups in Uganda,
Liberia, and Sierra Leone; Chechen combatants and terrorists; Somali militias; ruthless fighters of the Islamic State of Iraq and Syria; and many other
parties fighting in a non-Western way make use of psychoactive substances.
Thus they provide the continuity of the Assassin archetype.

As a result, more and more often regular troops have to face adversaries who
are under the influence of strong intoxicants. American Marines, for example, were forced to change their operational tactics after they had discovered
that many of the insurgents whom they fought in the second battle of Fallujah
in November 2004 had been drugged. Even severely wounded, they continued fighting. Standard firing procedure to focus on the body was, therefore,
unable to stop them, just like the British bullets found it hard to hold back
the fierce Zulu warriors. Hence the Marines had to refocus on head shots.
Amphetamines, cocaine, and piles of hypodermic needles and syringes were
found in houses and caches used by the irregulars in Iraq.[1] Americans discovered traces of methamphetamine production in insurgent hideouts. The rebels
of the Abu Musab al-Zarqawi's group very often fought drugged, which was
confirmed by findings (pipes, needles, and syringes) and randomly performed
autopsies of fallen fighters.[2]

The ten members of the Pakistani terrorist group Lashkar-e-Taiba (Army of the Righteous), who between November 26 and 29, 2008, carried out bloody attacks in Mumbai, labeled by the press the "Indian 9/11," leaving at least 172 fatalities and 300 injured, were strongly intoxicated.[3] Four commandos of terrorists simultaneously attacked various locations: a railway station, a Jewish center, and luxury hotels. Security services were taken by surprise by mobility of the terrorists who moved along Mumbai's streets shooting at random passersby, detonating explosives, killing rich tourists and business people. The bloody spectacle continued despite individual groups being eliminated, because the structure of the assault was of a network nature. The group that took over the five-star Taj Mahal Palace Hotel held out the longest: for sixty hours. Lashkar-e-Taiba terrorists spread death and terror, fought fanatically and with exceptional brutality, very much like the Assassins or the Moros. It is now known that they used steroids and cocaine, but also LSD, which was confirmed by autopsies and tests of needles and syringes found among the terrorists' personal effects. Psychoactive substances, particularly cocaine, made it possible for them to continue their struggle against Indian special forces for two and a half days without sleep or rest, and with little food.[4] Thus cocaine and steroids played a significant role in carrying out the attack. However, detecting traces of LSD is a bit of a mystery. After all, LSD is not a stimulant but a hallucinogen and psychedelic, and—as discussed—it is well known to cause hallucinations, euphoria, amusement, racing thoughts, problems with balance, lack of motor coordination, spatial orientation interference (especially incorrect distance assessment), and extraordinary sensory intensity. Perhaps, not only did the explosive mixes of psychostimulants and LSD boost and galvanize the terrorists into action but also put them in a wild hallucinogenic frenzy, not unlike the fury of berserkers.

Today, such dreadful, intoxicated "barbarians," as many would perceive them, are growing in numbers, and a phenomenon is particularly well demonstrated by the research conducted by Kan summarized in tables 12.1, 12.2, and 12.3. In the ranks of irregular armies, armed troops, and paramilitary groups, drugs play functions that are well known from history: they stimulate fighters, they are distributed as a reward for good combat performance, and they are also used in the recruitment of new fighters. Drugs, which are capable of reducing the stress accompanying warfare and making up for physical discomfort, are also a means of compensating for insufficient military training and discipline in the ranks of irregular units. At the same time, by rendering combatants fearless, ruthless, and fanatical, "they can increase the probability of winning for militarily weaker groups."[5] Thus drugs have become an important factor that contributes to the asymmetry, for it makes the enemy even more unpredictable for regular forces.

Table 12.1 **Degrees of drug use by irregular combatants**

Minimal	Haiti, Iraq (Sunni insurgents, Al Qaeda in Iraq) • leadership ignores drug use by individual fighters • fighters are often recruited via intoxication and addiction
Acute	Bosnia, Colombia, Congo, Peru, Philippines, Russia (Chechen rebels), Rwanda • leadership uses drugs as a reward • leadership encourages drug use as a motivation for atrocities against civilians • command and control problems occur among the ranks
Unrestrained	Liberia, Sierra Leone, Somalia, Uganda • heavy intoxication or addiction among troops who may conduct violent operations to support their habits • widespread drug use among fighters makes command and control nearly nonexistent

Source: Paul Rexton Kan, *Drugs and Contemporary Warfare* (Washington, DC: Potomac Books, 2009), p. 12.

Table 12.2 **Types of drugs used by irregular combatants**

	Traditional	*Transshipped*	*Looted*	*Manufactured*
Stimulant	marijuana, hashish, khat, mushrooms, coca	cocaine, ATS[*]	pharmaceuticals	ATS, *basuco*[**]
Reward	khat	heroin, cocaine	pharmaceuticals	ATS
Recruitment	marijuana, khat	heroin, cocaine	pharmaceuticals	unknown
Relaxant	marijuana, hashish	heroin, opium, marijuana	pharmaceuticals	prescribed medications for professional militaries

[*] amphetamine-type stimulants
[**] cocaine paste

Source: Paul Rexton Kan, *Drugs and Contemporary Warfare* (Washington, DC: Potomac Books, 2009), p. 54.

The drug known as Captagon or fenethylline has been a stimulant of choice for combatants on both sides of the civil war in Syria and the fighters of the Islamic State of Iraq and Syria (ISIS). This synthetic drug invented in 1961 is metabolized in the body to form two drugs—amphetamine and theophylline (a chemical of the Xanthine class). The UN Office on Drugs and Crime classifies it as an "amphetamine type stimulant" (ATS). It was prescribed for hyperactivity, narcolepsy, and depression but due to its high addictive potential was banned in most countries in the mind-1980s as demanded by the WHO. It has been a hugely popular and widely used illicit recreational drug in the Middle East but is nearly unknown elsewhere.

With the brutal civil war in Syria progressing, the country turned into a major producer of white pills of Captagon, thus supressing such main source countries as Lebanon, Qatar, Dubai, and Turkey. Radwan Mortada, an expert on extremist groups, observes that the manufacture and trade of Captagon gave rise to an enormous illicit war economy. A production of a bag containing 200,000 pills is reported to cost a few thousand dollars but its market value is about 1.2 million dollars.[6] Because Captagon is a popular recreational drug in the Middle East, it has become a lucrative source of business for the jihadists and a crucial means of funding of military operations and weapons. In August 2014, reports claimed that after the seizure of Aleppo by the jihadists, where pharmaceutical manufacturing laboratories are located, ISIS multiplied revenues from production and trafficking in Captagon.[7] In Lebanon and Saudi Arabia, some 55 million pills are reported to be seized a year.[8] It is a real fuel of war not only in terms of funding military operations but also propelling fighters into battle.

Captagon is a good combat drug. It induces the effects typical to amphetamine-like stimulants—it numbs the fear and supresses the pain, alleviates hunger, reduces the need for sleep, and induces strength. The jihadists fighting in Syria and with ISIS are reported to be given large amounts of Captagon. It is said that the drug turns them into ferocious and fearless fighters who easily perpetrate unusual violence. Therefore Captagon is often called a "tablet of horror."[9] Kurdish civilians who escaped Kobane recalled that ISIS fighters "are filthy, with straggly beards and long black nails. They have lots of pills with them that they all keep taking. It seems to make them more crazy if anything."[10] Their acts of savage atrocities can thus be explained as resulting not only from extreme jihad and Islamic State's ferocious culture, but also from drug-induced psychopathy. They are, in a word, high on two intoxicants: jihad and psychostimulants.

To an extent, ISIS's forces is an army of junkie jihadists. Counterfeit Captagon pills they take are often much more potent than the original Captagon, as they contain methamphetamine, ephedrine, and other drugs. Jihadist fighters are also reported to use other drugs such as cocaine, heroin, and hashish.[11] Strong

Table 12.3 **Substances used by combatants in selected contemporary conflicts**

Conflict	Supply	Demand	Type of drugs
Bosnia	transshipped	reward	heroin
	looted	stimulant	pharmaceuticals
Colombia	manufactured	stimulant	*basuco***
	traditional	relaxant	*basuco*
Haiti	transshipped	stimulant	cocaine
Iraq	manufactured	stimulant	methamphetamine
	looted	recruitment (Sunni insurgents)	pharmaceuticals
Liberia	transshipped	stimulant	cocaine
	transshipped	recruitment	cocaine
	traditional	relaxant	marijuana
Peru	traditional	stimulant	coca, base cocaine
Philippines	transshipped	stimulant	heroin
Russia	transshipped	reward	heroin
Sierra Leone	transshipped	stimulant	cocaine
	transshipped	recruitment	heroin
Somalia	traditional	stimulant	khat
	traditional	reward	
	traditional	recruitment	
Uganda	traditional	stimulant	khat
	traditional	reward	
	traditional	recruitment	

** cocaine paste

Source: Paul Rexton Kan, *Drugs and Contemporary Warfare* (Washington, DC: Potomac Books, 2009), p. 55.

psychoactive substances apart, warriors fighting in Syrian civil war consume large amounts of Red Bull. This popular energy drink shipped daily by Turkish traders to Syria helps them stay alert during grueling fighting.[12]

When on Captagon jihadists "ignore normal defensive fighting tactics," which makes them more unpredictable. An ex-Syrian fighter interviewed by the BBC confirmed: "It gives you great courage and power."[13] Drug-induced bravado may explain high death rates among "imported jihadists" which is twice as high when compared to the regular Syrian army and "five times the number of Hezbollah casualties."[14] A nineteen-year-old former ISIS fighter named Kareem, taken prisoner by the Kurdish forces, when interviewed by the CNN confessed: "They gave us drugs. Hallucinogenic pills that would make you go to battle not caring if you live or die."[15] When high on Captagon ISIS jihadists are utterly insensitive to pain. Like Zulu and Moro warriors they continue fighting even when seriously injured.

Since the mid-1990s the difference between a drug cartel and a guerrilla or terrorist group has been becoming blurry. Narco-guerrillas and narco-terrorists finance their operations by producing and trafficking illegal substances. They also protect producers and control transit routes. A case in point is the terrorists responsible for the Madrid train bombings in March 2004 who had obtained the money necessary to prepare the attacks by selling ecstasy.[16] Another example of an actor funding itself from drug trafficking comes from the Abu Sayyaf Group—an organization fighting to establish an independent Muslim province, a contemporary "Moroland" one might say, in the south of the Philippines. In 2002, together with the Philippine armed forces, Americans carried out Operation Enduring Freedom—Philippines against the group, which turned it into one of the targets of the global war on terror.[17] The United States Pacific Command described the Abu Sayyaf Group as an organization that employs "*ad hoc* strategies and activities that are determined by the mood swings of individual leaders, many with eccentric nicknames reflecting bizarre bandit camaraderie. Discipline is haphazard, and some are addicted to drugs."[18]

As a result of governments' actions in the frames of the war on terror, Al Qaeda has been significantly cut off from its sources of financing and turned to new ways of obtaining funds especially by trafficking drugs. Therefore, opium production in Afghanistan, after having been successfully routed by the Taliban regime, increased from 185 tons in 2001 to 8.2 thousand tons in 2007.[19] In March 2004 in a San Diego courtroom, Ilyas Ali and Muhammad Abid Afridi pleaded guilty to terrorist activities and trafficking in drugs and weapons. They had been arrested in Hong Kong while attempting to trade heroin and hashish in exchange for four Stinger missiles that Al Qaeda used against American forces in Afghanistan.[20] So, to sum up, it is fitting to quote Antonio Maria Costa, a former executive director of the United Nations Office on Drugs Control, who remarked, "A marriage of convenience between insurgents and criminal groups is spawning narco-cartels in Afghanistan linked to the Taliban."[21]

In turn, speaking of Latin America, the director of the Colombian national police observed, "One does not know if the drug trafficker is a guerrilla or if the guerrilla is a drug trafficker. The line is now blurred; it is a brotherhood community."[22] This phenomenon is particularly visible in the example of the Revolutionary Armed Forces of Colombia (Fuerzas Armadas Revolucionarias de Colombia, FARC). Despite a decrease in its revenues, which, according to the Colombian government's estimates, fell from 1.3 billion dollars in 2002 to approximately 500 million dollars in 2007, it is still recognized as the richest insurgent organization in the world.[23] It should not come as a surprise, given that 80 percent of cocaine consumed worldwide originates from Colombia, and FARC is responsible for about 50 percent of this supply.[24] Hence Johnny Carson's quip from the Film Academy Gala in 1981 has lost none of its topicality: "The biggest money-maker in Hollywood last year was Colombia. Not the studio, the country."[25]

Several factors have led to intensifying the use of drug trafficking as a means of financing activities of nonstate armed groups. The most important of them include (1) the end of the Cold War era rivalry and bipolarity, in the frames of which superpowers attempted to limit and control both production and smuggling of drugs; (2) changing trends in drug trafficking in the 1980s and 1990s; (3) the increasing "asymmetrization" of contemporary armed conflicts; and (4) globalization that works toward removing boundaries and barriers.

The fundamental effect of globalization is the forming of complex mutually interconnected networks and an immense freedom of flows in the world in which increasingly permeable borders and distances are losing in significance. In this context, Manuel Castells speaks of the dynamics of the "space of flows" (of people, goods, services, cash, investment, labor, technology, knowledge, and information) above state borders that has supplanted the traditional "space of places."[26] By abolishing boundaries and barriers, globalization renders activities of criminal actors, such as network-like international organized crime rings, terrorists, narco-guerrillas and other hybrid nonstate groups, substantially easier. By flattening, decentralizing, and deregulating the network, they expedite and facilitate their operations, bypassing traditional barriers and control points. The network constantly keeps redefining its structure, and thus it is characterized not only by incessant dynamics but also by a perfect adaptability. As a consequence of networking, codependency is growing, so that the world is, as declared by Thomas L. Friedman, becoming increasingly "flat."[27] Barriers are gradually disappearing both in the legal and illegal trades. As a result, drugs are inundating new, hitherto unexplored markets. Cocaine has become widespread, for example, in Africa where combatants receive it from drug traffickers in exchange for safe passage across territories under their control. In the 1990s the members of the Revolutionary United Front (RUF) in Sierra Leone were a good example of this.[28] Anyhow, cocaine was certainly used by combatants, among others, in Haiti, Iraq, Liberia, and Peru.[29]

Many groups also perceive drugs as an asymmetric weapon against the West. If it is, it is a perfidious weapon. By taking advantage of partiality to intoxicants, especially among the youth in developed countries, not only does it ruin lives but budgets as well, while simultaneously financing activities of illegal organizations. Americans and Europeans purchase substances that slowly consume and destroy them. At the same time, profits from drug trafficking make it possible for violent nonstate groups to continue military operations, thus contributing to prolonged conflicts which under different circumstances would perhaps subside in intensity or fizzle out altogether faced with the lack of funds necessary to pursue them. Therefore, as Kan aptly notes, "Rather than drugs being merely a generator of profit for organized crime, drugs have emerged as a strategic resource in politically motivated violence."[30]

Cocaine features as an enemy in the American war on drugs, waged especially against Colombian drug cartels. However, narcotic barons have also resorted to the rhetoric and language of war, perceiving their operations, that is, flooding the West, and the United States in particular, with a "white powdered plague," in terms of unorthodox warfare. Obviously, they display an inclination to exaggerate, glossing over and inventing ideology for their profit-oriented criminal ventures. Yet, in their own way, they have contributed to the fulfillment of the legendary prophecy of the Inca Sun God; they have been helping "turn the white men into brutes and idiots," weakening Western societies this way.[31] Insofar as white colonists distributing coca to the natives exploited them ruthlessly, drawing profits from their toil, nowadays Latin American drug cartels dealing cocaine to whites damage their health and undermine their social fabric, at the same time deriving colossal profits from their weaknesses, vanity, and pursuit of pleasure.

The deeper sense, allegedly unrelated to financial gain, that supposedly guides drug trafficking, was spoken of by Carlos Lehder, one of the cocaine kings of what was later to become the Medellin cartel, who created a great system for transferring the drug to the United States to virtually flood the country with the drug. Lehder, who served as the model for Diego Delgado, one of the main protagonists of the movie *Blow* (2001), considered himself a freedom fighter whose actions were to put a stop to American imperialism. In this spirit, when interviewed by an American TV station, he stated that cocaine, in American slang known as "blow," was "Latin America's nuclear bomb" that he planned to drop on the United States.[32] Also Cuba's involvement in drug trafficking has a supposedly ideological background. From the very beginning of the conflict with the United States, Fidel Castro supported producers and smugglers of drugs. He found that in this way one may weaken American society while financing weapon purchases and revolutionary activities in Latin

America. In 1975 Castro even entered an alliance with Colombian cartels, so that Cuba turned a blind eye on ships carrying drugs across its territorial waters and refueling on the island.[33] Hezbollah has operated following the same motives. Not only does it import to Lebanon raw materials and chemicals critical for the manufacture of heroin and cocaine to later distribute the market-ready product onto the streets of American and European cities, but it is also involved in trans-African drug trafficking. The network of centers and smuggling channels scattered throughout many countries allows Hezbollah to continue its war against Israel and the West by—to paraphrase Clausewitz—other, intoxicating means.[34] In fact, a fatwa declares: "We are making these drugs for Satan America and Jews. If we cannot kill them with guns, so we will kill them with drugs."[35] In the recent years, Hezbollah has activated operations in Latin America, especially in Mexico. Its agents cooperate with Mexican drug cartels: they work at boring tunnels under the Mexican-American border that are used to smuggle drugs into the United States; they also train narco-combatants in technologies for production of explosives and methods of carrying out car bomb attacks.[36]

To sum up, the use of psychoactive substances among combatants of non-state groups financing their activities from the drug trade and fighting in long-drawn contemporary wars constitutes one of the substantial factors that contributes to the increasing asymmetry of conflicts. An asymmetric adversary is an adversary whose attacks are erratic or very difficult to predict. And intoxicants further maximize the ominous unpredictability of irregular combatants. Anesthetizing effects of narcotics have the result that even when shot and wounded, they do not feel pain and continue fighting—just like the Moro warriors—although they should withdraw. Drugs increase a tendency for bravado and risk-taking; they make combatants accomplish tasks that, according to more or less rational calculations, they should not engage in. Moreover, habitual use of hard drugs like amphetamines or cocaine causes psychophysical changes, especially in behavior, such as paranoia, sense of loss, confusion, or heightened sense of fear. It may lead to excessive irritability, excitability, frustration, loss of control, and intensified violence. The body and brain chemistry of a drug addict is not the same as that of a nonaddict. In turn, cessation of substance use or a lack of drugs results in withdrawal, characterized not only by severe physical pain but extreme aggression as well. For example, the Russian Prosecutor General's Office confirmed that almost all Chechen terrorists who had seized a Russian school in Bieslan on September 1, 2004, were addicted to heroin and morphine. Many of them were considerably intoxicated during the assault, yet in the course of the three-day siege some of them ran out of supplies and were suffering withdrawal effects which can account for their peculiar brutality.[37]

Therefore, intoxicants consumed by irregular armies substantially compli-cate the tactical and strategic landscape of contemporary drug-fueled armed conflicts, whereas addiction to psychoactive substances, financing groups' operations through drug trafficking, and transforming the economy into a narco-economy when the fighting finally subsides render introduction of sta-bilizing and peaceful solutions more difficult.

Intoxicated Child Soldiers

They were not afraid of anything, because cocaine was working in
the system. . . . They slaughtered people like chicken.
—Mariatu from Sierra Leone quoted in Chris Coulter,
*Bush Wives and Girl Soldiers: Women's Lives
Through War and Peace in Sierra Leone*

In August 2000, during its military training mission in Sierra Leone, a British
Royal Irish Regiment patrol was captured by the West Side Boys, a formation
of fearless young male fighters. The unit surrendered and was taken hostage
because its commander was unwilling to order fire on the boys, of whom the
oldest was fifteen and the youngest seven years old. Humanitarianism, empathy, and traditional Western concepts of childhood appeared to be signs of
weakness and dangerously backfired. The rescue mission (Operation Barras)
undertaken by the British special forces was not a piece of cake. The West Side
Boys "seemed to be completely fearless. Some were likely on drugs or believed
that they were protected by magical amulets. Whatever the reason, the men,
women and boy soldiers of the West Side Boys fought hard and seemingly
without care of being killed."[1] The SAS soldiers performed without a twinge
of conscience, and the operation left between twenty-five and 150 youngsters
killed.[2] The Sierra Leonean boys were undaunted fighters largely due to their
use of intoxicants. The lesson learned from this embarrassing British experience is that the Western military must be carefully trained and psychologically
prepared for a confrontation with children in arms. Fighting juvenile soldiers
high on drugs may indeed be frustrating and culturally confusing.

Many non-Western styles of war would neither limit the active participation
of children in combat nor protect them "from the illicit use of narcotic drugs
and psychotropic substances" as prohibited by the 1989 UN *Convention on the
Rights of the Child* (Article 33).[3] While in postmodern societies teenagers have
been searching for novel ways to recreationally alter their states of consciousness, children in Africa, Asia, and Latin America have been intoxicated for a
very pragmatic purpose: to turn them into good combatants. While Western

youngsters have recently been experimenting with digital drugs (i.e., halluci-nogenic music files downloadable from the Internet), child soldiers have been given classic hard drugs such as amphetamines, cocaine, and heroin.

The Old-New Phenomenon

UNICEF defines "child soldier" as "any person under 18 years of age who is part of any kind of regular or irregular armed force or armed group in any capacity."[4] According to estimates at the turn of the twenty-first century, there were over 300,000 child soldiers fighting in more than thirty countries around the world. In the late 1990s about 40 percent of them operated in Africa.[5] The spread of the post–Cold War epidemic of child soldiering, which in the 1990s became a distinctive feature of wars in Africa, Asia, and Latin America, decreased in the first decade of the twenty-first century. Thus the number of child soldiers declined to about 250,000 minors actively involved in combat in almost twenty countries.[6] Despite this reduction, however, juve-nile fighters will remain an unavoidable feature of the strategic landscape for years to come.

The participation of children in war is not a new phenomenon. Drafting minors has a long history: Athenians and Spartans recruited boys into ranks; thousands of boys and girls marched with a Christian religious zeal in the Children's Crusade of 1212; during the American Civil War, between 10 and 20 percent of the Union and Confederate forces were under eighteen; and in 1945 the Hitler Youth units defended Berlin.[7] This list of historical examples of children's direct involvement in war could well be expanded, but overall, as Peter Singer makes us realize, they were incidental. They were departures from a norm that did not permit child soldiering.[8] What is, however, new, appalling, and far-reaching in its tactical consequences is the deliberate intoxication of children-at-arms. More disturbing still, this phenomenon of drugged young combatants has been on the rise since the 1990s.

The innocence and vulnerability traditionally attached to childhood are, in the context of war and violence, unsettling because youngsters are perceived as dangerous killers. The image of children high on drugs who kill without hesitation, like precisely programmed lethal war machines, is truly disturbing. But this is one of the realities of war. Yet how to explain such an appalling phe-nomenon? Let us begin with a somewhat simplistic but usefully quintessential depiction of child soldiers offered by John Pearn. He captures its essence as a triad of "anarchic civil war, high technology and lightweight weaponry, and drug or alcohol addiction."[9] So let me start with a short discussion of these three factors.

The Triad of New Wars, Smaller and Lighter Arms, and Drugs

Since the 1990s much has been written about a new type of war. Authors agree on some of its fundamental defining features, yet they differ in describing the phenomenon and giving it a name. Thus we read about "new wars,"[10] "wars of the third kind,"[11] non-Clausewitzean or "non-trinitarian wars,"[12] or "fourth generation warfare."[13] So what are the main distinguishing marks of new wars? They are intrastate (civil) rather than interstate conflicts. They usually break out in the aftermath of the failure of a state and are often driven by ethnic and religious disputes. They are, then, endemic to weak, failed, or falling states, and above all to "lawless zones," usually in the postcolonial and poorest areas of the world. They are the wars of various violent nonstate actors (such as insurgents, rebels, bandits, terrorists, etc.) against each other and against government authorities. In terms of tactics these conflicts are hybrid as they incorporate a range of different modes of warfare. Because they almost entirely blur the distinction between combatants and noncombatants, deliberately targeted civilian populations make up almost 80 percent of all casualties.[14] War making is not bound by, to follow Geoffrey Parker's phrase, any specific "etiquettes of atrocity," that is to say by the rules of engagement or the code of conduct.[15] Writing in 1991 on "the transformation of war," Martin van Creveld aptly diagnosed the coming convergence of crime and war by remarking: "Crime will be distinguished as war, whereas in other cases war itself will be treated as if waging it were a crime."[16] On the one hand, low-intensity conflicts are often fought for criminal interests because the warring groups capitalize on the very chaos they create. On the other hand, these wars are funded mostly by criminal activities, usually drug trafficking. Whereas the dynamics of child soldiering might have been accelerated by the great intensification of new wars, it is the young combatants who often significantly add to their very characteristics. They make them more brutal, unpredictable, protracted and—in Western eyes—more "barbaric."

The advancements in small and light conventional arms (machine guns and assault rifles, but also mortars, hand grenades, and other portable explosives) along with the forces of globalization have made small arms cheap and easily available across the world. They naturally became the weapons of choice in the numerous conflicts that have broken out since the Cold War. With the application of plastics, aluminum, and new designs, arms that traditionally used to be heavy and complicated to operate became light and relatively simple to use. In a phrase, the developments in design and manufacturing, which have made small arms child-portable, have enabled "the transformation of children into fighters just as lethal as any adult."[17] Small arms now fit well into small hands. The Polish journalist and writer Ryszard Kapuściński captured this transformation well in his book *The Shadow of the Sun*: "Today, handheld automatic weapons are short and light, the newer models increasingly resembling children's toys. . . . The dimensions of weapons are now perfectly suited to a boy's physique, so much so that in the hands of tall, massive men, the new guns appear somewhat comical and childish."[18] The Russian-designed Kalashnikov AK–47 assault rifle, the most popular weapon in the world, is manageable for children. Combatants as young as eight to ten years old can operate it after only a few hours of training. The rifle is very cheap too. Although between 1986 and 2005 the average international price for an AK–47 was 471 dollars, in 2001 it cost merely fifteen dollars in Mozambique, while in Afghanistan it could be purchased for as little as ten dollars.[19] Thus the "Kalashnikov Age" has given rise to the "Kalashnikov Kids," who very often go to battle high on drugs.

If the global proliferation of cheap and lethal small arms has been the most important tactical reason for the immense increase of children's participation in war, then the use of psychoactive substances has enabled the turning of underage recruits into highly effective, determined, and formidable combatants. Thus the consumption of drugs by young fighters has not only been widespread but also massive, which makes intoxication a substantial feature of the children-at-war phenomenon. It is not to contend that the use of drugs is the only nor even a major factor of turning children into soldiers, as one cannot downplay the crucial role of military training, but it is an important and disturbing measure. As globalization has facilitated the spread of illicit drugs, making them easily obtainable around the globe, a rich assortment of substances has been used worldwide in child armies for various but interlinked purposes.

The reasons for intoxication are common among irregular fighters, but with regard to young people we have to bear in mind at least two essential points. First, we are talking about drugging children whose minds and bodies are much more intensively affected than those of adults. Minors are highly vulnerable to habit-forming substances and subsequently more prone to developing addiction. This has grave psychosocial and physiological consequences for their future lives, and in particular threatens their successful demobilization and return to the civilian world. So the use of drugs by children also contributes to the more general problem of postconflict settlement and reconciliation. Second, intoxicants devastate the body, especially the nervous system; yet in the case of young persons, the harm is faster and more severe. Not only is the brain damage caused by drugs more serious in children than in adults, but the excessive use of psychoactive substances by minors has a harmful impact on their cognitive, emotional, and physical development. Of course, these concerns do not bother the commanders, because what matters is youngsters' effectiveness and the utmost exploitation of their battlefield advantages.

Advantages of Using Child Soldiers and the Role of Drugs

The employment of young fighters is highly beneficial. First, children are easily available and effortlessly recruitable. For example in 2006, in the majority of sub-Saharan countries, persons under eighteen constituted half the population and over 40 percent were below the age of fifteen.[20] Juveniles are thus seen as a readily accessible resource subject to exploitation by various warring parties.

Second, having a vast number of youth combatants is a very cost-effective solution simply because children are less expensive than adults. They eat and drink less, do not need special shelters or clothes, use cheap arms, and do not depend on sophisticated logistic systems in their operations. Most importantly, however, they do not need financial rewards and hardly ever receive any payment. An additional benefit is that after their recruitment children can be sent to the front line very quickly following only rudimentary training. As Ishmael Beah, probably one of the most famous former child soldiers from Sierra Leone and now an international activist working to stop the military use of youngsters, comments, "usually it takes a year to train before you can go to the front to fight. With us it was a week. All you have to know is to point the gun away from you and know the commands to crawl and know when to attack in ambush. That was it. After a week we were on the front."[21] Cruel and inhumane as it sounds, due to their capacity for quick adaptation minors are a "low-cost way to generate force."[22]

Third, because children lack a proper understanding of hazards, they are more prone to bravado. They will usually do what adults would not risk doing, for example, run in a frontal assault to clear a minefield. Children not only have nothing to lose, but they also have not developed a proper comprehension of the value of life. What is more, during adolescence young people tend to carelessly approach dangers, and "their instinct for self-preservation, especially in puberty, is considerably less marked than among adults."[23] For these reasons juveniles are of exceptional combat utility.

Fourth, being small, fast, agile, and less likely to arouse suspicion, youngsters can undertake tasks that would be challenging and risky for adults. Thus minors are often used for reconnaissance, espionage, and infiltration missions. A former boy soldier recalled that at the age of sixteen his "job was to run out into the 'Killing Fields' [no man's land] and grab weapons, watches, wallets and any ammunition from the dead soldiers, and bring it back to the bunkers . . . This was a difficult job as you could see the enemy and they could easily pick you off as you ran out and back again."[24]

Fifth, juveniles are much more obedient than adults; they follow orders without asking too many questions and, being highly vulnerable to indoctrination, are more susceptible to manipulation and conditioning. Therefore, children can be made into truly loyal combatants, usually much easier to lead into battle and command than adults. This is not, however, to assert that child soldiers are better combatants as compared to adult (professional) soldiers.

Sixth, minors can disconcert adult regular troops who may find themselves at a critical ethical crossroads and hesitate to fire or take other firm action at a crucial moment as the example of a British Royal Irish Regiment shows. Hence by bringing tactical surprise, young fighters can give their forces a battlefield edge.

All the advantages of employing children, which make them easy prey for the factions, are significantly multiplied through the use of drugs. Thus psychoactive substances turn young combatants into even better fighters and make them even more attractive subjects for recruitment. Overall, there are three main purposes of intoxicating child soldiers:

- recruitment, training, and building loyalty;
- enhancing morale, bravery, and cruelty; and
- rewarding good performance and dedication.

Let me now turn to these functions of drugs in child armies.

Recruitment, Training, and Building Loyalty

Armed groups, both government and resistance, draft minors either voluntarily or coercively. The motives for a child freely joining a military group are often multiple and interconnected.[25] In the highly insecure and frightening conditions of civil war, youngsters enlist to escape poverty and hunger, to break away from domestic violence, or to look for survival and safe havens when deprived of their family. They also seek to avenge the death of their relatives. Still, some join for adventure, prestige, or respect. Ricardo, who enlisted in a Colombian guerrilla army, is representative here: "What attracted me the most was the power of having a gun in my hands."[26] It is indeed not without reason that the AK–47 has been referred to as the "African credit card."[27] In 1992 Carolyn Nordstrom came to the astonishingly telling conclusion that the "least dangerous place to be in a war today is in the military."[28] Although she was referring to adults, her observation has become accurate for children too.

In some regions the majority of youngsters join voluntarily (it was esti-mated, for example, at the turn of the twenty-first century up to 60 percent of minors in the ranks of FARC joined of their own free will).[29] Nevertheless, it is forced recruitment that dominates worldwide, and at this point intoxicants are often used to incapacitate, dupe, and soften the young in order to kidnap, reluctantly enlist, and retain them. Armed commandos may raid streets, mar-ket places, schools, football fields, houses, and refugee camps, as well as pick-ing up children and driving them away. Units enter villages, kill people, burn homes, and abduct kids.

Once in a camp, recruits undergo brutal initiation rites. They are manipu-lated through humiliation, fear, and violence. What are the goals of these ritu-alistic rites of passage? The newcomers have to be transformed into obedient, loyal, fearless, and fierce soldiers with a strong identification with the group. In many African states, belligerent forces co-opt traditional tribal initiation rituals and use them for the "baptism of fire."[30] In the initiation process, which aims at instilling a new militarized identity, boys and girls are not only brutal-ized by their superiors but are at the same time forced to brutalize civilians. Thus they develop dual identities as both victims and perpetrators. The goal of the initial military training, in essence, is to completely disconnect newly enlisted youths from their past life. Various methods of conditioning are used, depending on the country and military organization: fear, exposure to vio-lence, beatings, introduction to prostitution and sexual abuse, slaughtering animals and drinking their blood, occult rituals, magic charms, voodoo tech-niques, alcohol, drugs, and—rarely—even ritual cannibalism.[31]

Conscripts are frequently manipulated, desensitized, and acclimated to vio-lence by the administration of psychoactive substances that help them cope with shattered emotions, induce forgetting former identities, and make killing easier. Marijuana, hashish, or a mix of cocaine or heroin with bullet-powder (known as "brown-brown" and very popular during the conflicts in Angola, Liberia, Mozambique, and Sierra Leone) are also used to imprint an ideological frame-work onto the minds of new draftees. When the initiation process is complete, children are transformed into combatants who are prepared to fight and die for the group, its leaders, and the cause; who are willing to kill without hesitation or regret; and who are ready to spread fear and commit unimaginable atrocities.

But there is something else involved that explains why new boy or girl recruits are intoxicated from the very beginning. Commanders want them to be habitual substance users. Addiction automatically makes them reliant on their leaders, the suppliers of drugs. Thus loyalty and devotion are created but also sustained through intoxicants. In 1957, in his important book on brain-washing, Joost Meerloo recognized such a strategy, grounded in the cruel exploitation of the weakness resulting from the physical and psychological symptoms of substance withdrawal. He wrote:

> In criminal circles addicting drugs like cocaine or heroin are often given to members of the gang in order to make them more submissive to the leader who distributes them. The man who provides the drug becomes almost a god to the members of the gang. They will go through hell for him in order to acquire the drug they so desperately need.[32]

When reading accounts of the deeds of child soldiers, especially in Africa, one has the impression that they not only went through hell to get the drugs they had become dependent on but, when doped, also committed horrific atrocities that made civilians' lives pure hell.

Intoxication plays an important and usually underestimated role in accommodating boys and girls into "an institutional structure of repressive patrimonialism in which their subordination to adults is based on a cruel mixture of brutality, personal benevolence, and reciprocity."[33] William Murphy, writing on young fighters in Liberia and Sierra Leone, uses the Weberian model of patrimonialism—a "traditional" form of domination—to explain the logic of dependency of child soldiers (clients) on their commanders (patrons). His is an important contribution to the study of child soldiering and goes well beyond the usually simplistic models of underage combatants pictured as passive victims, revolutionary rebels, or opportunists exploiting social and political chaos. Murphy shows how youngsters are incorporated into the new patronage structures that replace their previous family-based arrangements. Commanders substitute for parents or tribal elders and perform an important role in initiating children into adulthood. In the specific political and social culture of child soldiers, "patrons create conditions of dependency which drive people to seek survival and protection through clientalist labor and services."[34] In exchange for fighting, adults provide young combatants with the instruments of power/coercion and with material goods such as food, clothes, looted items, and drugs. The administration of intoxicants for initiation and ritual practices or on a daily basis not only tightens ties and the dependency between children and their military patrons but also facilitates youngsters' socialization into a specific patrimonial "stylistics of power."

Enhancing Morale, Bravery, and Cruelty

While for many young soldiers the gun is a real source of power, drugs can be more: a source of adult-like or even superhuman might. And indeed, before combat and in the heat of battle, many military groups habitually boost child fighters pharmacologically. Depending on the region, belligerent group, and substance availability, various intoxicants are used, but the most common are amphetamines, cocaine, marijuana, and gunpowder (mixed with drugs or used solely). A popular substance of choice is also khat (*Catha edulis*), a flowering plant containing an amphetamine-like stimulant: the cathinone alkaloid. In the East Africa region and in the southern Arabian Peninsula it has been traditionally consumed by both farmworkers and warriors and was highly popular, for example, during the Ethiopian-Eritrean war of 1998–2000.

The practice of regular intoxication of child combatants was reported in conflicts such as Afghanistan, Angola, Burma/Myanmar (which at the beginning of the twenty-first century was believed to have more young soldiers than any other country in the world), East Timor, Iraq, Lebanon, Liberia, Mozambique, Sierra Leone, Somalia, Sri Lanka, and the Democratic Republic of Congo (DRC). Let me now turn to the two textbook African cases: Sierra Leone and Liberia.

During the Sierra Leone civil war (1991–2002), both the government military and rebel militias (RUF) prepared their adult and child soldiers for battle by dispensing amphetamines (known as bubbles), crack (a cheap, impure, and very powerful type of cocaine), brown-brown, marijuana, and some local herbal intoxicants.[35] Before combat children were forcibly given drugs that turned them into little killing machines. Stimulants were often served mixed with food (be it rice or porridge), sniffed, or injected. The stories of former boy soldiers reveal the extent of substance consumption. Ishmael Beah, who fought in the government army, well remembers plain white capsules liberally distributed by the corporals that he soon became addicted to: "After several doses of these drugs, all I felt was numbness to everything and so much energy that I couldn't sleep for weeks." He goes on to recall:

> We walked for long hours and stopped only to eat sardines and corned beef with *gari* [manioc meal], sniff cocaine, *brown brown*, and take some white capsules. The combination of these drugs gave us a lot of energy and made us fierce. The idea of death didn't cross my mind at all and killing had become as easy as drinking water. My mind had not only snapped during the first killing, it had also stopped making remorseful records, or so it seemed.[36]

And a former junior RUF soldier reported: "We smoked weed [marijuana] and took so many pills [amphetamines]. When we went into combat, we felt no fear—I mean no fear!"[37] When there were no needles at hand, as was often the case, the commanders forcefully applied intoxicants under the boys' skin by cutting them and sprinkling wounds with the powdered psychostimulants. Former RUF members recall that before fighting the commanders would cut their temples, pectoral muscles or arm veins, apply amphetamines, and dress the wounds.[38] A young ex-rebel, Zakaria Turya, confessed: "This is where they would cut and put the 'brown-brown' [heroin mixed with gun powder]. [He shows a raised welt on his left pectoral.] We would then inhale cocaine. During operations, I sometimes would take it two or three times a day. I felt strong and powerful. I felt no fear."[39] Another boy combatant remembered how "[b]efore a battle, they would make a shallow cut here [on the temple, beside his right eye] and put powder in, and cover it with a plaster. Afterward I did not see anything having any value. I didn't see any human being having any value. I felt light."[40] In this way the warlords guaranteed that their troops were suitably high on stimulants and well prepared for duties. There was no chance of refusing to be put on drugs because such a "technical sabotage," as the RUF leaders called it, would mean the immediate execution of the insubordinate.[41]

Juveniles were simultaneously terrified and intoxicated. The testimony of a twelve-year-old boy, coercively enlisted by RUF, makes us realize the extent of the dreadful pressure under which junior soldiers had to operate: "After they gave me drugs, I started killing. I killed a lot of people. I don't know how many. While I was shooting, I had no idea how many people I was killing. I chopped of hands. I killed. But I wasn't myself when I was doing it. They would have killed me if I'd refused."[42] Under the influence of this highly explosive mixture of drugs and threats minors committed the worst atrocities.

Former child soldiers who participated in the civil war in Liberia (1989–2003) presented similar recollections. Consider a boy nicknamed FW, who in 1990–1992 fought with the Independent National Patriotic Front of Liberia (INPFL) and admitted being given "bubbles" (cheap amphetamines) to make him "strong and brave."[43] Both government and rebel forces issued their young combatants alcohol, amphetamines, cocaine, marijuana, and cane juice mixed with gunpowder (a drink that "made them high and was supposed to give them the courage to go and fight at the front").[44] Another member of the INPFL, Ram Dee, recited a rhyme that proves the widespread use of uppers:

I am a rebel
I fought off the trouble
I took in the bubble [amphetamines]
I said double trouble. I'm a man who's not stable.[45]

Solomon F., who fought in the ranks of government militia in the 1990s, gave the following testimony:

We smoke grass, cigarettes, *dugee* (tablets), *cokis* (mashed tablets in a powder). It all makes you brave to go on the front. The commanders give it out. . . . Anytime you go on the frontline, they give it to you. Just got to do something to be strong because you don't want the feeling of killing someone. You need the drugs to give you the strength to kill.[46]

In an extreme method of desensitization, sometimes children had drugs put into their eyes, so they could not clearly see the people they slaughtered.[47] In short, intoxicants enabled easy and emotionless killing.

Children are fearless fighters not merely due to the psychopharmacological effects of regular drugging but primarily because they strongly believe in their immortality. To reinforce this conviction, commanders tell minors that the medicines they are given make them bullet resistant. They are also persuaded to believe, just like the Zulus or the Moros, that magic incantations and amulets render them untouchable. A former member of the rebel group Liberians United for Reconciliation and Democracy explained that "if a bullet hit you, it would bounce right off."[48] During the civil war in the Congo, the warring factions organized special initiation rituals for junior recruits. These, foregrounded in traditional indigenous magical rites and ceremonies, involved the forced ingestion of drugs, which was "claimed to induce a spirit of manhood, a military character."[49] Children were made to expect that magic substances would give them extraordinary might. Overall, young soldiers are indoctrinated to think that drugs and amulets grant them divine protection; the strong anesthetic effects of intoxicants only tend to confirm these convictions. As a young warrior explained, "even if you are wounded, you don't feel anything."[50] But despite being a merely virtual protection constructed through drugs and beliefs, it makes children fight fiercely irrespective of high risks.

Underage combatants significantly add to the lethality and cruelty of civil wars. Indoctrinated, conditioned under the severe pressure of brutal force, terrified with constant threats, and often intoxicated, children become subservient killers. There are a number of explanations as to why they are much more ruthless and atrocious in their deeds than adults.

First, they are, as Singer notes, "willing to carry out the most dangerous and horrifying assignments" because they do not fully understand the consequences of their actions.[51]

Second, children are not fully aware of danger in general, thus they take more risks than is considered acceptable by a majority of adults. Having an "underdeveloped death concept," youngsters do not understand the fatal consequences of their precarious behavior.[52] The crux of the matter was well expressed by Graça Machel, a widow of Mozambique's president Samor Machel and Nelson Mandela's wife, in her report on the *Impact of Armed Conflict on Children* issued in 1996. The document notes, "The youngest children rarely appreciate the perils they face. A number of case studies report that when the shelling starts the children get overexcited and forget to take cover. Some commanders deliberately exploit such fearlessness in children, even plying them with alcohol or drugs."[53]

Third, intoxication makes them more angry and savage, desensitized, and obedient. Indeed, many attribute the enormous levels of children's bestiality to pharmacologically induced mania. Young combatants turn into what Chris Coulter calls "drug-crazed tribal desperados."[54] Writing on women and conflict in Sierra Leone, Coulter quotes one of her interviewees saying: "That is how they are brave to do all these things, without the drugs they cannot do it. Because I cannot stand and see my mother and kill her! But because of the drugs you can't recognize who is standing in front of you."[55] Mind-altering substances not only considerably change the perception of reality, but they also leave children, as Singer aptly observes, "almost operating on another plane of reality."[56] A former member of the Mai Mai militia, a group fighting with government forces during the civil war in the DRC (1996–2002), confessed that "after taking a spoonful of porridge [with hallucinogenic herbs], I cannot see the difference between men and animals."[57] Thus unstoppable teenage armies have often slaughtered people like cattle. In Sierra Leone the Small Boys and Small Girls Units performed some of the cruelest killing in the war and inflicted awful terror on the civilian population. Local people always feared rebel attacks but were literally scared to death when young fighters approached their homes. Michael Wessells reports that the villagers he interviewed recalled traumatic memories of the RUF junior soldiers who were "pumped up on drugs and had 'that crazy look' in their eyes, which signalled they would kill everything in sight or commit mutilations such as cutting off people's arms or hands."[58] The aggression inhibitors that normally operate in most people do not work in stoned, youthful combatants. Thus "intoxicated violence" knows no restrictions.

Altered states of mind build up what Denov and Maclure describe as the "collective illusion of omnipotence."[59] Some children in uniform perform completely irrational and commit suicidal acts that seem fanatical and mad. Young soldiers conducting human wave attacks are usually navigated to such deeds with alcohol, drugs, or frequently by the explosive mixture of both. Using children to clear the land of mines was so prevalent in some countries that in Guatemala, for example, they were known as "mine detectors."[60] In Sri Lanka and Burma/Myanmar, child soldiers were forced to take amphetamines or tranquilizers before being sent into human wave attacks that almost always produced vast numbers of casualties.[61] During major offensives against rebel positions in the 1990s, the government army often used human wave tactics. The resistance forces believed, and some army medics confirmed, that most of the boy soldiers in the ranks of the Myanmar units were fighting drugged, "probably on methamphetamines."[62] In 1995 one of them, nicknamed "Aye Myint," confessed:

> We also distributed tranquillizers to the soldiers in the various camps around our unit. Before battles, we would take tablets the size of goat pellets and mix each with a lemon. Then they would be given to the soldiers out behind the barracks where no one could see. In the Ho Pang area, they ground 5 of these tablets and mixed them with army rum and gave them to 30 porters. The porters were sent to mined areas to sweep for mines. All of them died.[63]

Anesthetized by uppers or downers, minors are also used as decoys or additional targets in order to provoke the enemy to waste ammunition. According to one account, "there were a lot of boys rushing in the field, screaming like banshees when they rushed the barbed wire (barricade in the field). It seemed at first like they were immortal or impervious or something, because we shot at them but they just kept coming."[64] It is striking how much this description recalls the image of the fighting Zulus or Moros. To sum up, with their senses and survival instincts dulled by drugs, young fighters are sent into frontline combat as cannon fodder or used simply as disposable human land-mine detectors on a trial-and-error basis.

Let me now, finally, turn to the third main reason for getting child soldiers intoxicated.

Rewarding

In every military organization rewards are as important as punishments for maintaining high troop morale, for boosting motivation, and strengthening loyalty. Combatants need to be energized with benefits, otherwise their zeal for fighting will sooner or later deteriorate. In other words, to follow Scott Gates's typology, they need to be given a mixture of pecuniary and nonpecuniary rewards.[65] The former are tangible and these can be money, food, looted goods, extra free time, longer passes, alcohol, tobacco, or drugs. On the other hand, benefits distributed as nonpecuniary rewards are "incorporated into the agent's utility through the value associated with performing the task as assigned" or "stem from camaraderie among members of an armed rebel group."[66] Drugs are among the most important and frequently used pecuniary rewards given to child soldiers. Soon after joining the formation, whether voluntarily or by being forcefully drafted, children learn a great survival principle—it is much better to be rewarded (usually for good killing) than punished. Insubordinates can receive a variety of penalties, including execution. The horrifying vision of cruel punishments coupled with memories of pleasant drug-induced states works as an effective compliance mechanism.

Above all, it is important to recognize two key and hidden reasons for the distribution of intoxicants as reward in the aftermath of battle. First, it strengthens addiction among children and thereby their dependence on the supplier of the drugs, that is, the group and its leaders. Second, prizing young fighters for their good combat performance with pleasure-inducing substances shapes their attitude by making them grateful and ipso facto more associated with the organization. Rewarding is essentially an instrumental activity by means of which loyalty is transferred to the person who holds the power to reward and punish.

Apart from being rewarded by a superior, many young fighters self-reward with drugs. A telling example is that of the Sierra Leonean West Side Boys. They used mostly crack, heroin, and psychotropic pharmaceuticals such as ephedrine and diazepam (which is generally known as Valium but in Sierra Leone is referred to as "top-up" or "UNAMSIL" as it was brought to the country by Pakistani soldiers on a UN mission).[67] In fact, the truly fearless West Side Boys were almost always high on self-rewarded drugs in the course of fighting.

Intoxicants used as reward, both given out and self-prescribed, turn the majority of minors into addicts, which in the short term is highly desirable for the group they fight for, but in the long term has severe consequences for the children and their societies.

Addiction as an Obstacle to Demobilization and Reintegration

The reintegration of homecoming soldiers has always been a challenging and painful experience. However, the problem is incomparably greater when those who are demobilized are underage combatants. While it is much easier to turn children into soldiers than their adult counterparts, it is much more difficult to unmake them and for them to readjust to civilian life because, as the UNICEF representative Ian Levine observed, "the entire moral universe of the child has to be reversed 180 degrees; this is a huge undertaking."[68] And this is their second conversion—or perhaps *re*conversion.

Usually, they are very fluent in the language of violence and know nothing but the culture of the gun; hence, when released from military service, they feel robbed of their identity and disempowered. Their relations with family, the community, and society have been destroyed because of their enlistment in armed groups. Demobilization yet again endangers their identity, which had been brutally rebuilt through the extreme hardship of soldiering and had been maintained by the strong bonds with their unit. Reintegration—that is turning a soldier back into a child—is a long-lasting and immensely difficult process made even more difficult by war trauma and substance dependence on alcohol and drugs. Both combat stress reaction and addiction are terribly toxic obstacles to a former child soldier's psychosocial transition to civilian life and emotional recovery.

Detoxing former child soldiers and helping them overcome their addiction is one of the most serious tasks facing the Disarmament, Demobilization and Reintegration (DDR) programs. Young veterans suffer from acute withdrawal symptoms after being cut off from their comrades, leaders, and drugs. They become emotionally raw, depressed, aggressive, and violent. The severe loss of the previous way of life also fosters substance abuse. Intoxication offers a mock mechanism for coping with the uneasy process of transition and (re)adaptation to a new and unfamiliar situation. At the same time, however, addiction hinders reintegration by strengthening former soldiers' feelings of isolation from society and rejection by the community. This often creates a vicious cycle because, as former soldier from the DRC Erick Kenzo explains: "We have used drugs, and often the addiction lasts after we have been demobilized. Some continue to take drugs because of neglect. They are not helped to reintegrate into society, or to understand what has happened to them."[69] Ishmael Beah's story well illustrates this point. Beah describes what he and his fellow ex-soldiers did when they ran out of cocaine and marijuana in a demobilization camp:

> We broke into the mini-hospital and stole some pain relievers . . . and red and yellow capsules. We emptied the capsules, ground the tablets, and mixed them together. But the mixture didn't give us the effect we wanted. We got more upset day by day and, as a result, resorted to more violence. In the morning, we beat up people from the neighborhood who were on their way to fetch water at a nearby pump. . . . We began to fight each other day and night.[70]

Life in the DDR camps is difficult, and the drug problem crosses the gender divide. Denov and Maclure recount the story of demobilized RUF girl soldiers who turned to violence against the DDR staff after not receiving financial benefits on time. To build up courage before the attack, they used the "same technique that they were taught as RUF fighters," that is, they took drugs.[71] In countries like Angola, Liberia, Mozambique, and Sierra Leone many young female ex-combatants have turned to intoxicants, crime, and prostitution as a common postconflict survival strategy. One girl confessed: "I now live on prostitution . . . I live in the street exposed to all kinds of danger and I am tired of living in the street. To cope, I take drugs; either cocaine or brown-brown. [When I take the drugs] I feel relieved and I don't think of any problems, no bad memories of the war, and no sadness."[72] Addiction is a vast problem, as drug use is often linked to crime. In fact, the widespread lawlessness in Liberia, for example, has been attributed precisely to heavy substance abuse.[73]

Program coordinators working for international NGOs estimate that almost 95 percent of children employed during the war in the Congo had been introduced to drugs.[74] According to UNICEF, toward the end of the Sierra Leone civil war over 80 percent of the RUF rebels "had used either heroin or cocaine."[75] Whereas before the conflict drug abuse had been more of a local than a widespread problem, in the years since the war the country has been experiencing serious epidemics of substance abuse among demobilized child soldiers.[76] Major Phil Ashby, an officer in the British Royal Marines and the UN military observer in Sierra Leone, stirringly described his experience with the former RUF juvenile fighters whom he met in 2000: "They're so drugged up they don't often know their own names, let alone that there's a Peace Process."[77] In Africa the problem is almost universal. According to Edward Grant, a psychiatrist who ran the clinic for addicts in Monrovia, almost 70 percent of Liberia's "40,000 combatants, most of them child soldiers, continue to be drug users."[78]

Substance dependence is the long-term legacy of children's participation in war; it has obviously been a serious obstruction to their successful rehabilitation but also to the whole process of postconflict settlement. Nevertheless, in a somehow ironic twist, the drug factor can also play a positive role in the social unmaking of former child soldiers. Many of them take advantage of what Susan Shepler calls the "discourse of abdicated responsibility." They defend themselves in front of their communities by arguing that they cannot be held accountable for the atrocities committed, simply because they were coercively recruited, compulsorily given drugs, turned into addicts, and forced to kill. Shepler observes that "these claims of innocence ease children's reintegration into their communities and also make it easier for community members to live with former fighters in their midst."[79] Thus forceful intoxication is sometimes perceived as an effective measure or excuse for clearing juveniles of blame.

A Challenge to Regular Armed Forces

Sergeant Nathan Chapman of the United States Army Special Forces was the first American serviceman reported to die in action during Operation Enduring Freedom (OEF) in Afghanistan. He was killed on January 4, 2002, probably by a fourteen-year-old Afghan boy armed with an AK–47. The Department of Defense did not confirm this information.[80] Maybe because it was not true, maybe because the sniper's age could not be verified, but maybe because the Pentagon did not want to admit that the adult elite soldier, a Ranger, was shot by an amateur adolescent who could well have been wired on drugs. Would not this be regarded not so much as a sign of weakness but of dishonor? In terms of military operations, the challenges that American troops face as well as the character of war, it makes, I think, a difference whether Sergeant Chapman's killer was forty or fourteen.

The employment of minors has become a deliberate strategy by many insurgent, terrorist, criminal, and hybrid violent armed groups. They are, Romèo Dallaire vividly explains, "a commander's dream coming true: the perfect low-technology, cheap and expendable weapon system, which can perpetuate itself ad infinitum."[81] Children hooked on drugs bearing AK–47s have become an inescapable, distinctive, and emblematic feature of contemporary warfare. And inevitably, regular armed forces will run into the problem in the future. The following examples illustrate the challenge.

In 2005 the American media disseminated some hot news: the Taliban was abducting eight- to twelve-year-old boys and girls and sending them to madrasas in Pakistan, where they were indoctrinated and trained to become insurgents and suicide bombers or instructed in the planting of roadside bombs. Children were "brainwashed" to such an extent that they would do anything, even kill their parents.[82] According to UNICEF, in 2004 the insurgent forces could have included as many as 8,000 young fighters.[83]

On another front of the war on terror, during Operation Iraqi Freedom (OIF) in 2003, the American forces encountered child soldiers in at least seven cities.[84] Saddam Hussein recruited youngsters into his armed forces, and following the American intervention, minors become tempting targets for enrollment into insurgent and terrorist organizations. Both Sunni and Shia fighters made use of child soldiers who "were paid between 200 to 300 dollars to plant bombs and were glorified in Web stories that feature child martyrs."[85] Some 2,400 juveniles were captured in Iraq after the American invasion in 2003.[86] Al Qaeda was using girls as young as fourteen to carry out suicide attacks in Iraq. Rania was one such would-be suicide bomber. In August 2008 she was searched by a police patrol, and it was discovered that a window frame was nailed to her back and the girl was strapped with a vest containing fifteen

. kilograms of explosives. According to a policeman, "she seemed drugged by a sedative, though it was not clear."[87] Indeed, Rania confessed that she had been intoxicated and turned into an unwilling terrorist. Girls were put on drugs and forcefully made into suicide bombers who blew themselves up or were remotely detonated. Some of these would-be female assassins were sentenced to years in prison because it was assumed that only imprisonment could effectively protect them from the insurgents and terrorists.

In yet another war, that currently rends famine-ravaged Somalia, it is estimated that up to 60 percent of soldiers are children recruited by Islamic militias—some as young as eight "are drugged, others brainwashed."[88] And during the civil war in Libya in 2011, both Gaddafi and the rebel forces employed young fighters, who to some extent might have been pharmacologically hopped-up.[89]

For the same reasons that juveniles are exploited by military groups, they have become temptingly attractive to Latin American drug cartels and narco-insurgencies, in Mexico and Brazil in particular. Bands of "urban child soldiers" have turned into specific violent branches of drug cartels, becoming an intrinsic element of Latin American gangs. The participation of children in gang wars further blurs the already disappearing distinction between war and crime, so that the phenomenon can be discoursed in terms of "high-intensity crime" and "low-intensity conflict." In fact, it is both—a peculiar combination of crime and war.

An estimated 5,000–6,000 armed children fight for cartels and their factions in drug trafficking wars waged in the favelas of Rio de Janeiro.[90] In Mexico as many as 30,000 children may be working for various drug syndicates.[91] Youngsters are pushed into the arms of gangs by lack of education, employment, and opportunities, that is to say, by desperate indigence (20 percent of Mexicans live below the extreme poverty line).[92] One of the underage "gang soldiers," Edgar Jimenez Lugo of dual Mexican-American citizenship, began killing for the Beltrán Leyva cartel at the age of eleven. This "hit boy" became emblematic for the horrific nature of the drug war in Mexico, a conflict which from 2006 to 2012 cost the lives of perhaps as many as 60,000 people. Arrested in December 2010, he was sentenced to three years for killing and mutilating four people, carrying illegal weapons, and trafficking in cocaine. According to the Mexican army's statement, "he acknowledged having killed at least seven people under the influence of drugs provided by a cartel leader."[93] Hit boys and hit girls are not only regularly well paid but, due to the peculiarity of their job, are also boosted and rewarded with intoxicants. Because many use alcohol, marijuana, crack, or sometimes pure cocaine, they can be easily manipulated and navigated by the narcos (drug gangsters). Unique in this respect is La Familia Michoacana, Mexico's most dangerous, deadly, and bizarre cartel.

Having a very biblical and almost missionary character, it focuses on poor and marginalized young people. La Familia usually enlists youngsters from rehabilitation centers and "recruits must clean up their lives by throwing off any drug and alcohol addiction they may have."[94] Thus the use of intoxicants is strictly prohibited in its ranks. Although La Familia's approach to drugs is distinctive in the underworld of Latin American cartels, it only confirms the complexity of Mexico's "multi-sided narco-insurgency."[95]

Despite some intensive campaigns by various activist groups, government, and nongovernment organizations, there is very little prospect for eliminating child soldiering in the near future. For that reason, regular armed forces must be well-prepared for the threats and dilemmas they will face when confronted with "Kalashnikov children" often hopped-up on drugs. Let me list three ways in which intoxicated young combatants pose a challenge to professional militaries. First, underage soldiers significantly add to the mess, confusion, and chaos of war. Children in uniform are themselves erratic, but when drugged they become even more aberrant. The employment of young fighters greatly increases the unpredictability of war, which Western militaries, the American in particular, have been desperately seeking to eliminate, mostly through new high-tech combat systems. Contrary to these attempts, intoxicated child soldiers greatly increase the randomness of the battlefield, only confirming the Clausewitzian vision of war as an uncontrollable event governed by chance.

Second, it follows that young fighters do not play by the rules of engagement or respect humanitarian law. While professional soldiers often have some understanding of the laws of armed conflict, child soldiers, as Ignatieff pointed out writing on irregulars, "know nothing of Dunant's code of honor."[96] Thus operating outside the generally accepted norms of war, unrestrained, fanatically determined, and crazy on drugs, they generate high levels of slaughter and pose great dangers for Western forces that have been increasingly operating under the pressure of the doctrines of "force protection" and humanization. Therefore, they may seriously slow down the progress of regular troops.

Third, because child soldiers, especially when high on drugs, can inflict heavy casualties, they should be quickly neutralized or eliminated. However, professional soldiers are often reluctant to shoot children. They usually see them in the way they perceive youngsters in their own societies—as innocent and harmless. Children must be protected not killed, and should be given candies not bullet holes. Although these moral dilemmas are completely understandable, they could lead to fatal consequences because if a serviceman hesitates, he and his colleagues might be dead. The legal status of child soldiers or the rules of engagement that would permit killing them is not the point here. As Jeff McMahan observes, it is "permissible to fight against them in exactly the same way one would fight against adult combatants."[97] Easy to say, yet killing a child, even if he or she is the fiercest of fighters, may result in acute mental disorders for a soldier, which could develop into severe combat trauma. Indeed, as David Grossman reminds us, "the killing is always traumatic," but when you have to kill children, "the horror appears to transcend description or understanding."[98] An American soldier in Iraq, who encountered young combatants during the fighting in Karbala, perfectly captured the essence of this phenomena: "Anybody that can shoot a little kid and not have a problem with it, there is something wrong with them."[99] Thus the ethical dilemmas experienced by adults on the front line give children a significant advantage that explains, writes Münker, why "[w]arlords tend to rely on child soldiers when they are faced with UN peacekeeping troops; this regularly causes great distress to the blue helmets, who hesitate to open fire and even prefer to surrender rather than become involved in fighting."[100] This was not the case only with the British Royal Irish Regiment in Sierra Leone, as described at the beginning of this chapter, but also, for example, with the Indian troops during the peace operation in Sri Lanka in 1987–1990. When it turned out that the soldiers would have to fight with the Tamil Tigers' young combatants, they flatly refused, demanding an end to the intervention.[101] A few years later, in 1997, the Tamil Tigers' Leopard Brigade, a unit comprised mainly of child orphans, surrounded and killed about 2,000 Sri Lankan army commandos. This example of children defeating elite state formations severely deflated the army's morale.[102] Thus confronting child soldiers can have a serious demoralizing effect on regular troops.

To conclude, using child soldiers hopped-up on drugs is the antithesis of the contemporary Western strategic culture, which is focused so much on the value of the individual human life. The "barbarian" utilization of young fighters and the multiplication of their effectiveness through psychoactive substances violate, at least in axiological terms, the principles of the Western "humane way of war."[103] Because the phenomenon of intoxicated child soldiers will likely persist in plaguing future wars, regular armed forces must be well prepared and equipped with specific rules of engagement and tactics for confrontations with young fighters in states of drug-induced mania.

Drugs in the Contemporary American Armed Forces

Wearing down the enemy in a conflict means using the duration of
the war to bring about a gradual exhaustion of his physical and moral
resistance.

—Carl von Clausewitz, *On War*

Speedy War and the "Violence of Speed"

Speed is the essence of war.

—Sun Tzu, *The Art of War*

In one of the scenes in a 1986 movie, *Top Gun*, Lieutenant Pete "Maverick"
Mitchell, played by Tom Cruise, walking up to his F-14 fighter jet shouts: "I
feel the need—the need for speed!" Today Americans could refer to their military operations using a modified version of the slogan: "We feel the need—the
need for greater speed!" Military operations conducted by the United States
since the Gulf War (1990–1991) until the intervention in Iraq (2003) are remi-
niscent of, to use Paul Virilio's comment on politics uttered in 1977, "a police
pursuit at greater speed."[1]

During Desert Storm (January–February 1991), the initial period of
operations was recognized to be crucial for winning a quick tactical victory,
whereas the fundamental role was played by the air force—the most precise,
most effective, and fastest type of armed forces. Over the first few days of OIF
(Operation Iraqi Freedom), launched March 20, 2003, the U.S. Air Force conducted between 1,500 and 2,000 combat missions a day.[2] In 2001 General John
P. Jumper, acting as the air force chief of staff (2001–2005), hit the nail on the
head when he stated that long-term and incessant operations prosecuted "24
hours a day, 7 days a week" were of strategic importance in guaranteeing the
United States victory in contemporary warfare.[3] Conducting 24/7 missions

incessantly serves not only to surprise the adversary but also to wear the enemy down and substantially lower their combat worthiness and ability to offer resistance.

For the tactics based on a forced wear and tear of enemy troops to bear fruit, while simultaneously managing the fatigue of one's own units, one must prevent the boomerang effect, so that the excessive speed of operations does not adversely impact the combat capabilities of American forces. Since the initial period of hostilities is condensed in time and extremely intensified, the air force has a key role to play in strategic air campaigns, which already traditionally open American military interventions. All this amounts to a challenge of an exceptionally tiring task faced by pilots: very long missions, the so-called CONOPs (continuous operations) that often last without breaks for more than twenty-four hours are interspersed with shorter missions, the so-called SUSOPs (sustained operations) that last more than twelve hours. Therefore, pilots must maintain persistent combat readiness and regenerate quickly. In 2001, during OEF (Operation Enduring Freedom), long-range B-2 bombers flew sorties to Afghanistan from Whiteman Air Force Base located in the vicinity of Knob Noster, Missouri, some 17,000 kilometers from targets in the theater of conflict. The B-2's missions ranked as the longest in the history of aviation: occasionally they continued for up to forty-four hours. Two years later, during OIF, the B-2's missions were shorter with an average duration of thirty-five hours in the case of planes taking off from Whiteman and less than twenty-four hours in the case of bombers stationed at forward operating locations (FOLs), such as Diego Garcia.[4] Nevertheless, it was during the Iraqi war that the record was beaten, as one of the sorties was fifty hours long.

Since operations are conducted at a breathtaking speed, at a manic "operational tempo" (OpTempo), nonstop, and usually at night, soldiers, and pilots in particular, experience an immense pressure of what Virilio referred to as the "violence of speed."[5] The murderous pace of an increasingly impulsive war requires military personnel to function not only on the verge of physiological capacity of the human body but also well beyond it.

Risky Combat Fatigue and Operational Sleep Deprivation

> Man was not made for endless activity; Nature destined him for interrupted existence.
> —J. A. Brillat-Savarin, 1825 quoted in Paul Martin, *Counting Sheep: The Science and Pleasure of Sleep and Dreams*

Continued intense effort, stress, and sleep deficits cause immense combat fatigue. Colonel Daniel B. Allyn, commander of the 3rd Brigade Combat Team, 3rd Infantry Division during OIF recalled that since he undertook his duty on March 21, he and his men "slept for about half an hour at the assault position and did not rest again until March 24."[6] A commander of a detachment of Marines confessed: "I didn't get my first hour of sleep until after 48 hours, and I have been catching 20-minute catnaps ever since."[7]

Paradoxically, the influence of fatigue caused by sleep deficit on the human body is comparable to the effects of alcohol consumption and intoxication. Psychomotor ability and alertness tests, as well as simulator driving results, allowed researchers to conclude that a negative impact of activity which continues incessantly for twenty to twenty-four hours on human performance has effects similar to a blood alcohol concentration of 0.08–0.10 percent.[8] Symptoms following forty-eight hours of sleep deprivation correspond with the body's physiological reaction to alcohol at the concentration of 0.15 percent. What conclusion may be drawn from this? We have to realize that there is only a slight difference between a person driving a car when suffering from great exhaustion and sleep deprivation and a person driving under the influence of alcohol.[9]

Meanwhile, despite severe and chronic sleep deprivation, long-lasting military operations conducted at high speed require concentration, alertness, and great efficiency. Each twenty-four-hour period of continuous activity without sleep means that operational ability decreases, on average, by 25 percent; although, in some subjects and in the case of tasks requiring heightened attention, this drop may be even 30 to 40 percent. The research into the influence of fatigue on F-117 fighter jet pilots revealed that the sleep deficit of twenty-seven to thirty-three hours had weakened their performance ability by more than 40 percent when compared with normal conditions.[10] After forty-eight hours of activity, the performance capacity of the person deprived of sleep decreases by 50 to 70 percent. Under such circumstances soldiers may become almost dysfunctional.[11] Obviously, it is an individual matter and depends on the length and quality of sleep before the mission, the time passed since the previous task, physical condition of the body, mood, and individual psychophysical characteristics (the so-called sleep profile).

Fatigue may kill, metaphorically and literally, since it is paramount to an increased risk of errors that can lead to unfortunate events.[12] It has been calculated that sleep deficit and sleepiness contribute to approximately 10 percent of traffic accidents in the United States.[13] Many studies demonstrate that also working night shifts is related to an increased risk of accidents.[14] Fatigue and nighttime operations constitute a serious risk factor in the military setting too. During the first seven days of OIF in March 2003, Americans and British lost forty-four soldiers, 64 percent of whom perished not in combat but as a result of accidents (51 percent) and friendly fire (13 percent). Retired Army Special Forces major Andy Messing Jr., executive director of the National Defense Council Foundation in Alexandria, Virginia, forecasted that as soon as troops get used to the new combat environment, the number of fatal accidents would drop, yet it would rise again with "fatigue and combat stress" because "the biggest killer is fatigue, and right now we have a whole Army running toward Baghdad on zippo hours of sleep."[15]

To limit the destructive influence of fatigue and sleep deficit in aviation operations, various strategies of alertness management have been developed.[16] They can be divided into nonpharmacological and pharmacological. The former include adequate training (i.e., the ability to appropriately distribute strength) and tactical naps, which are used during long two-person flights (such as B-2 bomber planes). During the war in Kosovo in March–June 1999, B-2s flew long sorties from airbases located in the United States. The commanders were so concerned that pilots would fall asleep that garden lawn chairs, purchased from Walmart (for less than nine dollars per piece), were arranged behind their seats.[17] Thanks to this solution, when an opportunity presented itself, pilots had a chance to take a regenerating nap. Tactical naps are the most effective nonpharmacological method for sustaining alertness and counteracting fatigue. The U.S. Air Force allows its pilots to take preplanned power naps in the cockpit; they are recognized as a significant instrument in fatigue and risk management.[18] However, there is a certain disadvantage to naps: immediately upon waking up the so-called sleep inertia lingers for approximately half an hour. This is characterized by decreased alertness, impaired action, and a sense of numbness[19] After waking up, mental performance may be down by 20 percent than normal, which could adversely impact the reaction time and speed of performed tasks.[20]

In short, nonpharmacological methods do not guarantee fully overcoming fatigue and sustaining efficacy. They are helpful but fail to deliver a satisfactory victory in the struggle against sleepiness and exhaustion. This is why Americans have been set on finding a psychopharmacological substitute for sleep.

"Go Pills" and Pharmacological Management of Fatigue

> [T]he manipulation and understanding of human sleep is one part of human performance modification where significant breakthroughs could have national security consequences.
>
> —JASON, *Human Performance*

Pharmaceutical agents counteracting fatigue are divided into two categories: stimulants and depressants, that is to say, substances that either prevent or help falling asleep, or as American pilots themselves labeled them, "go pills" and "no-go pills."

Substances sustaining and bolstering the body's ability in the situation of exhaustion and sleep deficit are, in turn, divided into three categories: xanthines (caffeine, teobromine, and theophylline), amphetamines, and a new generation of synthetic agents. Caffeine is a traditional first-line, popular, and noncontroversial stimulant, though it is moderately effective. Currently, it is used in the form of tablets (100–200 milligrams, e.g., NoDoz pills), chewing gum (available since 2003 when Stay Alert chewing gum was created for the American military and advertised as "Stay Alive with Stay Alert"), or candies. Caffeine, whose effects are relatively short lasting (four to five hours), is not free of side effects such as anxiety, irritability, nausea, trembling, or increased heart rate.[21] Moreover, it is a diuretic, and as such it may contribute to excessive dehydration of pilots who face the challenge of maintaining adequate hydration during flights.[22] As used these days by the military, caffeine is not a sufficiently effective alertness and fatigue management tool; thus, it is worth taking a closer look at the other two categories of uppers: dextroamphetamine and a new generation of stimulants.

Dextroamphetamine

Dexedrine is an amphetamine stimulant created in the 1930s that significantly boosts the nervous system, alleviates symptoms of fatigue, and enhances concentration. It is used in the treatment of attention deficit hyperactivity disorder (ADHD) and narcolepsy (excessive daytime sleepiness). Taken off-label by healthy individuals for nontherapeutic purposes, it shows a strong stimulating action. Its influence on psychophysical performance ability may be described as sustaining (restoring abilities weakened or lost as a result of sleep deficit or disruptions in the circadian rhythms) and strengthening (improving efficiency of an individual functioning on the verge of their psychophysical capability). The boosting power of ten milligrams of Dexedrine is similar to that of at least four cups of strong coffee; it does not, however, entail unpleasant and undesired side effects caused by high doses of caffeine. Ingesting Dexedrine by sleep-deprived individuals at timed intervals allows them to sustain normal levels of performance capacity over the period of fifty to fifty-five hours on average, although research demonstrated that this period may at times be extended even to sixty-four hours.[23]

The life-saving stimulating action of dextroamphetamine became evident to the Apollo 13 astronauts. On April 17, 1970, the last day of the mission

troubled by problems and plagued by serious defects (mostly electricity shortages caused by an oxygen tank explosion), the crew was extremely exhausted,
and the commander, Jim Lovell, made computer errors rendering the preparations for the return flight to Earth difficult. NASA literally struggled to
bring the craft safely back to Earth. One of the elements of the rescue strategy
employed by the Space Center in Houston was ordering the astronauts to take
the Dexedrine they had been supplied.[24]

In Stanley Kubrick's cult movie *Dr. Strangelove or How I Learned to Stop
Worrying and Love the Bomb* (1964), Major "King" Kong is the captain of a
B-52 bomber plane, a part of a bomb flight dispatched by the mad General
Jack Ripper suffering from anticommunist paranoia, set to carry out a nuclear
attack against the Soviet Union. During the flight King scrupulously checks
the contents of his essential kit. In a black comedy convention, characteristic of the entire movie, the director has him find a 45 mm machine gun; two
packets of ammunition; food rations for four days; a packet of condoms; three
lipsticks; three pairs of nylon stockings; a miniature Bible and an English-
Russian dictionary; one hundred dollars equivalent in rubles; one hundred
dollars equivalent in gold; nine packets of chewing gum; and a first aid kit containing antibiotics, morphine, vitamins, pep pills, hypnotics, and sedatives.
It was not merely a movie fiction. As we know, when Kubrick was shooting
his motion picture, stimulants (popularly known as pep pills) indeed featured
in the kits of U.S. Air Force pilots. In 1960 the Strategic Air Command had
officially approved of the limited use of amphetamines, while the Tactical Air
Command followed in its footsteps two years later.[25]

Nevertheless, in the 1980s the public opinion was somewhat shocked
to find out that American pilots stationed in West Germany regularly flew
"on speed." In 1988 Colonel Russell B. Rayman, chief of Air Force Surgeon
General's Aerospace Medical Consultants Office, admitted in an interview for
the *Washington Times* that pilots were given amphetamines. It was, Rayman
argued, "a safe, sensible policy." He added, "We've never had an accident with
this, and it's smart." Whether pilots took the pills was entirely their choice
since using them was not obligatory. Besides, as Rayman concluded, "the great
majority don't even use them, but some say they feel good having them available, just in case."[26]

Dextroamphetamine was used by the crews of F-111 long-range aircraft during more than thirteen-hour-long missions in Libya in the course
of Operation El Dorado Canyon, carried out April 14–15, 1986. American
planes took off from Upper Heyford and Lakenheath bases in Great Britain.
Pilots were required to get proper sleep during the day, get prepared for the
duties in the afternoon, take off at 6:00 p.m., reach the target destination

around midnight, attack, return, and land the next day at about 7:00 a.m.[27] Despite significantly upset biological clocks, crews had to get enough sleep and rest. Military doctors in Lakenheath, Major Klaus O. Schafer, and Upper Heyford, Lieutenant Colonel Peter Senechal, independently of each other and without any guidelines from the headquarters, resolved to make sedatives (Secobarbital) and stimulants (Dexedrine) available to pilots.[28] These medications had been in standard use since the mid-1950s for the purposes of "crew conditioning" (or "fatigue management" in today's military parlance). Most pilots ingested Dexedrine already after accomplishing the mission, that is, on their return flight to the base. In a 1988 paper on his experience of preparing airmen for the mission in Libya, Peter Senechal noticed the great value of dextroamphetamine as an instrument of crew conditioning. He also postulated the use of "no-go pills" as a standard element for preparing pilots for missions and preventing fatigue.

Dexedrine was used again in December 1989 and distributed to F-15 fighter jet plane pilots participating in Operation Just Cause against Panama.[29] In turn, during the Gulf War in 1990–1991, 65 percent of fighter jet pilots participating in Operation Desert Shield and 58 percent in Operation Desert Storm enjoyed amphetamine support (with 17 percent regularly flying on go pills).[30] In units carrying out particularly intensive and long-lasting sorties, the proportion was even 96 percent. From among the pilots who had used pharmacological support, 61 percent found that go pills played a crucial role in completing their tasks.[31] As one pilot acknowledged, "without go pills I would have fallen asleep maybe 10 to 15 times."[32] As an anonymous squadron commander stated, availability of go pills had become a flight safety issue. Dextroamphetamine "doping" was taken advantage of not only by pilots on long-distance missions but also, particularly during Desert Shield, by F-15C crews whose flights were each time four- to six-hours-long, providing protection for AWACS planes that monitored the Iraqi air space for twenty-four hours a day.[33]

In March 1991, however, Air Force Chief of Staff General Merrill McPeak banned the use of go pills, arguing that "Jedi Knights don't need them" anymore.[34] The official justification held that with the termination of combat operations in the Gulf, pilots had returned to regular missions. Thus, because heightened readiness was no longer required, pharmacological support had been rendered unnecessary. Yet it seems that other factors were crucial to this decision. Some military doctors discovered that during the Gulf War there were pilots who used dextroamphetamine much too willingly. Furthermore, the entire affair stirred an inconvenient interest from the media, which were trying to investigate the circumstances of use of amphetamines by the air forces and presented the issue as particularly controversial.[35] After all, amphetamines featured on the list of controlled substances, and their extra-medical use was inadmissible. Still, according to many a pilot, expert, and military physician, the ban on using go pills was not only wrong but also outright detrimental. John Caldwell, Kory Cornum, and Rhonda Cornum offered the following critique of the prohibitive decision: "Unfortunately, the elimination of amphetamine use has put aircrews at increased actual risk for the sake of eliminating theoretical risk."[36] So in 1996 Air Force chief of staff John Jumper repealed the ban and with the beginning of the bombing mis-sions in the Balkans, the U.S. Air Force renewed the use of go pills. In 2001 the consent for the use of pharmacological enhancement during some excep-tionally long flights was further confirmed.[37] Currently, under specific cir-cumstances, the American military makes dextroamphetamine available to their pilots. The latest approval for the employment of stimulants was given in 2000 by the medical staff of the navy, while its pilots began to use Dexedrine only in November 2002 during the operation in Afghanistan, which had already been ongoing for more than a year.[38]

What are the requirements for using go pills? The air force fighter jet and bomber plane pilots embarking on missions longer than eight hours in the case of one-manned flights or exceeding twelve hours in the case of two-person crews can each time obtain ten-milligram pills of Dexedrine. Pilots are also entitled to receive go pills when their sorties are separated by less than twelve hours and as a method for combating jet lag to adjust to a new time zone.

Formally, it is up to the pilots to decide whether and when they want to use a stimulating pill. In a short "informed consent" form that they have to sign before being allowed to be issued pills, the declaration that they use go pills of their own free will appears several times. It reads, for example: "My decision to take Dexedrine is voluntary. I understand that I am not being required to take the medication. Neither can I be punished if I decide not to take Dexedrine." Yet there may be some pressure as attested by the fol-lowing fragment: "However, should I choose not to take it under circum-stances where its use appears indicated, I understand safety considerations may compel my commander, upon advise of the flight surgeon, to deter-mine whether or not I should be considered unfit to fly a given mission."[39] During extremely long sorties, which at times continue for more than forty hours, pilots have no choice, despite officially having the right to choose freely. They are aware that if they do not want to fall asleep or make an error due to enormous operational fatigue, in other words, if they want to return to their base safely, then in specific circumstances they should—for their own sake—resort to stimulants. Most frequently aircrews use go pills after completing a combat mission, that is, on their return flight to the base, and therefore when the risk of committing errors caused by fatigue is the highest. Jonathan Dowty thus remembers OIF:

> The pilots that had the greatest challenge were those who were on their way home from their tiring mission just as the sun started rising. The combined effects of the fatiguing sortie, the "relaxing" hour and a half flight home, and the rising sun provided a significant challenge to pilots who still had to navigate and land their aircraft. Anecdotally, the group of pilots who flew on that shift relied most heavily on medication, primarily near the end of their sortie to increase their alertness prior to landing.[40]

Go pills are not abused, since the majority of pilots treat them exclusively as a pragmatic solution to the problem of combat fatigue. The decision to dispense the tablets is taken by the commander of the air force unit (usually a squadron) in agreement with a military physician upon obtaining written consent from the higher command. At least twenty-four hours before the planned employment of the medication, the unit commander files with his direct combat command a written application for the use of psychopharmacological agents. The application must receive a positive opinion from the unit's flight surgeon and flight commander. The consent pertains to a single mission or a particular operation consisting of several missions. Pilots account for the go pills they take; return the unused ones; and fill in special forms providing the number of ingested tablets, time taken, and circumstances of their use.[41] A peculiar internal, collective, and informal control system has emerged: frequently all pilots in a given unit have access to these data—while filling in their forms, they can see their colleagues' forms. A U.S. Air Force pilot explains: "If all your companions so far used, say, two pills, and you took ten of them, then it raises suspicions not only of the command, but also of other pilots. It is a signal that there might be something wrong with you. You are being watched closely from now on."[42] Additionally, a military doctor completes the documentation related to the use of go pills, that is, issuing reports after the end of each operation and weekly accounts. Hence the use of stimulants is under strict control, covered by bureaucratic protocol with precise procedures and instructions.

Due to the fact that amphetamines cause longer lasting stimulation (with a half-life of approximately twelve hours), the pilots who use go pills often suffer from insomnia. To facilitate falling asleep and artificially balance the upset biological clock, physicians administer "no-go pills." No-go pills also facilitate an appropriate adjustment of the sleep and wakefulness rhythm to enable aircrews to sleep during the day and fly sorties overnight. Medications of this type also maximize the regenerative value of sleep. Since the Gulf

War, temazepam, known under its trade name of Restoril, has been the most popular psychotropic soporific agent.[43] From among 269 pilots participating in Operation Desert Storm who also took part in the study on the use of no-go pills, 54 percent confirmed having taken them, indicating as the main cause noise and difficult conditions unconducive to sleep.[44] Two other popular sleep-inducing agents are zolpidem (Ambien) and zaleplon (Sonata).[45] Temazepam, with a half-life of eight to ten hours, is used mostly to sustain sleep over relatively long periods of time. Zolpidem, with a half-life of two to two and half hours, is used to initiate sleep and facilitate short naps without the hangover effect. And the best agent inducing one- to two-hour naps is zaleplon, whose half-life is only an hour.

In the opinion of a physician serving on one of the F-15 fighter jet squadrons, because both Dexedrine and Restoril played a very beneficial role during Desert Storm, their use should become more common.[46] This was precisely what happened after the ban on stimulants was revoked in 1996. During the conflict in Kosovo in 1999, military doctors from the air force base in Whiteman recommended: "It is evident that these missions can be flown much more safely if we include stimulant medication [i.e., go pills] as an option for the aircrews as an additional tool to combat fatigue."[47] The war in Kosovo was said to have been the first postmodern war not only due to its humanitarian motives, boiling down to the famous slogan "saving strangers," meaning the protection of persecuted Albanians of Kosovo. The air campaign over Serbia was a momentous event in the process of the humanization of war in the West also because limiting one's own losses to the absolute minimum became the overriding political and military goal.[48] And pharmacology played a role in achieving this aim.

The studies conducted on a group of pilots who took part both in Operation Southern Watch in the years 1991–2003 (monitoring the no-fly zones over Iraq) and OIF in 2003 reveal that the majority of them used go pills and no-go pills. Surveys conducted among nineteen F-16 pilots who participated in flights of duration exceeding eight hours showed that sixteen of them used Dexedrine (all during the return flight and/or before landing), while eighteen of them took soporifics (zolpidem and temazepam).[49] During one flight, pilots were able to take more than one go pill because the command's guidelines assumed that if a pilot chooses to use Dexedrine, then it should be taken in regular four-hour intervals until landing. Moreover, the command's policy allowed pilots to take the second pill if within fifteen minutes from ingesting the first dose they did not feel any significant increase in alertness. The airmen from the group covered by the study would use, on average, almost two pills for a single mission.[50] During OIF, between March and May 2003, pilots received a ration of six ten-milligram or twelve five-milligram pills of dextroamphetamine before flights to be used as needed.[51]

Most of B-2 bomber plane crews also used stimulants. On average, sorties from the Whiteman base in Missouri lasted thirty-five hours, whereas those from Diego Garcia were on average seventeen hours long. What is interesting, dextroamphetamine was more often taken by crews flying from Diego Garcia (97 percent) than from Whiteman (57 percent). The decisive majority of pilots (97 percent) who used go pills confirmed their positive impact on maintaining alertness and concentration.[52] So, one might say that the employment of go pills and no-go pills in the U.S. Air Force has become so common that currently, under specific circumstances, it would be fitting to recognize it as a routine, although voluntary, procedure for operational risk management. In 2003 Colonel Peter F. Demitry, the then science and technology chief for the Air Force Surgeon General, commenting on dextroamphetamine, proclaimed: "Fatigue kills, this medicine saves lives."[53] Because cheap and simple-in-use stimulants save not only lives but also money (i.e., the costs of the loss of trained personnel and equipment), it was not without a good reason that Demitry labeled go pills as a kind of "insurance policy."

Critics, however, point out that the use of go pills may entail certain risks. Like other drugs, Dexedrine has side effects and may be a threat to one's health. The American Food and Drug Administration (FDA) classifies it, similar to cocaine, methadone, morphine, or opium, as a Schedule II drug on a five-grade scale and, therefore, a substance with a high risk of abuse and a narrow spectrum of therapeutic application. In comparison, Schedule I drugs include heroin and LSD. The most frequent side effects of Dexedrine include excessive excitation, nervousness, increased heart rate and blood pressure, dizziness, blurred vision, insomnia, and decreased appetite. Prolonged use of high doses may heighten one's level of aggression and/or induce amphetamine psychosis, which features as the most serious side effect, for it causes hallucinations, delusions, and bouts of paranoia. According to the drug's manufacturer, GlaxoSmithKline, it may adversely impact the ability to engage in high-risk activities, especially such as operation of machinery and vehicles.[54] A prolonged consumption of considerable quantities of Dexedrine may lead to substance tolerance and the need to take ever higher doses of the drug. Therefore, there is a risk of forming a habit that may lead to addiction. As mentioned, some squadron leaders during Desert Storm became so disquieted by the scale of dextroamphetamine use that they chose to prohibit it.[55] Moreover, as Dessa Bergen-Cico notes, the functioning of a human being in the cycle of pharmacological stimulation (go pills) and sedation (no-go pills) may result in disturbing the delicate biochemical stability of the brain equilibrium by interfering with the normal levels of neurotransmitters. This can, in turn, make the individual taking go and no-go pills "more susceptible to depression, anxiety and addiction."[56]

Yet the U.S. Air Force claims that no cases of adverse or dangerous effects of psychostimulants have been recorded, since pilots are administered low doses of dextroamphetamine: between thirty to sixty milligrams per twenty-four hours, that is more or less the same as the amount given to children with ADHD (forty milligrams per twenty-four hours).[57] To the contrary, it is the use of stimulants that allows increased crew safety by preventing the risk of accidents. Furthermore, before pilots are allowed to take advantage of the mind-boosting benefits of go pills, they submit to "ground testing" to be individually checked for possible side effects.

American public opinion learned about the air force's use of psychostimulants on the occasion of the Tarnak Farm incident that occurred on April 18, 2002, in the vicinity of Kandahar in Afghanistan.[58] Two F-16 fighter jets, operated by Major William Umbach (flight commander) and Harry Schmidt, took off from Kuwait headed for Afghanistan. While returning from a ten-hour reconnaissance mission, the pilots were, as it seemed to them, attacked. Schmidt asked permission to attack. In reply, he was ordered to withhold fire until AWACS identified the target, which usually takes up to five minutes. Schmidt, however, did not wait and dropped, in self-defense he claimed, a laser-guided bomb. Thirty-eight seconds later, the AWACS crew reported it to have been friendly fire. What Schmidt interpreted as a hostile attack had been, in fact, exercises in the former Taliban training camp in Tarnak Farm conducted by Canadian soldiers from the Alpha Company of the 3rd Battalion of Princess Patricia's Canadian Light Infantry Regiment. Four soldiers were killed and eight wounded. These were the heaviest losses caused by "blue-on-blue" fire suffered by Canadians in coalition operations since the Korean War.

The pilots were court-martialed, accused of a breach of discipline and violation of the "rules of engagement," and charged with involuntary manslaughter. Schmidt adopted the following line of defense: the tragic incident was caused by the "fog of war" and negative effects of amphetamines. An hour before the event, Umbach ingested five milligrams and Schmidt took ten milligrams of Dexedrine. Schmidt's counsel for defense claimed that dextroamphetamine, the use of which was in principle forced on the pilots by military authorities, caused impatience, excessive excitation, and aggression; and impaired their ability to rationally assess the situation and make correct decisions.[59] In the face of sensational media reports, the air force had little choice but admit that as a part of the "fatigue management program," American pilots were administered rations of small doses of dextroamphetamine. It was, however, an opportunity rather than coercion, since the use of the pills depended on the voluntary decision of the crew.

According to the report prepared jointly by American and Canadian brigadier generals Stephen T. Sargeant and Marc Dumais, the tragedy had precious little to do with Dexedrine. Schmidt, according to his statements, was experiencing amphetamine psychosis when he attacked the Canadians. Because it was administered in low doses, equivalent to drinking several cups of coffee, the stimulant could not have induced such a state. Other circumstances, and the human factor in particular, were of decisive nature in this case.[60] Namely, Umbach was an average pilot, unlike Schmidt—an outstanding top gun flight instructor, nicknamed "Psycho" by his friends. On that ill-fated day, Schmidt set out for his seventh mission over Afghanistan since his arrival in the Persian Gulf region.[61] Yet it was Umbach, whom Schmidt held in little esteem, who was nominated the flight commander, which seriously weakened the discipline of the team. In the situation during the Tarnak Farm incident it is, under the rules of engagement, the flight commander who issues the order to exit a dangerous area, wait for AWACS to verify the target, and, potentially, to use arms. Meanwhile, it was Schmidt who, quoting the need for self-defense, took the initiative. Refuting the thesis on Dexedrine's impact on Major Schmidt's decision, the air force representatives also pointed out that American pilots had flown hundreds of missions, and although they had used dextroamphetamine, no other such incidents had ever occurred. This stance is also confirmed by clinical tests which demonstrated that, contrary to popular opinion that stimulants contribute to an increased probability of risky behaviors, dextroamphetamine restores the disinclination to risk-taking that is characteristic of a rested person. Therefore, in controlled doses it does not increase bravado.[62]

The Tarnak Farm incident, causing a media storm and attracting the public's substantial interest, tarnished the image of the U.S. Air Force. It was so also due to further speculations whether go pills were the source of fatal errors and incidents of firing at civilians and other victims of friendly fire. Despite the groundlessness of these assumptions, the command ordered pilots to return all the go pills they had been issued. Lieutenant Colonel Michael "Zak" Franzak, a Harrier pilot in the Marine Attack Squadron 513, who in the years 2002–2003 participated in the operation in Afghanistan, provides the following account of the temporary ban on pilots' use of stimulants:

> AJ walked over, his face red. "You're not going to believe this, Zak, but we got to turn in our go pills."
> "What? What are you talking about?"
> "Grouper got an e-mail from the CG directing us to turn in our 'go' pills. It's fucking Tarnak Farms. That's what it is."
> "What about the no-go pills?" I asked.
> "Just the go pills, Zak. Everyone has to turn them in. Word came from the commanding general. We don't have a choice. It's the fucking asshole F-16 pilots who killed the Canucks last year. One of them

is now claiming that the air force issued him uppers, which made him overly aggressive and this resulted in his, quote, lapse of judgment, unquote." AJ rolled his eyes sarcastically. . . .

Every pilot in the squadron had the same opinion after reading the [Tarnak Farm] report: the two F-16 pilots were hell-bent on dropping their bombs on something in Afghanistan—anything. . . . The incident stood as a warning to us all of what could happen in combat if we choose to act recklessly. The incident also robbed us of a tool we used to maintain our operational tempo. I knew for a fact the go pills didn't make me aggressive—they helped keep me awake, and, for that matter, alive.[63]

Finally, Major Umbach was cleared of the charges, given a reprimand for neglecting command duties, and received consent for early retirement. In turn, the charges brought against Major Schmidt were significantly mitigated: he was found guilty only of neglecting his duties and given a sharp reprimand for "an astonishing lack of flight discipline," and a financial penalty just under $5,700.[64]

The media hype around go pills has become extremely inconvenient for the armed forces. After all, the United States is the only great power officially authorizing operational use of amphetamines to maintain the capacity of its military personnel. Therefore, for this topic to become less controversial, the Pentagon supports intensive research into developing a new generation of stimulants, which would be more effective and longer lasting than amphetamines; free of side effects; and, most importantly, given the high risk of potential public criticism, not classified as prohibited and addictive substances. The recently implemented Preventing Sleep Deprivation program managed by the Defense Advanced Research Projects Agency (DARPA), a follow-up to the previous Continuous Assisted Performance Program, is aimed to "prevent the harmful effects of sleep deprivation" and increase "soldiers' ability to function more safely and effectively despite the prolonged wakefulness inherent in current operations."[65] The agency has allocated tens of millions of dollars to finance the research into identifying a psychopharmacological nonamphetamine sleep substitute. Modafinil, discovered decades ago, has come forth as a miraculous, almost ideal agent.

Modafinil

A new generation of psychostimulants has been frequently labeled "eugeroics." This name, literally meaning "good arousal," was coined from the Greek words *eu/eus* (good) and *egeirein* (arousal). Eugeroics "arouse well," since they produce effects similar to amphetamines, but they do not cause inconvenient side effects, such as euphoria, increased heart rate, higher blood pressure, insomnia, and so forth.[66] Modafinil, adrafinil, and virgil are the most well-known eugeroics. Modafinil was produced in the late 1970s in France in Laboratoires Louis Lafon by Michel Jouvet, professor emeritus of experimental medicine and neurophysiologist. At present, it is produced under the name of Provigil by Teva Pharmaceutical Industries Ltd., an American biopharmaceutical company, which in 2011 bought Provigil's previous manufacturer, Cephalon. Modafinil constitutes an attractive alternative to traditional uppers, because in a dose of 300 milligrams it has a stimulating effect similar to fifteen to twenty milligrams of dextroamphetamine, that is, it energizes, awakens, and maintains mental acuity and efficacy despite a lack of sleep.[67]

What are its advantages?[68] Firstly, it promotes a natural sense of wakefulness with insignificant risks normally associated with ingestion of traditional uppers. Secondly, modafinil also enhances mood and short-term memory, boosts mental acuity, sharpens attention and concentration, and supports planning and decision-making processes. Thirdly, from the research conducted to date, it follows that the substance has a low potential for abuse. Both in subjects taking modafinil over a period of nine weeks and in narcolepsy sufferers who used it occasionally for periods of up to ten years, no addiction or increased tolerance were detected.[69] Fourthly, modafinil has surprisingly few side effects. Usually, they do not depart from the symptoms related to ingestion of a placebo, although some research at times recorded certain adverse events such as irritability, dizziness and headaches, gastrointestinal disorders, nausea, heartburn, and loss of appetite.[70] The maximum safe dose of modafinil is 600 milligrams per day but to limit the probability of its undesirable effects this can be reduced to 300 milligrams—the amount demonstrated effective in clinical trials in subjects deprived of sleep for periods between forty-eight and sixty-four hours.[71] Some researchers proposed a thesis that unwanted effects of modafinil are not related to its action, but rather result from long-term sleep deprivation and chemically suppressed fatigue.[72] Fifthly, modafinil does not impact the body's circadian cycle, since it does not bind to receptors related to the sleep and wakefulness cycle.[73] Because it affects only specific areas of the central nervous system responsible for wakefulness, it does not disturb the process of falling asleep. Modafinil is therefore an "intelligent" agent that stimulates only when the person under its influence wants to stay alert. And that is precisely one of the greatest advantages of this eugeroic when compared with amphetamines, which induce nonselective stimulation usually making falling asleep impossible without the help of soporifics. Sixthly, the application of modafinil does not cause "wakefulness overdraft," hence it does not require incurring a sleep debt and the need to repay it. As a rule, after thirty to sixty hours of persistent wakefulness, one needs approximately fourteen hours of sleep, but with modafinil this is not so, and a mere eight hours suffice.[74] It is, indeed, an exceptional characteristic.

At the same time, this wakefulness-promoting drug continues to remain a mysterious substance as the mechanism of its action has not been fully identified yet. For a long time it was thought not to influence the process of absorption of dopamine by neurons, which was, in turn, linked to the lack of risk for abuse and addiction. However, the research conducted by Nora Volkow and colleagues demonstrated that modafinil is, in fact, a dopamine reuptake inhibitor, which means that it may have a certain potential for addiction.[75] By suppressing neuronal absorption of dopamine, a neurotransmitter responsible for, among others, the states of wakefulness and intense concentration, modafinil increases its levels in the brain, resulting in greater alertness. The drug also reabsorbs another neurotransmitter called noradrenaline.[76] Therefore, in essence, its mechanism of action is not general, for it results in an exceptionally selective stimulation of the central nervous system, to a minimal degree affecting the peripheral nervous system. This explains why the drug does not cause undesired adverse events and painful hangover effects characteristic of the majority of traditional stimulants.

In 1998 the FDA allowed the use of modafinil in the treatment of narcolepsy and sleep apnea as well as sleeping disorders accompanying diseases such as Parkinson's or Alzheimer's. In 2004 it also approved its use by shift workers struggling to stay awake. In turn, in 2007 a longer acting version of modafinil—armodafinil—was allowed on the market available as Nuvigil.[77]

Although in the United States modafinil is still a controlled substance classified as a Schedule IV drug—similar to Xanax, Ambien, or Valium—and, moreover, it is not designed to be used by healthy people, it quickly became one of the most popular "smart" or "designer drugs." In 2006 Cephalon, then Provigil's manufacturer, was for the first time ever listed by *Fortune* magazine in its ranking of America's 1,000 biggest companies. It came as no surprise because global profits from sales of modafinil increased from five million dollars in 2005 to one billion dollars in 2009, with a prognosis of ten billion dollars in 2018.[78] It is estimated that in 90 percent of cases the drug is used for extramedical purposes.[79] Commonly known as the "zombie pill" and "Viagra for the brain," it has developed into a very popular lifestyle drug—"a cognitive enhancer" that does not treat but enables people to live and work faster and harder. This is why it is increasingly more often used by healthy individuals who seem to lack time for sleep.[80] Perhaps modafinil and its newer improved versions will soon become a great liberator for sleep, just as the contraceptive pill was for sex.

In 1989 Michel Jouvet, the discoverer of modafinil, predicted that this medication "could keep an army on its feet and fighting for three days and nights with no side-effects."[81] Two years later, during the Gulf War, the French army tested the drug, administering it every six to eight hours to the soldiers of the Foreign Legion.[82] In the following years, the French conducted a variety of experiments on infantrymen and pilots. They confirmed the effectiveness of modafinil in maintaining efficiency on a level close to normal during intense work, ongoing for sixty to sixty-four hours nonstop.[83] Obviously, Americans became interested in modafinil as an agent capable of counteracting the adverse effects of serious and onerous sleep deprivation during long-term military operations. Their first tests were conducted in 2000, when the drug was administered to helicopter pilots training in flight simulators. They were given a 200-milligram dose three times a day. The experiment proved a great success. The eugeroic perfectly eliminated fatigue, while pilots had no difficulties in performing maneuvers requiring high precision (such as taking the course and maintaining flight direction or precise turns). Advantageous influence of modafinil was observed in particular between 3:30 a.m. and 12:00 p.m., that is, when exhaustion related to the lack of sleep is the most severe. After thirty hours without sleep, pilots' efficacy remained on a level close to normal. And, astonishingly, after forty sleepless hours their performance decreased only insignificantly.[84]

Then, in 2001 Americans tested the effects of modafinil on pilots performing forty-hour-long missions during OEF. And the team led by Greg Belenky of the Walter Reed Army Institute of Research in Silver Spring, Maryland, conducted promising experiments with modafinil in the conditions of the longest sleep deficit ever recorded. Soldiers participating in the study were deprived of sleep for the extraordinary period of eighty-five hours. Nonetheless, the optimum time of maintaining mental and psychomotor performance capacity on a level close to normal with the use of modafinil is approximately up to forty hours.

Since 2000 Americans have conducted a host of experiments aimed at carrying out comprehensive research into the military usability of modafinil. Their scale is attested to not only the number of publications in scientific journals but also by the variety of specific research areas. For example, when scientists discovered that systems in the brain responsible for regulation of the sleep-wakefulness cycle and hunger are interconnected, the Pentagon financed a four-year program directed at estimating the risk of increased obesity among pilots using modafinil.[85]

To sum up, the results of the majority of studies confirmed modafinil's usefulness in combat conditions.[86] The stimulant is deemed highly advantageous for it almost painlessly alleviates most of the problems related to decreased performance capacity and mood deterioration resulting from total and chronic sleep deficit. It is an ideal psychopharmacological instrument for managing alertness, sleep, and fatigue; and it is safe, easy to use, devoid of serious adverse effects, nonaddictive or, at the worst, of low habit-forming potential, characterized by small toxicity; and it does not tamper with the body's circadian cycle. Another important feature of modafinil is that it does not interfere with the process of falling asleep, so that after their mission, soldiers do not have to take no-go pills, and sleep is possible whenever an opportunity arises. Short unexpected breaks may occur during any military operation, thus giving servicemen time for brief, regenerating power naps. In such cases, unlike dextroamphetamine, modafinil guarantees high flexibility and allows one to control sleep, which makes it an exceptionally attractive combat booster. Not only is it, therefore, a wakefulness-promoting agent but also a peculiar "nap in a pill." Given all this, it comes as no surprise that the American military found it to be a wonder go pill and a potentially worthy successor to dextroamphetamine. In 2001 a committee on military nutrition research recommended the use of modafinil, which "compared with other well-known stimulatory substances such as caffeine and amphetamine, . . . appears to have the advantage of combining wakening and stimulating properties, with an appreciable absence of unwanted side-effects."[87] In December 2003 the American Air Force sanctioned the use of modafinil during specific sorties. Two-hundred-milligram doses (400 milligrams per day maximum) were approved to be distributed to bomber pilots for missions longer than twelve hours and to pilots of two-pilot fighter jets for flights lasting more than eight hours. In August 2006 the use of modafinil for one-pilot fighter jets was also authorized.[88] Overall, the same rules and procedures that apply to dextroamphetamine apply to modafinil.[89]

Toward a New Generation of No-Go Pills?

The problem of sleep deprivation is universal in the military. It has its roots not only in the lack of time for rest during combat operations but frequently also in the disruption of the biological clock by changing time zones, an unfriendly and alien climate, emotions (stress and fear), unfavorable environmental conditions (such as noise), and general discomfort. Circumstances permitting soldiers to grab a nap in the war zone may appear unexpectedly and suddenly; therefore, one must know how to use them effectively. Soldiers often have to sleep during the day, which can be difficult since it stands in contradiction with the circadian clock rhythm. Soporifics help optimize sleep and, as we know, their controlled distribution to servicemen is approved by the American military.

A peculiar revolution in the quest for medications capable of altering sleep architecture is, we are told, presently occurring in pharmaceutical laboratories.

On one hand, the works on soporifics inducing sleep for a specific period of time—say four, five, or six hours—and then causing subjects to wake up are under way. This type of agent would be widely applicable during military operations as they would allow soldiers to condense portions of sleep in uncertain combat conditions. On the other hand, medications that allow a more effective and regenerating sleep are visible on the horizon. As is well known, sleep consists of four phases: immediately after falling asleep a several-minute-long period of shallow sleep (half-sleep or drowsiness) occurs, to be followed by the time of transition to deep sleep, and the slow-wave deep sleep phase (NREM, total rest and regeneration) then moves to the stage of paradoxical sleep (REM) in which visual and emotional dreams appear. New hypnotic drugs are supposed to eliminate "redundant" phases of the sleep cycle leaving only NREM, that is, the most recuperative for the body. This would reduce minimum sleep time by increasing its quality. Thanks to new pharmaceuticals, it will be possible to obtain the level of alertness and efficiency, which is normally achieved after six to eight hours of sleep, within only three to four hours. The first experimental medication of this type facilitating the change of sleep architecture and lengthening the slow-wave sleep came as Gaboxadol, a drug developed by Merck and Lundbeck. This highly promising agent was examined under advanced clinical trials, but in 2007 they were discontinued due to unexpected side effects, like disorientation and hallucinations.[90]

The laboratories of pharmaceutical companies are working on developing a new generation of soporifics. In the "24/7 society" (to use the term coined in 1993 by Ede Moore), sleep has been becoming out of fashion, thus, the race to conquer it gathers momentum.[91] Even a newer generation of traditional medications, such as zolpidem, act like alcohol on neurotransmitter GABA (gamma-Aminobutyric acid), which constitutes an activity switch, a peculiar "brake fluid" of the brain. GABA-stimulating compounds decrease neuronal activity, thus allowing one to fall asleep. Future medications will be equipped with a different mechanism of action, as exemplified by Merck-marketed Suvorexant (trade name Belsomora) that was approved for sale in the United States in 2014. It is an orexin receptor antagonist. By blocking the action of orexin, a hormone playing a crucial role in stimulating alertness and energy burning, the medication induces good-quality sleep and causes none of the side effects characteristic of traditional hypnotics. Peter Kim, president of Merck Research Laboratories, admitted: "Suvorexant selectively targets an important pathway involved in helping to promote sleep" and is "a new, first-in-class treatment for patients with insomnia."[92] It will certainly be of great value to the military too.

Experts agree that the future of sleep pharmacology belongs to new hypnotics that not only will be able to initiate sleep, program its length, detect and intensify slow-wave sleep, but at the same time will also be safe and almost nonaddictive. Armed forces, of course, dream of such perfect no-go pills.

Conclusion

Looking forward to the future, given the developments in neurobiology and psychopharmacology and the eager interest of the American military in research into newer and better eugeroics, we may well imagine that psycho-pharmaceuticals will enable soldiers to boost their "brain processors," prevent their persistent "overheating," and improve or substitute sleep.

Two, in my opinion, possible tendencies are worth drawing attention to. First, today, maybe except for some special forces, only air forces implement a fully fledged policy of psychopharmacological management of alertness, sleep, and fatigue, but in the future it is going to extend to other services. Second, while at present neuropharmacological agents are used to compensate for the effects of sleep deficit and fatigue, in the future, the military will resort to chemical support, and perhaps even mostly, to significantly enhance soldiers' performance. The goal will not be limited to sustaining combatants' efficiency but will extend to boosting their capacity. Thus the American armed forces will be implementing a form of cosmetic psychopharmacology. In his bestselling book *Listening to Prozac* (1993), the American psychiatrist Peter Kramer introduced the idea of "cosmetic pharmacology" to describe the use of psy-choactive medications by healthy people who require no therapy for enhancing mood and efficacy, in a word—for feeling "better than well."[93] The concept captures the blurring distinction between the therapeutic and enhancing effects of drugs, between restoring a disease-afflicted body to its natural condition and bestowing supernatural possibilities on humans. And so, the science fiction visions of superman seem to become less and less fantastic.

Substance Use and Abuse by Soldiers

Due to the asymmetric character of the wars in Afghanistan and Iraq, American servicemen experienced severe stress, which, in turn, gave rise to the drug problem. Compared with 1998, illicit substance use among American military personnel recorded an almost twofold increase by 2005, reaching 5 percent.[94] In the years 2002–2004, the Veterans Health Administration diagnosed 277 cases of substance dependence; in the years 2005–2007 there were 3,057.[95] These statistics should, however, come as no surprise because given the character of the combat environment and enemies employing highly irregular methods of warfare, OEF and OIF abounded in multiple stressors. Insurgency and urban warfare, the lack of clear front lines, and traumatic images of massacred soldiers and civilians resulted in a significant increase in the number of servicemen suffering from serious mental disorders (on average 11 percent of those returning from Afghanistan and 17 percent of those serving in Iraq).[96] In April 2008 approximately 303,000 Afghanistan and Iraqi veterans suffered from PTSD or other severe disorders.[97]

Soldiers with mental problems were routinely administered psychotropic drugs that were supposed to quickly render them combat worthy again. Thanks to pharmacology, psychologically injured servicemen could be sent to serve their second or third tour. It was a short-sighted and detrimental policy. In effect, PTSD sufferers, with their invisible wounds barely healed, went back to Afghanistan and Iraq, which not only led to the worsening of their condition but at times also resulted in tragic incidents: suicides, homicides, or substance overdoses. Between 2006 and 2009, 47 percent (188) of army deaths classified as "incidental or cause unknown" were due to drug or alcohol abuse, of which 74 percent (139) were related to prescription medications. In 2009 the army recorded seventy-four cases of soldier's deaths caused by drug overdose.[98]

What was recorded was a massive increase in prescription medications issued to military personnel. In 2009, approximately 106,000 of ground force soldiers were prescribed analgesics or antidepressants. In 2010, 14 percent of American servicemen received potent opioid analgesics, mainly oxycodone. Steve Robinson, an intelligence analyst working for the Department of Defense under President Bill Clinton's administration, thus reported: "Soldiers I talked to were receiving bags of antidepressants and sleeping meds in Iraq, but not the trauma care they needed."[99] Medical personnel were, in general, ill-prepared to diagnose and treat PTSD and other mental disorders. According to research conducted in the years 2003–2005, as many as 90 percent of military psychiatrists, psychologists, and social workers had received no formal training in basic PTSD therapies recommended by the Department of Defense and Department of Veterans Affairs.[100] Therefore, the opinion expressed by Thomas Kosten, a psychiatrist from the Michael E. DeBakey VA Medical Center in Huston, that the methods of treating mental disorders in soldiers did not substantially differ from the techniques employed during the Vietnam War should not be surprising.[101] Hence to make depression, anxiety disorders, and insomnia somewhat bearable, soldiers frequently resorted to alcohol and drugs. As a result, many also developed psychotropic and analgesic agents dependency, as these substances were readily and liberally prescribed to them.[102]

At the same time, a black market for prescription medications emerged.[103] Valium (diazepam), a psychotropic medication that at high doses has intoxicating effects, was particularly popular among troops in Iraq. One veteran, John Crawford, confessed: "We were so junked out on Valium, we had no emotions anymore."[104] Soldiers also turned to substances commonly used for doping in sports, that is, steroids, which became hugely popular since they pass routine urine drug tests undetected. In 2005 Italian police in Trieste busted a criminal ring supplying American forces deployed in Iraq with steroids (nandrolon, among others). The group sold their wares over the Internet.[105]

Another factor contributing to the increase in the illicit use of psychoactive substances by servicemen, especially on duty, was relaxing the American armed forces recruitment requirements. Due to the careful selection of candidates and military discipline, rates of drug use in the military are, as a rule, lower than in the general population. Relaxing entry requirements entails the risk that substance habits common in the general population will spread to the military. Yet the Pentagon was faced with a serious challenge; namely, the shortage of those willing to enlist. Given that the wars in Afghanistan and Iraq were losing social support, maintaining recruitment standards hitherto in force would mean a serious manpower deficit. Therefore, youths with criminal records involving illegal substances and related offenses were accepted to the armed forces.[106] For example, a boy named Sean Thomas enlisted in the Marines, hoping he would be able to put an end to his past: membership in a New York street gang and drug taking.[107]

As an example of brutality triggered by the abuse of intoxicants, take the incident of five U.S. Marines who, in March 2006 in Al-Mahmudiyah south of Baghdad, gang-raped a fourteen-year-old girl whom they later murdered. The Marines had taken whisky fortified with codeine-containing cough syrup and painkillers.[108] This was their manner of coping with the psychological burden resulting from the nature of their mission: hopelessness, depression, and constant fear. Their main task was patrolling roads in search of planted explosive devices. During missions of this type, one never knows whether the soldier's next step triggers a land mine, whether a sniper will fire at him, or whether a civilian approaching the control point carries a hidden bomb, and on and on. The stress is enormous, first and foremost due to the fact that the adversary remains invisible until it is too late.

To conclude, if an increase in the unauthorized use of drugs by military personnel is a common feature of war, it may be particularly disquieting in the case of conflicts in Afghanistan and Iraq. It is worth remembering, however, that it was not illicit drug use that was the greatest problem during OEF and OIF, but alcohol, psychotropic prescription medications, and analgesics. Overall, as has been the case throughout the centuries, prescription and self-prescription of intoxicants remains intrinsic to military life.

Conclusion

Quod licet Jovi, non licet bovi.
—A Latin phrase, literally, "What is permissible
for Jove is not permissible for an ox."

Almost every war was accompanied by some psychoactive substance, be it tobacco, alcohol or drugs. When analyzing the history of drugs in warfare— see table C.1 for the summary of the main examples of the military use of intoxicants discussed in the book—it is possible to arrive at the following conclusions.

1

War has been a powerful force popularizing intoxicants and their consumption. On one hand, marching armies "exported" them to new territories; on the other hand, soldiers deployed and fighting away from home came into contact with local psychoactive substances and intoxication practices, frequently "importing" them on their return. Sometimes veterans would disseminate information on wondrous effects of stimulants they had received on the front line, this way promoting their use within society. In short, the specific character of military service has been conducive to consumption of drugs, whereas the high mobility of armies facilitated their proliferation. Therefore, war has been a significant factor contributing to the globalization of a variety of intoxicants; an entire gamut of their intake methods; and frequently, also addiction, as illustrated by examples given below.

Roman legionaries returning from their conquests, especially from Egypt and the Middle East, brought the knowledge of opium. Later, the Islamic conquest of Europe was accompanied by Arabization of the conquered territories, including establishment of the opium trade.[1] In turn, another factor that contributed to the popularization of opium in Europe came between the eleventh

Table C.1 The use of psychoactive substances in war

Warriors, armed forces or state/war	Psychoactive substance*			
	Administered by the military	Self-prescribed by combatants	As a potential psychochemical weapon	Used to finance military operations/political agenda and/or jeopardize enemy forces/society
Homeric warriors		lotus, opium ("nepenthes")		
Hannibal's army; war against the revolted African tribes (200 BC)			mandrake (atropine)	
Inca warriors, traditional use	coca leaves**			
Siberian tribes (Chukchi, Yakuts, Yukaghirs, Kamchadals, Koryaks, and Khanty)		Amanita muscaria		
Scandinavian berserkers	Amanita muscaria or Amanita pantherina			
Indian warriors, traditional use		hashish (bhang)		
Warriors of the peoples of West Africa; traditional use	cola nuts			
Sotho warriors, traditional use		cannabis		
Massai warriors, traditional use	thorny olkiloriti tree			
Yanomami Indians, traditional use	hauma			

Otomac Indians, traditional use	yupe (*Piptadenia peregrina*)	
Turkish soldiers, 16th century	opium	
Indian warriors; anti-Spanish Rebellion of Túpac Amaru II (1780–83)	coca leaves	
French soldiers; Napoleon Bonaparte's expedition to Egypt (1798–1801)	hashish	
Swedish soldiers; Swedish-Norwegian war (1814)	*Amanita muscaria*	
Great Britain; Opium Wars (1839–42, 1856–60)		opium
Chinese soldiers; Opium Wars (1839–42, 1856–60)	opium	
Sikh warriors; traditional use	opium	
Union and Confederate soldiers; American Civil War (1861–65)	"laudanum," morphine, opium	"laudanum," morphine, opium
Prussian soldiers; Prussia's wars with Austria (1866) and France (1870–71)	morphine	
Zulu warriors; traditional use; Anglo-Zulu war (1879)	*Amanita muscaria, Boophane disticha,* cannabis (*dagga*), *intelezi*	
French soldiers deployed in West Africa (19th century)	cola nuts	

(*Continued*)

Table C.1 Continued

Warriors, armed forces or state / war	Psychoactive substance*			
	Administered by the military	Self-prescribed by combatants	As a potential psychochemical weapon	Used to finance military operations/political agenda and/or jeopardise enemy forces/society
American soldiers; Philippine-American war (1899–1902)		opium		
American soldiers deployed in the Panama Canal Zone (after 1914)		marihuana		
German and French soldiers (mostly pilots); First World War	cocaine	cocaine		
Australian soldiers; First World War	cocaine	cocaine		
British and Canadian soldiers; First World War	cocaine	cocaine		
Used against British soldiers by Germany; First World War				cocaine (according to British propaganda)
Wehrmacht soldiers; Spanish Civil War (1936–39)	methamphetamine (Pervitin)			
Wehrmacht soldiers; Second World War	methamphetamine (Pervitin)	methamphetamine (Pervitin)		
British soldiers; Second World War	amphetamine (Benzedrine)	amphetamine (Benzedrine)		

American soldiers; Second World War	amphetamine (Benzedrine)
Japanese soldiers; Pacific War	methamphetamine
Used by Japan against its occupied territories, particularly China	cocaine, heroin, morphine, opium
Finnish soldiers; Winter War (1939–41)	cocaine, heroin, morphine, opium
Finnish soldiers; Continuation War (1941–44)	cocaine, heroin, methamphetamine (Pervitin), morphine, opium
Soviet soldiers; Second World War	valerian, vodka mixed with cocaine
American soldiers; Korean War (1950–53)	dextroamphetamine, methamphetamine; heroin, heroin mixed with amphetamine (*speedballs*)
American Army; during the Cold War (1953–75)	mainly anabasine, BZ, LSD, MDA, MDMA, mescaline, scopolamine
British Army; during the Cold War (the 1950s and 1960s)	LSD
Czechoslovak Army; during the Cold War (the 1970s)	LSD

(Continued)

Table C.1 Continued

Warriors, armed forces or state / war	Psychoactive substance*			
	Administered by the military	Self-prescribed by combatants	As a potential psychochemical weapon	Used to finance military operations/political agenda and/or jeopardise enemy forces/society
American soldiers; Vietnam War (1965–73)	dextroamphetamine, neuroleptics (e.g., chlorpromazine), opiates (codeine), sedatives, steroids	amphetamines, barbiturates, cocaine, LSD, marijuana, morphine, opium, sedatives		heroin (according to American propaganda and media)
Soviet soldiers; Afghan War (1979–89)		cocaine, hashish, heroin, marijuana, opium and local opium products (e.g., *koknar*)		
United States, Afghan mujahideen, Pakistan, the Soviet Union; Afghan War (1979–89)				cocaine, hashish, heroin, opium
American pilots; Gulf War (1990–91), Kosovo War (1999)	dextroamphetamine, sedatives and soporifics (mostly temazepam, zolpidem, zaleplon)			

American pilots; OEF (2001) and OIF (2003)	dextroamphetamine, sedatives and soporifics (mostly temazepam, zolpidem, zaleplon)	cocaine, codeine, diazepam (Valium), marijuana, opioid painkillers, steroids (e.g., nandrolon)
terrorists, insurgents, jihadists, rebels	amphetamine, ATS (amphetamine-type stimulants) (e.g., Captagon, cocaine paste, hallucinogenic mushrooms, hashish, heroin, khat, LSD, methamphetamine, morphine, painkillers, sedatives, steroids)	cocaine, heroin, opium
child soldiers; wars in African and Asia	amphetamines, gunpowder (and mixtures of cocaine or heroin with gunpowder, e.g., *brown-brown*), hashish, khat, local herbal intoxicants, marihuana, psychotropic drugs, (barbiturates and benzodiazepines)	

* Alcohol and tobacco excluded; in alphabetical order
** Merging of columns means that the consumption of intoxicants was customary and it is impossible to distinguish between prescribed and self-prescribed drug use

and thirteenth centuries along with returning crusaders who, owing to Arabs, had become familiar with the forms of the drug's use.[2]

Tobacco found its way to the Old Continent thanks to members of Christopher Columbus's voyages, and "[t]he first group to use tobacco in Europe were," as Rudi Matthee reminds us, "the soldiers and sailors who set out on military expeditions and commercial ventures from the ports of Lisbon, Genoa and Naples."[3] Hence both trade and war together played a decisive role in the spread of tobacco use. Yet in continental Europe it gained in popularity only during the Thirty Years' War (1618–1648). For, as Matthee writes, "English troops put at the disposal of Frederick of Bohemia in 1620 were seen smoking as they marched through Saxony. Before long, Germany was cultivating its own tobacco and served as a springboard for the spread to Austria and Hungary" and then further to eastern, northern, and southern Europe.[4] And the popularization of high-proof spirits in Europe probably had to do with the wars conducted in the second half of the seventeenth century and in particular with the campaign waged by Louis XIV against Holland in 1672.[5]

On their return to France, the soldiers who had participated in Napoleon's Egyptian expedition (1798–1801) brought not only a substantial supply of hashish but, more importantly, the habit of its consumption that became an extremely fashionable way of entertainment in the bohemian world of Paris. Subsequently, hashish overflowed to other European countries, while in the wake of the conquest of Algeria (1830–1847) it became established in the French society for good and ceased to be a pastime reserved for higher circles of society and artists.

A massive use of opium and morphine in treatment of the sick and wounded during the American Civil War (1861–1865), Austro-Prussian War (1866), and French-Prussian War (1870–1871) left entire swathes of veterans addicted, many of whom had developed the habit trying to cure the "soldiers' disease," frequently using laudanum, opium, or morphine until the end of their days. The veterans' habits were believed to contribute to higher rates of addiction in societies at large.

The First World War resulted in the increased use of cocaine not only among soldiers but also among civilians. Finally, the scale of its consumption and risks related therewith forced Great Britain to adopt firm antidrug measures first in 1916 and then in 1920.

The Second World War made the use of amphetamine stimulants commonplace, especially in American, British, Finnish, and Japanese societies, mainly due to the demobilization of troops and the vast stores of such substances gathered by pharmaceutical companies to meet army demands. In defeated Japan, for example, military supplies of methamphetamine, which found their way to legal and illegal circulation, resulted in an outbreak of Japan's first drug epidemic (1945–1955). And in the Finnish society, the proliferation of drug use came as a result of the Continuation War (1941–1944) against the Soviet Union.

During the Korean War (1950–1953) American soldiers discovered a method allowing them to substantially boost the effects of amphetamines by mixing them with heroin. These speedballs soon became popular in American society, similar to other drug mixtures, especially heroin and cocaine.

To sum up, the convergence of drugs and war has frequently led to the shaping of new relations between warfare and society. Paraphrasing Charles Tilly's famous remark, "War made the state, and the state made war,"[6] one may say that to a lesser or greater degree drugs shaped warfare, while warfare shaped the society, often by spreading and popularizing intoxicants.

2

Historians have dedicated little or no attention to the use of psychoactive substances by combatants, armies, and states since not only was the topic rather inconvenient, but it was also a sort of taboo. As a rule, state authorities kept military use of intoxicants a secret. Knowledge of pharmacological means allowing for the maximization of troops' combat efficiency had to be protected to maintain a strategic edge. The secrecy was dictated also, especially in the twentieth century, by the desire to avoid an inconvenient public debate, inquisitive questions, and journalist investigations, particularly in times when the very same state that supplied military personnel with drugs banned the general public from consuming them. Along with the greater role of the media and an increased influence of public opinion on politics in democratic countries, questions inquiring why drugs are generally bad but when put to political use they are deconstructed or rehabilitated have become inconvenient, too. The ongoing process of proscription of mind-altering substances, initiated in the years of the First World War, was accompanied by their military use that, in turn, was becoming an increasingly awkward subject for authorities. Secrecy, therefore, masked contradictions in policies: penalizing social consumption of intoxicants while at the same time providing military personnel with psychopharmacological boosters to gain a tactical advantage. The Third Reich and the United States from the 1950s on are textbook examples of that.

3

Throughout history, the use of psychoactive substances by warriors was surrounded by many myths and stereotypes rooted deeply in social awareness

shaped either by the atmosphere of secrecy or by cultural and social reproduction of false or exaggerated ideas. What is important, these myths have
always had a negative and sinister undertone, and they have also been frequently used for political and propaganda purposes. They served the goals
of legitimizing antidrug measures adopted by authorities and penalizing
social consumption of intoxicants, fomenting hatred toward the enemy and,
to a degree, dehumanizing the adversary, bolstering patriotism and national
identity, and justifying a defeat of one's military or not achieving victory.
Examples of such myths are

1. the legend of the Assassins;
2. the soldiers' disease after the American Civil War;
3. the cocaine panic in Great Britain during the First World War;
4. a vision of opium-crazed Chinese soldiers during the Korean War;
5. communist brainwashing techniques, in particular the myth of the
   Manchurian candidate; and
6. a threefold myth related to the Vietnam War: not only the myth of the
   American army losing due to the habitual use of marijuana, heroin, and
   other drugs, not only the myth of the addicted veteran (the other) dangerously spreading addiction and its effects in American society upon their
   return from Indochina, but also the myth of communists using drugs to
   weaken American operational capacity and devastate the very social fabric
   of the nation.

In the United States certain substances, such as marijuana and heroin, were
portrayed as exceptionally dangerous. The use of drugs was presented as
the enemy's perfidious assault threatening the nation's vitality. The image of
a junkie veteran was sometimes accompanied by drumming up social fears
and emotions, as was the case during the Civil War and the war in Vietnam.
It would also be worth connecting this phenomenon to outbreaks of "moral
panic" occurring in the United States and other countries; that is, the sense
"that there is something wrong with our society because of a moral failure on
the part of specific individuals. This moral failure is linked to the use of various
substances called drugs."[7] Oftentimes these moral panics were used in a highly
instrumental fashion. As Ann Dally observes,

> Governments and doctors capitalize on collective fantasies. They
> publicize the drugs in a way to induce horror and fear. This policy
> costs governments and nations dearly, but it provides other politi-
> cal benefits, including to the medical profession. The dangers of

these substances are both created and emphasized with zeal rather than evidence.[8]

What of it, if it turned out to be an effective tool in the hands of politicians.

4

At times the pursuit of a tactical or strategic advantage over the adversary resulted in attempts to create a magic pill that would make it possible to transform soldiers into organic combat machines, or developing a new category of a psychochemical weapon, or discovering a truth serum. Such research frequently necessitated risky medical experiments on humans, such as in the Cold War era in the United States. This in turn stirred and keeps stirring serious ethical doubts. They were, however, largely ignored as insignificant, since the research served the higher goal of national security. Such reasoning was prominently inscribed in the realist way of thinking about politics, which is characteristic in the so-called ethics of responsibility.

The essence of the difference between private and public ethics was expressly articulated by Niccolo Machiavelli. The point is not that politicians or state officials enjoy greater freedom, but that they act, or at least should act, according to a different moral system than the one followed by individuals in private and social life. Political responsibility flows along a completely different circuit from that of individuals' morality. It is so, since the survival of the state, community, and their safety are the highest values. Politicians, and leaders in particular, are first and foremost responsible for citizens who entrusted them not only with power but, what nowadays is frequently forgotten, also their safety. To realize these fundamental goals, at times rulers must resort to lying, cheating, torturing, and even killing. As Machiavelli and an entire host of realists following in his footsteps endeavored to persuade, they do not do so only to further their particular interests, that is, to hold onto power, but for the greater good of the community. Plato wrote of a "noble lie": "It's likely that our rulers will have to use a throng of lies and deceptions for the benefit of the ruled."[9] An example of ethics of responsibility can be the suspension of the habeas corpus principle, one of the foundations of the American political system, in relation to people suspected of terrorist activities after 9/11. Actions immoral from the perspective of private ethics become morally justified in terms of public safety. Therefore, is subjecting a small group of people to medical experiments involving considerable risk indefensible, especially if it could contribute to the development of a wonder weapon? A weapon that would bring victory and save not only our soldiers' lives but also those of the enemy's army and population?

Proponents of the ethics of responsibility consider it an unquestionable axiom. Yet some grave doubts remain when dealing with cases of supreme emergency and the principle of necessity which assumes "that when conventional means of resistance are hopeless or worn out, anything goes (anything that is 'necessary' to win)."[10] Albert Camus's play *The Just Assassins* (1949) is based on the failed attempt on the life of a tsarist official, the Grand Duke Serge Alexandrovich, by Narodnaya Volya (People's Will), a group of Russian revolutionaries and terrorists. When the assassin notices that the duke is accompanied by his two small children and a woman, he hesitates and aborts his mission, walking away without using a bomb hidden under his coat. In the mouth of one of his companions who applauded the decision to withdraw from the assault, Camus puts the following words: "Even in destruction, there's a right way and a wrong way—and there are limits."[11] Hence, if we find like General William Tecumseh Sherman that "war is hell," even in the midst of the hell of war there is, as Camus reminds us, a way that is more right and one that is less right—there are limitations. Engaging in polemics with Machiavelli, this is to say that not all goals justify the means. On the other hand, it is worth remembering an important but not sufficiently known remark by Reinhold Niebuhr, the American Protestant theologian, holding that moral choices are not made between the moral and the immoral, but rather between the immoral and less immoral.[12] This should be kept in mind when it comes to state experiments with psychoactive substances on humans, which may imply a clash between private morality and the ethics of responsibility. All in all, however, one must be very careful here, as quite too often public good, national security, or supreme emergency have been used to justify ethically dubious and, as history teaches us, unnecessary actions.

5

Intoxicating substances, especially hallucinogenics, were originally used for religious purposes since they facilitated and sometimes even enabled communication with the world of deities and supernatural powers. It was in this strictly cultural context that they were initially used by warriors. Yet in time they were stripped of their traditional cultural meaning. Along with the desacralization of hallucinogens and their growing use for purposes other than ritual, shamanic, and religious—mainly hedonistic—not only did their perception and functions change, but also the possibilities for collective control of their consumption were lessened. Sacred plants and psychoactive substances stripped of their religious sanctions, prohibitions, and commandments controlled by a given community have found their way to the realm of the *profanum*. As a result, their use, mostly in the pursuit of pleasure ("without internal brakes" and social control), has bred addiction, terminal illnesses, and deleterious social and economic consequences.

Rigorously framed within premodern cultures, intoxicants were therefore governed by exceptionally strong religious sanctions that effectively prevented their use for purposes other than those socially recognized and accepted. It was thus thanks to the social control over the customs of drug use that these substances were extremely rarely misused or abused. Such control prevented taking them for pleasure, and it was highly effective since it connected the intoxicant to the symbolic and ritual content, to the *sacrum*. This being such, then no grave social problems of addiction and substance abuse existed. Opium or coca in their unrefined form and administered in a traditional mode constituted no serious threat to human health. Along with their refinement, however, their addictive potential became gradually stronger, thus rendering them more treacherous. Opium concentration in laudanum (widespread in the 1770s), then in morphine (synthesized in 1804 and marketed in 1817) and heroin (synthesized in 1874 and marketed in 1897), transformed a mildly addictive substance capable of bringing relief and well-being into dangerous drugs. Depending on the degree of refinement and purity, morphine may be ten times stronger than opium, while heroin is two to three times stronger than morphine. The possibilities of increasing potency can be scary, as illustrated by etorphine, known as M99 or immobilon, a substance synthesized in 1960 that is 10,000 times stronger than morphine. It is used as a sleeping agent for capturing elephants and rhinoceroses: two milliliters of etorphine are capable of knocking down an adult rhinoceros, whereas a drop of it on human skin may cause death in mere minutes.

Coca leaves faced a similar fate. The isolation of a single alkaloid (1859) gave rise to the production of highly addictive cocaine. Developments of modernity transformed the potential inherent in the leaves of *Erythroxylum coca* into a powerful drug. As David Courtwright astutely observes, "The history of psychoactive substances resembles that of the arms race."[13] Ever more powerful substances with the effects ever increasing in intensity (the so-called hard drugs) are also more addictive and dangerous as their "destructive potential" is expanding. The processes of concentration, refinement, and synthesis accompanied the beginnings of industrial production of drugs for commercial purposes. This was the route explored earlier by alcohol: what cocaine is to coca, morphine is to opium, and high-proof spirits are to wine. Along with the popularization of recreational and escapist use of increasingly more purified and hence more addictive substances, which have crossed from the sphere of the *sacrum* to that of the *profanum*, the social problem of drug dependency began to feature more and more prominently also in the armed forces.

6

The main principle organizing life in the era of modernity, to summon Max Weber's authority, came as the domination of instrumental, or formal, rationality spread to all areas of life, this way gradually "demagifying the world." Rationalization extended its reach also to the processes of obtaining, manufacturing, and consuming drugs. The instrumental rationality signifies a utilitarian approach to life and reality. It is a pragmatic orientation aimed at immediate and effective attainment of the intended goal by appropriately selected means. The economics of action, that is, making such decisions—adopting such norms, models, and solutions that yield more gain than loss—plays a key role in this respect. Therefore, calculation and impersonality have become the characteristics of the modern organization of social, economic, and political institutions. The systematic application of scientific and technological knowledge has equipped human beings with constantly improving and more effective means. In the case of warfare, the main motives of instrumental rationality are weapons systems, organizational machine, logistics and transportation, medical care, and so forth. However, Weber's rationalization can be seen expressed also in the armed forces' use of increasingly stronger and more effective psychoactive substances, aimed at enhancing the performance and operational capacity of soldiers, but also in attempts to create a psychochemical weapon. Thomas Szasz aptly observed:

> Until the advent of the machine, most men had to labor most of the time to survive. Hence, most of the major drugs that affect behavior— in particular, marijuana, opium, and cocaine—were used to enable men to work better, harder, and longer. These drugs were to pretechnical man what machines are to technological men: they helped him to increase "productivity" or "output."[14]

This remark is also pertinent in the context of war, with the reservation that combat productivity and killing efficiency were enhanced both exogenously (equipping soldiers with new weapons) and endogenously (boosting them pharmacologically). At the same time, the intensified mechanization of warfare contributed to increasing the stress experienced by combatants and thereby causing a rise in unauthorized consumption of drugs by military personnel, who use them as a panacea for the horrors and traumas of the modern technologized battlefield. Unlike in the case of productive work, the mechanization has not resulted in reducing the soldiers' need for pharmacological support. To the contrary. Rationalization, for Weber constituting the essence of the modern Western civilization, pertained to various spheres: economy, law, political community, city, religion, art, and so on. Its overwhelming influence extends to war as well. It could hardly be otherwise, considering the remarkable expansiveness of modernity.

Disenchantment-breeding reality creates systems stripped of mystery, mysticism, and magic, where everything seems to revolve around efficiency and good performance. A demagified system is gaining in significance at the expense of the individual who is reduced to the role of one of many impersonal and nameless elements thereof. Insofar as Weber wrote about the "demagification of the world" as an inseparable outcome of rationalization, I would rather speak of the "demagification of war" as an inseparable outcome of its instrumentalization, resulting from continuous implementation of new technologies. Psychopharmacology may be seen as a "disciplinary technology of the body" (or political technology), to evoke one of Michel Foucault's key notions. Regarding disciplining, Foucault refers to "[t]hese methods, which made possible the meticulous control of the operations of the body, which assured the constant subjection of its forces and imposed upon them a relation of docility-utility."[15]

In 1982, two years before his demise, "Foucault raised the possibility of writing 'a study of the culture of drugs or drugs as culture in the West from the beginning of the nineteenth century.'"[16] What would be the guiding thesis of such a book were it to ever come into being? I think the main theme of Foucault's work would, in general, be the use of the body as an instrument of power and object of experiments and the political and cultural definition of what is right and legitimate, and what is wrong and illegitimate. For Foucault, drugs, on one hand, constituted a form of political control (penalization) and on the other, the individual's resistance to authority (substance use and abuse). After all, he took them himself. His partner of many years, Daniel Defert, confessed: "I don't know if he injected," but his drugs were "stronger than mere alcohol or hashish."[17] Sadie Plant notes:

> Perhaps Foucault was always writing on drugs, and didn't need to write the book at all. The figure of the addict walks silently through the corridors of his hospitals, his asylums, and his prison cells, and drugs are implicit in all his work, bound up with his studies of medicine, psychiatry and the penal code, his studies of the shifting definitions and treatments of sickness, insanity and crime.[18]

Next to the administration of justice and prison systems, in modern times state control over the body has never been more important and stronger anywhere else than in the army. The soldier's disciplined, efficient, trained, and effective body is a precondition for military success and, hence, for the defense of society. Armed forces embody the principles of "the control of bodies and individual forces . . . exercised within states."[19] Foucault writes in *Discipline and Punish*:

> What was then being formed was a policy of coercions that act upon the body, a calculated manipulation of its elements, its gestures, its behavior. The human body was entering a machinery of power that explores it, breaks it down and rearranges it. A "political anatomy," which was also a "mechanics of power," was being born; it defined how one may have a hold over others' bodies, not only so that they may do what one wishes, but so that they may operate as one wishes, with the techniques, the speed and the efficiency that one determines. Thus discipline produces subjected and practiced bodies, "docile" bodies. Discipline increases the forces of the body (in economic terms of utility) and diminishes these same forces (in political terms of obedience).[20]

And so, by distributing drugs to soldiers, authorities (or more broadly speaking, "state-the-dealer") implemented the repressive form of subjugating their bodies. In reality, this practice may be found to constitute a peculiar "pharmacological drilling." In the name of economics and enhanced performance, in the name of rationalization of their operations, armies chemically disciplined the bodies of their fighting men. Already shaped by a rigorous drill and training, they could be controlled also from inside. Soldiers' bodies were optimized and their minds tuned through psychopharmacological means. According to Foucault, authorities treat individuals as permanent energy supplies to be used by the state when the need arises. If so, then when enforcing its power to manage citizens' bodies through the use of stimulants, especially cocaine and amphetamines, this energy may be accumulated and extracted from the body, thus transforming the military man into a boosted and significantly more efficient chemical quasi-cyborg. Stimulants, constituting a "technology of disciplining the body," increase soldiers' strength (enhancing their energy capacity and thus their usefulness on the battlefield), while simultaneously weakening this strength (speeding up the burning of energy stored in the body, but supplying nothing in exchange). At the same time, the tacit consent of superiors for individual consumption of self-prescribed drugs also constituted a form of managing servicemen's bodies. It is so, since intoxicants mitigate negative psychological effects of participation in war, so that they may delay or even prevent the occurrence of battle trauma and PTSD. In this way they allow the maintenance of body economics, because a useful soldier is a combat-worthy soldier, the one who did not lose the fight against stress and his own nerves. Thanks to the knowledge about the mechanisms of action of psychoactive substances, the state was able to produce a pliant body, thus turning its own energies upon itself. This knowledge is power (Foucault would have approved), for it increases the body's performative and productive capacity. Therefore, in this context, drugs in warfare might be perceived as a political and military "technology of the body," and as such they are nothing else but an emanation of Weber's march of instrumental rationality. Furthermore, also antidrug policies and regulations penalizing the consumption of intoxicants may be analyzed from the perspective of technologies for disciplining of the body—both individual and collective because the misuse of psychoactive substances, adversely impacting morale and operational capacity, can lead to a deterioration of the army. In this case disciplining in the form of bans, orders, and punishments aims to prevent or counteract the drug problem in the military.

7

The shaman differs from mountebank, medic, and magician in his ability to directly contact spiritual forces by altering his state of consciousness through ecstasy. Using a variety of techniques, the shaman transcends the normal state of mind. He embarks on journeys between various realities to gain hidden knowledge and powers but also to help people. Practiced in many non-Western cultures, shamanism "represents the most widespread and ancient methodological system of mind-body healing known to humanity."[21] Mircea Eliade claims that true shamanism is possible exclusively without any artificial stimulation. According to him, the use of hallucinogens to attain ecstasy came as a symptom of the decline of shamanism. He writes:

> Intoxication by mushrooms also produces contact with spirits, but in a passive and crude way. But, as we have already said, this shamanic technique appears to be late and derivative. Intoxication is a mechanical and corrupt method of reproducing "ecstasy," being "carried out of oneself"; it tries to imitate a model that is earlier and that belongs to another plane of reference.[22]

In yet another place, he even more emphatically claims:

> Narcotics are only a vulgar substitute for "pure" trance. We have already had occasion to note this fact among several Siberian peoples; the use of intoxicants (alcohol, tobacco, etc.) is a recent innovation and points to a decadence in shamanic technique. Narcotic intoxication is called on to provide an *imitation* of a state that the shaman is no longer capable of attaining otherwise.[23]

Eliade's view has incited controversies and has been questioned because hallucinogenic substances have been used by shamans since ancient times not only as the easiest and fastest but also as an effective technique (one of many) leading to supernatural visions and experiences.[24] Despite criticism, Eliade's claim can be used, I think, as a starting point for formulating an analogical thesis on the "pharmacologization" of warfare: the growing use of increasingly more refined and synthetic psychoactive substances by the military has contributed to the intensification of processes that come as products of modernity (such as the instrumentalization of warfare and the dehumanization and objectification of soldiers). In consequence, this might have in part led to the decline of the "warrior spirit" and precipitated the weakening of the existential dimension of war in the West. Intoxication of soldiers helps stimulate their courage but in an artificial manner. By boosting their strength, it facilitates their transformation into heroes, yet it is not a natural but pharmacologically mediated process. As Christopher Coker notes, "For true warriors, war-making is not so much what they do but what they *are*."[25] War is their calling, vocation, their spiritual and existential experience, a specific way to simultaneously test and affirm their humanity, a constant overcoming of the body's weaknesses stemming from our biological limitations. All these characteristics combined form "warrior's existential virtues." War and combat shape warriors' identities—the very source of their heroism. And a concept of heroism "includes everything from risk taking to selflessness and fearlessness, but not foolhardiness."[26] Foolhardiness and temerity are characteristics contrary to courage since spiritual power manifests in the ability to control oneself. A true warrior will not recklessly disregard danger or take risks for matters of little importance. So, how about the following paraphrasing of Eliade? The military is "no longer capable of attaining" warrior qualities such as high spirits, courage, and heroism otherwise than through the means of excessive stimulation with increasingly more synthetic (i.e., artificial) psychoactive compounds. Or perhaps this argument is equally flawed as that of Eliade, for, as I have tried to demonstrate in this book, the use of drugs—more or less powerful, more or less organic— has been intrinsic to warfare.

Whatever the issue, the existential dimension of war has been waning and disappearing because of technological, social, economic, and organizational, but first and foremost cultural and mental changes. In the twentieth century, and particularly in its second half, a Weberian-like rationalization of warfare in the West transformed war into a phenomenon of an almost exclusively instrumental nature. It has been stripped of its existential dimension. Long ago the soldier became an element of the system or, as Foucault would put it, "Man-the-Machine."[27] Nowadays, however, the American military perceives servicemen as the weakest element in the machinery of war. Equipped with super-modern weapons systems, American armed forces keep searching for new neuropharmacological compounds to facilitate transforming humans into super-effective machines. Man has to better fit the system. Thus a disturbing dream of Frederick Winslow Taylor comes true. In his *Principles of Scientific Management* Taylor wrote: "In the past man has been first; in the future the system must be first."[28] As the former director of Defense Advanced Research Projects Agency Tony Tether put it in June 2001, one of the basic challenges that the American military faces in the twenty-first century "is preventing human performance from becoming the weakest link on the future battlefield."[29] The human link must therefore be strengthened to enhance its effectiveness, for example, by neuropharmacology.

Epilogue

War as a Drug

> In the beginning war looks and feels like love. But unlike love it gives nothing in return but an ever-deepening dependence like all narcotics, on the road to self-destruction. It does not affirm but places upon us greater and greater demands. It destroys the outside world until it is hard to live outside war's grip. It takes a higher and higher dose to achieve any thrill. Finally, one ingests war only to remain numb.
> —Chris Hedges, *War Is a Force That Gives Us Meaning*

Historians have given the nineteenth century many a name: the age of industrialization, the era of colonialism, the age of nationalism and liberalism, "the era of triumphant modernity," or, following Lenin's analysis, the period in which imperialism was born. "The age of machine" is yet another frequently and aptly used label. However, why is "the age of intoxication" mentioned so seldomly? After all, the century witnessed a widespread use of opium, morphine, cocaine, hashish, ether ... Some exceptions apart, the period did not know serious nor systematic prohibitions, since the above-mentioned substances were not generally considered harmful; on the contrary, they ranked among the most popular remedies for a host of ailments and diseases.

Yet the nineteenth century can be spoken of as the age of intoxication also in a metaphorical sense. Other heady, and oftentimes also highly addictive, factors included, in particular, industrialization, colonialism, nationalism, liberalism, and Marxism. Earlier centuries had also induced a certain level of intoxication, but they had not done that on such a large scale and with the intensity of the nineteenth century. Industrialization meant humankind's intoxication with technology and an advancing process of rendering humans addicted to and dependent on the machine. Progress, in the era of modernity identified with scientific and technical development, was measured by the construction of ever more advanced mechanical devices. Originally, machines were to make the lives of humans easier, to enable them to conquer the environment.

Yet, similar to drugs in its action and therefore offering only apparent liberation and freedom, the machine ultimately restricted freedom of the individual,
rendering humans dependent on it. Colonialism, in turn, intoxicated with the
power and exploitative rule over other peoples and conquered territories. For
the European powers colonies were like a heady drug: possessing them was
the precondition for great power status. Liberalism, on the other hand, with its
ideas of freedom, private ownership, and free trade would intoxicate a growing
number of intellectuals, businessmen, politicians, and societies. And the country to become intoxicated with the (neo)liberal philosophy the most was the
United States. Imperialism, in turn, seduced capitalists and rich countries with
the idea of financial capital, its accumulation and multiplication, exports, and
gaining access to new markets. A new source of intoxication and addiction was
also on the rise: Marxism, defined by Raymond Aron, who was paradoxically
paraphrasing Marx speaking of religion, as "opium for intellectuals." Many
twentieth-century thinkers were deluded by their faith in leftism, revolution,
and the proletariat as a potential source of a just transformation.[1] In this context
it is worth quoting Carl Gustav Jung's observation: "Every form of addiction is
bad, no matter whether the narcotic be alcohol or morphine or idealism."[2]

Speaking of narcotic metaphors, one of the most powerful, exceptionally
graphic and suggestive is, however, that of "war as a drug." I contend that it
is interesting and useful to invoke here Avital Ronell's "narcoanalysis" of literature. In her thought-provoking book *Crack Wars: Literature and Addiction
Mania* (1992), she interprets writing and reading (hallucinogenric) literature
in terms of addiction, drawing on Martin Heidegger's analysis of the addictive structure of human existence. For Ronell "being-addicted" is "a primary
ontological mode that includes all forms of addiction to something, each of
which has its own way of being."[3] It is not only nor necessarily an intoxicant
that makes humans dependent. In Heideggerian terms, "being-in-the-world"
(*Dasein*) can indeed be seen as a certain type of "being-on-drugs." Thus in re-
reading Gustave Flaubert's *Madame Bovary*, Ronell shows via the example of
Emma Bovary how reading literature is not that much different than taking
a drug. An addictive compulsion (i.e., the need to intoxicate oneself, to hal-
lucinate and dream) is joined at the hip with literary obsession. Ronell makes
us notice the correlation not only of reading and drugs but also of writing and
drugs, for, in essence, "the horizon of drugs is the same as that of literature."[4]
If literature and drugs happen to be conjoined, then the same is even truer of
war and drugs. So, let me try to unpack the metaphor of war as a drug by taking
a look at the collective (i.e., national) and, most importantly, individual (i.e.,
warrior's) dimensions of the narcotic of war.

Firstly, in the era of modernity, communal intoxication with war is closely
related to nationalism. The vision of a victorious struggle that may be a source of

national pride would push societies into a state of collective elation and euphoria. Emotions of this type accompanied, for example, the Japanese during the war with Russia (1904–1905); the Germans, the French, and the British at the outbreak of the First World War (1914); the Argentineans during the Falkland War (among many anti-Western incidents and attacks, in June 1982, crowds took to the streets of Buenos Aires demanding weapons to continue the struggle against the British); or Serbs during the war in Bosnia and Herzegovina (1992–1995). The First World War was particularly telling in this respect: upon Great Britain's declaration of war against Germany crowds of cheering Londoners marched to the Buckingham Palace to close it in a festive siege for several days. When on April 6, 1917, the show in progress in the New York's Metropolitan Opera House was suddenly interrupted to announce that the Congress had just declared war on Germany, the audience welcomed the news with "loud and long cheers."[5] The American psychologist George Everett Partridge observed that the mood induced by the war resembled "ecstasy" or "social inebriation."[6] One might add intoxication too. To a large degree, not only was the First World War a consequence of nationalist ideas, it was also their ultimate expression. Nationalism intoxicates with a sense of communality, separateness, exceptionality, and frequently also superiority. Societies intoxicated with nationalistic fervor are ready for unparalleled sacrifices and ruthlessness, too. Throughout history, and excepting religion, nationalism has provided the strongest stimulus to give one's own life in the name of an abstract, metaphysical idea of a nation. As Marx attempted to persuade, religion is opium for the masses, and the very same could be said about nationalism. Inducing an altered state of consciousness, it facilitates the sense of dedication and supreme loyalty to the community that in many cases verges on the irrational and, under a different set of circumstances, would be difficult to comprehend.

Secondly, and most importantly for this book, for many warriors, war was and continues to be the most powerful intoxicant. Despite all its horrors, brutality, and stress, combat is highly addictive for many. It is so because only combat can stimulate the body into releasing such enormous doses of hormones, adrenaline in particular, or trigger such complex emotions or experiences. In terms of adrenaline stimulation of the brain and body, no sport, even the most extreme, equals battle. This comparison of war to a drug, oftentimes appearing in film and literature, especially in war memoirs of soldiers and veterans, was superbly relayed by James Hillman, who quite remarkably wrote of "a terrible love of war."[7] The nature of this addictive sensation was exposed, among others, by Francis Ford Coppola in *Apocalypse Now* (1979) in the example of Captain Benjamin Willard (played by Martin Sheen). And the entire closing part of the movie is kept in a psychedelic atmosphere: hallucinogenic movements of one of the main characters, Lance Johnson, and a hypnotizing oriental track by The

Doors (the band whose name was borrowed from the title of Aldous Huxley's famous book *The Doors of Perception*, which describes his experiences of taking mescaline). Not only is war intoxicating and addictive, not only is it a hallucinogenic experience from the fringes (of existence), at times it may also be a powerful metaphysical experience, a true experience of humanity.

In her film *The Hurt Locker* (2008) Kathryn Bigelow also draws on the metaphor of war as a drug. Sergeant Major William James (played by Jeremy Renner) becomes a new commander of an elite sapper unit in Iraq. Despite the extreme danger, unlike his tragically deceased predecessor, he prefers to diffuse explosives without the assistance of highly specialized life-saving robots. At times, he works without his sapper's overalls. He is a risk-taker who really likes what he does. James epitomizes the existential dimension of war, more and more a seldom characteristic of military operations conducted by the United States. He understands war, and he feels its existential appeal, while the stress and the risk do not serve to merely mobilize him to do the job but are essential to his very existence. James is also an oddball who collects pieces of explosive devices he disarmed and sleeps in the sapper's protective suit. Although war is accursed, although there are moments when James is fed up with all this Iraq and the conflict with militants resorting to exceptionally drastic methods of combat, deep inside he loves his profession and cherishes a strange emotion toward war. Upon his return home, to his girlfriend and little son, he has great problems adapting to everyday life. And the issue is not merely the lack of social understanding for soldiers coming back from an unpopular war. The main reason is that in normal conditions, in the peacetime society of consumption, James does not know how to live; he feels forlorn. In one of the most moving scenes of the film, we see the protagonist completely lost in a supermarket where he is faced with the need to purchase breakfast cereal. A simple daily activity of choosing one product out of many alternatives is an extremely difficult decision for him. At war, possibilities of choice are usually limited. Additionally, discipline, regulations, and training make servicemen form conditioned responses. What is most important, however, is that life in society may not be able to supply a sufficient dose of emotions for a person addicted to an adrenaline rush, and therefore to stress, tension, and danger. Samuel Hynes writes superbly about it, confirming the universal nature of this phenomenon: "What is it, exactly, that war lovers love? Not the killing and the violence, I think, but the excitement, the drama, and the danger-life lived at a high level of intensity, like a complicated, fatal game (or a Wagnerian opera)."[8] Quiet life provides no stimuli that could immerse the brain in a chemical bath of hormones. This is why James so much misses the accursed Iraq, the awful war he got addicted to. He became entrapped in the hurt locker from the film's title. Like any true junkie, he finally finds a way to supply his body with what it craves. He enlists again, trying to escape the quiet monotony of life. He prefers combat zone to his family. Being a danger and risk addict, James clings to the reality of battlefield much like a moth unable to stay away from the fire. So he goes back to Iraq because of "a terrible love of war."

Research in fact confirms that soldiers often return from war with a higher level of excitement motivation than they had before their initial deployment. Active participation in combat, and being exposed to danger in particular, often pushes their optimum tolerance for arousal upward. Thus they become adrenaline junkies who go on to be redeployed for no other reason but to have their growing desire for sensation and excitement satisfied. "It is very likely," Morten Brænder writes persuasively,

> that adrenaline junkies—just as real drug addicts—build up men-
> tal (if not physiological) tolerance as a result of their thrill-seeking
> behavior. What goes for the consumption of alcohol, medicine, and
> euphoriants also goes for the consumption of adrenaline: The more
> you take, the more it takes to gain the same effect next time. If we
> translate this to the sphere of soldiers, this implies that an initial level
> of excitement motivation may actually be "pushed upward."[9]

Redeployment means putting oneself voluntarily at risk, and this is also pre- cisely what addiction is about. Avital Ronell captures it particularly well: "The *toxic maternal* means that while mother's milk is poison, it still supplies the crucial nourishment that the subject seeks. . . . Emma [Bovary] is absorbing medicine that nourishes by poisoning."[10] Could not the same be said of soldiers and war? Getting back to Bigelow's motion picture, it offers a positive answer to this question. The message conveyed by the film is simple, and it is announced in the opening quotation of the film: "The rush of battle is often a potent and often lethal addiction, for war is a drug." This sentence has been taken from an exceptionally inspiring book authored by lifelong *New York Times* journalist, foreign correspondent, and war reporter Chris Hedges: *War Is a Force That Gives Us Meaning* (2002), which discusses war as a source of a collective but, first and foremost, personal identity, meaning, and sense. Hedges suggestively shows how war seduces both masses and individuals; he proves what a mighty intoxicant it is.

Yet why, in the first place, would young people want to partake in war, in this "bizarre and fantastic universe that has a grotesque and dark beauty"?[11] Well, contrary to what Jeremy Bentham or John Locke would have us believe, happiness is neither the main nor the only thing humans crave. We also, and perhaps above all else, seek sense and meaning. And "war is sometimes the most powerful way in human society to achieve meaning."[12] For "it can," argues Hedges, "give us purpose, . . . a reason for living."[13] It is so, since it creates an opportunity to rise above human narrow-mindedness, predilection for conflict, and egoism. War is a borderline event that in its own peculiar way allows the human to acquire self-knowledge. Combat becomes the ultimate test in humanity, vesting lives of participants with the highest of values. They experience human fragility, they come to realize the accidental nature of their own existence, and they see how trivial their lives were before the war. Many have the sense of being involved in events of historic significance. Thus war, as Hillman captures the essence of it, "begs for meaning, and amazingly also gives meaning, a meaning found in the midst of its chaos. Men who survive battle come back and say it was the most meaningful time of their lives, transcendent to all other meanings."[14] Soldiers and veterans insist "that war expands and extends what is possible in life for an ordinary man, that for once he need not be simply a man mending shoes in Soho, or an insurance salesman. War offers experiences that men value and remember: shoes and insurance don't do that."[15] In 1906 William James put it particularly well: "Showing war's irrationality and horror is of no effect" on modern man. "[T]he horrors make the fascination. War is the *strong* life; it is life *in extremis*; war taxes are the only ones men never hesitate to pay, as the budgets of all nations show us."[16] For young boys, war brings associations with a sense of power that stems from carrying a gun and being able to decide about others' lives. A military surgeon who took part in the Soviet intervention in Afghanistan quoted a verse that evocatively captures this forcibly seductive allure of war:

> Women and wine
> Are all very fine
> But a real man needs more:
> The sweet taste of war![17]

From time immemorial war has been the source of male identity—in fact, as an exceptionally male occupation, it defined masculinity and constituted an initiation, a rite of passage from boyhood into manhood. Barbara Ehrenreich puts it particularly well:

> Men make wars for many reasons, but one of the most recurring ones
> is to establish that they are, in fact, "real men." Warfare and aggressive
> masculinity have been, in other words, mutually reinforcing cultural
> enterprises. Warmaking requires warriors, that is, "real men," and the
> making of warriors requires war. Thus war becomes a solution to what
> Margaret Mead termed "the recurrent problem of civilization," which
> is "to define the male role satisfactory enough."[18]

A warrior, therefore, impersonates the characteristics of "true masculinity"—above all else, strength—and as Simone Weil argued in her landmark essay *The Iliad or the Poem of Force* (*L'Iliade ou le poeme de la force*), written in the summer and autumn of 1940 just after the fall of France, "force is as pitiless to the man who possesses it, or thinks he does, as it is to its victims; the second it crushes, the first it intoxicates."[19] What is highly intoxicating is the satisfaction found in visiting destruction on others, which for John Glenn Gray seems to be "peculiarly human, or, more exactly put, devilish in a way animals can never be."[20] In *The Good Soldier* (2009), a film by Lexy Lovell and Michael Uys, James Massey, a veteran who served in the 2003 Iraq war, confesses: "I can honestly tell you that there is no other feeling in a world that comes close to hunting another human being. That's what you are trying to do. The drawback to it is the fact that you want to do it again. Because you enjoyed it. That's almost kind of like a drug. You become addicted to it." The consequences of being intoxicated with power and—as Ardant du Picq, a nineteenth-century French officer and military theorist put it—with "the dark beauty of violence," which is related to participation in war, tend to be cruel.[21] Hedges notes: "The myth of war sells and legitimizes the drug of war. Once we begin to take war's heady narcotic, it creates an addiction that slowly lowers us to the moral depravity of all addicts."[22] Besides, for many non-Western militants in irregular units, paramilitary formations, terrorist cells, guerrilla organizations, and, in particular, for child soldiers, war is everything—a way to live their lives and a lifestyle to which they are addicted.

Arthur Rimbaud preached that intoxication brings love and poetry but also their negation, thus leading to madness and decadence. In 1999 the British journalist Anthony Loyd published a book *My War Gone By, I Miss It So*. It is a tale of his cross-addiction—to heroin and to war in Bosnia. Loyd poignantly demonstrates the auto-destructive impulse feeding on war and narcotics. Just like Michael Herr in *Dispatches*, Loyd depicts war as the ultimate drug experience. A brutal borderline experience that may bring either *catharsis* or annihilation. War has always been, continues to be, and will remain a powerful drug. For both Herr and Loyd experiencing war was "like taking drugs, like being stoned."[23] Intoxicants have the ability to momentarily transform monotonous, depressing, or terrifying life into delightful, fascinating, and blissful. Yet it is but a fleeting illusion. The return to reality, which frequently becomes even harder to bear, is painful. A yearning for an apparent escape emerges. The artificial paradise quickly becomes paradise lost and narcotics play, as Stanisław Ignacy Witkiewicz, a Polish writer, painter, and philosopher who experimented with substances, put it, a role of damaging and "deceitful comforter."[24] Pain accompanies pleasure; the momentary liberation is often followed by a state of permanent addiction. Such is the essence of a habit. And such is the essence of "a terrible love of war," which "is a love sublime, a love in terror. It is unspeakable. The veteran does not, cannot talk about these moments both because it was so terrible and because it was so loving."[25] This peculiarity of the drug-like nature of war was perfectly captured by Franklin J. Schaffner in his movie *Patton* (1970), a biographic tale of George Patton, a great American general and a hero of the Second World War. In one of the scenes the general strolls around a battlefield after the fighting is over. We see broken ground, burnt tanks, and dead bodies. Patton raises a dying officer, kisses him, and looking at the destruction in the aftermath of an exceptionally bloody fight, says: "I love it. God help me, I do love it so. I love it more than my life." How much Patton in this scene resembles Clearchus, the veteran Spartan soldier, described by Xenophon in his *Anabasis* as *philopolemos*, a "lover of war."[26]

Social and cultural myths constructed and reconstructed for years on and fueled by the heat of political rhetoric and propaganda reinforce this dark allure of war. Societies and states raise their future soldiers, instilling in young men ideals of glory and nobleness surrounding the willingness to sacrifice themselves for their community. It was in this spirit that soldiers marching to the front lines of the First World War had been molded. This in particular pertains to German volunteers who for years had been fed with narcotic visions of valiant heroes struggling and winning. The incomprehensible willingness of millions of young European men to sacrifice their lives in the trenches made Sigmund Freud attempt to explain it by a specific thrill-seeking behavior which he famously called the "death drive." It was also precisely in this spirit of patriotism and national glory that American young people were mobilized during the Second World War: in February 1943 *The Magazine Publishers of America* released a taboo-breaking photograph of a dead soldier lying on his belly with a caption saying: "What did *you* do today . . . for Freedom?"[27] Not only did pop culture and film stars, such as John Wayne and Audie Murphy in particular, idealize the war, but they rendered it outright sacred. Philip Caputo in straightforward words comments on Wayne's impact on the forming of his own romantic vision of war: "Already I saw myself charging up some distant beachhead, like John Wayne in *Sands of Iwo Jima*, and then coming home a sun-tanned warrior with medals on my chest."[28] Raised on the tales of the greatest generation of soldiers fighting in a noble war in defense of freedom, shaped by the Hollywood, brought up in the spirit of civic virtues and duties, the baby boom generation was going to war. They were sons of the very same men who had fought in the Second World War, and they were departing for Vietnam with heads full of figments of a good war: "They expected to do in Vietnam what their fathers had done in Normandy and Italy and Guadalcanal—enter a struggle on the right side, fight hard and win, and be praised for it."[29] Many young boys responded to the seductive appeal from President Kennedy: "Ask

not, what your country can do for you. Ask what you can do for your country." Similarly, indoctrination and propaganda persuaded young Russians that
the war in Afghanistan was not merely a service to their motherland but the
communists' true international duty. The literature and film about the Great
Patriotic War created a fantastic picture of war not only as an exciting adventure, but also as something noble and worthy—a lofty defense of fundamental values. Thus, in essence, the authorities and society construct, reinforce,
and take advantage of the fetching image of war, which becomes an even more
"enticing elixir" fed to boyish minds susceptible to this type of influence.[30] The
old generation, in short, would prepare the young to be ready and willing to
fight.

Soldiers are often doped by war in a twofold manner—not only can war
itself be a true narcotic for them but an engagement in combat may also result
in their becoming addicted to real drugs. Especially when the romantic and
heroic fantasies guiding young men are painfully shattered when confronted
with the realities of the battlefield. This, in turn, entails yet another aspect of
the metaphor of war as a drug. Veterans suffering from PTSD live in war constantly and against their own will. One may say that they are in a way addicted
to their memories. A Soviet nurse thus commented on the Afghan war: "No
one likes this war. And yet I still cry when I hear the Afghan national anthem.
I got to like all Afghan music over there. I still listen to it, it's like a drug."[31] War
memories are usually extremely vivid, but if soldiers were exposed to a strong
stressor, if they survived a traumatic experience, then frequently these recollections will remain impressed deep in their emotional memory. They are too
often unable to free themselves of the images from the past that return at the
least expected moments of their lives. Their combat-induced mental illness,
like addiction, destroys the ability to live in society: they become dysfunctional and frequently also destructive in their personal relationships. Since
PTSD is not fully curable and medications alleviate symptoms only temporarily, sufferers very often resort to intoxicants that give them an apparent sense
of regaining control of their brain and memory, of fighting the demons of war
lurking in their heads. Drug use can be seen as a simulated expression of indi-
viduality, an apparent realization of their personal freedom. In this way, the
war's addictive potential continues long after the war is over. To paraphrase
Clausewitz, for many addicted veterans is intoxication not a continuation of
their participation in war by other, that is, psychopharmacological, means? In
times of peace, drugs become, in a way, a substitute for the thrilling war. Or
perhaps this is an overinterpretation.

American military psychologists and psychiatrists attempt to discontinue
veterans' participation in war by experimentally treating PTSD sufferers with
MDMA, a drug commonly known as ecstasy. This semisynthetic psychoactive

methamphetamine derivative (3,4-methylenedioxymethamphetamine) was created in 1912 and patented two years later by the German Merck. It is both a stimulant and hallucinogenic agent, conducive to evoking feelings of empathy, closeness, and emotional warmth. It has been called, writes Matthew Collin, a "psychedelic amphetamine," "yet it neither induces hallucinatory visions nor encourages the same soul-searching and potentially scary mental manifestations as LSD. To stress the difference it has been called an 'empathogen' (empathy-generating)."[32]

MDMA did not escape the attention of the American military. Already in the 1950s and 1960s, it was tested on animals at Edgwood Arsenal as one of the potential combat agents of the Cold War. Given the effects of ecstasy, it is not surprising that military experiments did not yield the expected results. A certain popular myth has, however, become associated with the drug, a myth according to which during a cease-fire in no man's land in the midst of the First World War "British and German soldiers laid down their guns, came out of the trenches and had a friendly game of football together—of course, the myth insists, they had taken the newly invented MDMA beforehand."[33] Thus was the pharmacological narration employed to explain the cases of brothers-in-arms bonding on the Western Front. And it was not improbable. In the 1980s and 1990s ecstasy became a street drug, so popular that in combination with dance music and clubs putting on acid house, it was a factor fueling the youth culture of the chemical generation (especially in Great Britain and the United States). Youths partying on ecstasy were going through what soldiers of the First World War may have experienced: "holding hands with new soulmates, telling their life stories and their most intimate emotions to people who seemed to *really understand* for the first time."[34]

Ecstasy was made illegal in Great Britain in 1977. In the United States only in 1985 did the Drug Enforcement Administration include it within the Schedule I category of controlled substances comprising the most addictive and dangerous agents of little therapeutic value. In 2001, however, a permit for conducting an experimental study with MDMA on PTSD sufferers was granted. For already in 1976 Leo Zeff discovered that the "psychedelic amphetamine" helped patients express emotions more easily and deal with criticism.[35] Since 2010 a team of researchers headed by Michael Mithoefer has been conducting research on American veterans suffering from war trauma.[36] Ecstasy turns out to be very helpful in psychotherapy: by enhancing intimacy it makes it easier for former soldiers to recount their traumatic experiences. The drug allows patients to overcome the psychological defense mechanisms that prevent one from gaining a deeper understanding of one's self. In essence, the therapeutic goal has a lot in common with the tenets of the ecstasy youth culture of the 1980s: "At its heart was a concerted attempt to . . . conjure from sound and chemistry, however briefly, a kind of utopia—what anarchist philosopher Hakim Bey has described as a *temporary autonomous zone*."[37] Those who suffer from PTSD would give a great deal to recapture such an autonomous zone in their brains oppressed by traumatic emotional memories.

If further studies confirm the optimistic preliminary results, then in the future ecstasy will assist soldiers and veterans in extricating themselves from painful mental states they experience following their participation in war. Brad Burge, director of communication at the Multidisciplinary Association for Psychedelic Studies, which coordinates the research into the use of ecstasy in psychotherapy, admits that the question is no longer whether but when MDMA becomes a legal prescription drug to be used in PTSD therapy. He believes that it is a matter of the near future, say by 2025.[38] Popular among the youth and sometimes dangerous, this club drug will be used to help a veteran's PTSD-troubled brain combat its addiction to the demons of war. Thus chemical ecstasy will make getting rid of negative effects of a traumatic ecstasy of war even more possible. The history of drugs in warfare abounds and will abound in paradoxes of this type.

NOTES

Preface

1. Clausewitz, *On War*, p. 85.
2. Szasz, *Ceremonial Chemistry*, p. 19.
3. Nicolai, *The Biology of War*, p. 250.
4. Keegan, *A History of Warfare*, p. 251.
5. Courtwright, *Forces of Habit*, p. 91.
6. Robson, *Forbidden Drugs*, p. 198.
7. Courtwright, *Forces of Habit*, p. 189.
8. Szasz, *The Myth of Mental Illness*.
9. Quoted in Robson, *Forbidden Drugs*, pp. 248–9.
10. Szasz, *The Myth of Mental Illness*.
11. Shay, *Achilles in Vietnam*, p. 62.
12. Derrida, "The Rhetoric of Drugs," p. 20.
13. Robson, *Forbidden Drugs*, p. 249.
14. Nietzsche, *The Birth of Tragedy*, p. 17.
15. Lewin, *Phantastica*, p. 1.
16. Quoted in Robson, *Forbidden Drugs*, p. 8.
17. Huxley, *The Doors of Perception*.
18. Weil, *The Natural Mind*.
19. Quoted in Booth, *Opium*, p. vii.
20. Lingis, "The Will To Power," p. 52.
21. Walton, *Out of It*, p. 2.
22. Walton, *Out of It*, p. 12.
23. Znaniecki, "The Object-Matter of Sociology."
24. Keegan, *A History of Warfare*; Gray, *Postmodern War*; Coker, *Waging War*; Jandora, "War and Culture"; Porter, *Military Orientalism*.
25. Quoted Virilio, *Speed and Politics*, p. 88.
26. Quoted in Holmes, *Acts of War*, p. 7.
27. Plant, *Writing on Drugs*, p. 248.

Prologue

1. Mead, "Warfare Is Only an Invention"; Ehrenreich, *Blood Rites*; Grossman, *On Killing*.
2. Ehrenreich, *Blood Rites*, p. 11.
3. Quoted in Keegan, *A History of Warfare*, p. 95, from Fried, Harris, and Murphy, *War*.
4. Keegan, *A History of Warfare*, p. 95.

5. Quoted in Granier-Doyeux, "Native Hallucinogenic Drugs Piptadenias," http://www.unodc.org/unodc/en/data-and-analysis/bulletin/bulletin_1965-01-01_2_page006.html, accessed June 1, 2014.
6. Quoted in Holmes, *Acts of War,* p. 142.
7. Hynes, *The Soldiers' Tale,* p. 62.
8. Jünger, *Sturm,* p. 10.
9. Gray, *The Warriors,* p. 12.
10. Lazarus, *Psychological Stress.*
11. Jünger, *Storm of Steel,* p. 232.
12. Courtwright, *Forces of Habit,* p. 139.
13. Rosenthal, *The Herb,* p. 109.
14. See Shephard, *A War of Nerves.*
15. Jünger, *Sturm,* p. 30.
16. Gabriel, *No More Heroes,* pp. 130–31.
17. Williams, *Rum,* p. 248.
18. Paris, *Pharmacologia,* p. 111.
19. Quoted in Gately, *Drink,* p. 175.
20. Hanson, *The Western Way of War,* p. 131.
21. Gately, *Drink,* p. 12.
22. Gately, *Drink,* p. 36.
23. Courtwright, *Forces of Habit,* p. 140.
24. Gately, *Drink,* p. 38.
25. *The Works of Tacitus,* http://oll.libertyfund.org/simple.php?id=787, accessed July 29, 2015.
26. Sun Tzu, *The Art of War,* p. 77.
27. Samuel B. Griffith, "Introduction," in Sun Tzu, *The Art of War,* p. 37.
28. Holmes, *Acts of War,* pp. 246, 244.
29. Holmes, *Acts of War,* p. 247.
30. Quoted in Holmes, *Acts of War,* p. 247.
31. Williams, *Rum,* p. 227.
32. Williams, *Rum,* p. 227.
33. Wilson, *Alcohol and the Nation,* p. 270.
34. Wilson, *Alcohol and the Nation,* p. 270.
35. McCallum, *Military Medicine,* p. 8.
36. Quoted in Courtwright, *Forces of Habit,* p. 141.
37. Wilson, *Alcohol and the Nation,* p. 26.
38. Courtwright, *Forces of Habit,* p. 12.
39. Dunn, *Frontier Profit and Loss,* p. 178.
40. Quoted in Kopperman, "The Cheapest Pay," p. 448.
41. Quoted in Gately, *Drink,* p. 196.
42. Burns, *The Spirits of America,* p. 16.
43. Williams, *Rum,* p. 228.
44. Williams, *Rum,* p. 173.
45. Walton, *Out of It,* p. 148.
46. Courtwright, *Forces of Habit,* p. 141.
47. Quoted in Gately, *Drink,* p. 313.
48. McCallum, *Military Medicine,* p. 8.
49. Myerly, *British Military Spectacle,* p. 73.
50. Kopperman, "'The Cheapest Pay,'" p. 445.
51. Stanley, "Army Temperance Association," p. 55.
52. Kiernan, *European Empires,* p. 129.
53. Quoted in Williams, *Rum,* p. 225.
54. Bushnell, "The Tsarist Officer Corps," p. 755.
55. Bushnell, "The Tsarist Officer Corps," pp. 755–6.
56. Bushnell, "The Tsarist Officer Corps," p. 756.
57. Keep, *Soldiers of the Tsar,* p. 186.

58. Segal, *Russian Drinking*, p. 72.

59. Herlihy, *Alcoholic Empire*, p. 56.

60. Keep, *Soldiers of the Tsar*, p. 186.

61. Tolstoy, *War and Peace*, part 3, chap. 9, p. 338.

62. Herlihy, *Alcoholic Empire*, p. 54.

63. Herlihy, *Alcoholic Empire*, p. 55.

64. Quoted in Herlihy, *Alcoholic Empire*, p. 61.

65. Herlihy, *Alcoholic Empire*, p. 53.

66. Czubiński, *Historia Powszechna XX wieku*, p. 48.

67. Quoted in Herlihy, *Alcoholic Empire*, p. 52.

68. Quoted in Segal, *Russian Drinking*, p. 149.

69. Quoted in Segal, *Russian Drinking*, p. 149.

70. Herlihy, *Alcoholic Empire*, p. 61.

71. Segal, *Russian Drinking*, p. 75.

72. Segal, *Russian Drinking*, p. 149.

73. Bushnell, "The Tsarist Officer Corps," p. 756.

74. McGowan, "Alcohol," p. 82.

75. Herlihy, *Alcoholic Empire*, p. 63.

76. Segal, *Russian Drinking*, p. 102.

77. Quoted in Herlihy, *Alcoholic Empire*, p. 66.

78. Herlihy, *Alcoholic Empire*, p. 67.

79. Reese, *Soviet Military Experience*, p. 59.

80. Quoted in White, *Russia Goes Dry*, p. 17.

81. Figes, "The Red Army," p. 196.

82. Lewis, *Babbitt*, p. 87.

83. *U.S. Army "Prohibition,"* http://druglibrary.org/schaffer/alcohol/prohibit.htm, accessed July 30, 2015.

84. Quoted in Gately, *Drink*, p. 357.

85. Quoted in Gately, *Drink*, p. 357.

86. Quoted in Gately, *Drink*, p. 370.

87. Quoted in Gately, *Drink*, p. 364.

88. Gately, *Drink*, p. 364.

89. Quoted in Greenaway, *Drink and British Politics since 1830*, p. 93.

90. Holmes, *Tommy*, p. 329.

91. Quoted in Holmes, *Tommy*, p. 331.

92. Quoted in Holmes, *Acts of War*, p. 249.

93. Fussell, *The Great War*, p. 46.

94. Quoted in Gately, *Drink*, p. 360.

95. Quoted in Fussell, *The Great War*, p. 47.

96. Quoted in Fussell, *The Great War*, p. 47.

97. Holden, *Shell Shock*, p. 11.

98. Prestwich, *Drink and the Politics of Social Reform*, pp. 167–8.

99. Prestwich, *Drink*, p. 168.

100. Prestwich, *Drink*, p. 172.

101. Quoted in Prestwich, *Drink*, p. 172.

102. Quoted in Mulholland, "Mon docteur le vin," p. 79.

103. Quoted in Mulholland, "Mon docteur le vin," p. 77.

104. Quoted in Gately, *Drink*, p. 461.

105. Barthes, *Mythologies*, pp. 58–9.

106. Quoted in Toussaint-Samat, *A History of Food*, p. 164.

107. Quoted in Toussaint-Samat, *A History of Food*, p. 164.

108. Quoted in Gately, *Drink*, p. 304.

109. Quoted in Mulholland, "Mon docteur le vin," p. 84.

110. Mulholland, "'Mon docteur le vin," pp. 83–4.

111. Prestwich, *Drink*, p. 246.

112. Holmes, *Acts of War*, p. 250.
113. McCallum, *Military Medicine*, p. 9.
114. Kittel, "Alkohol und Wehrmacht."
115. Bergen-Cico, *War and Drugs*, p. 42.
116. Quoted in Ulrich, "The Nazi Death Machine," http://www.spiegel.de/international/the-nazi-death-machine-hitler-s-drugged-soldiers-a-354606.html, accessed June 16, 2012.
117. Sajer, *The Forgotten Soldier*, p. 98.
118. Merridale, *Ivan's War*, p. 139.
119. Reese, *Stalin's Reluctant Soldiers*, p. 161.
120. Quoted in Gabriel, *The New Red Legion* p. 153.
121. Merridale, *Ivan's War*, p. 271.
122. Ohnuki-Tierney, *Kamikaze Diaries*, pp. 177–8.
123. Quoted in Ohnuki-Tierney, *Kamikaze Diaries*, p. 122.
124. Ohnuki-Tierney, *Kamikaze, Cherry Blossoms, and Nationalism*, p. 19.
125. Kuzmarov, *The Myth*, p. 35.
126. Kuzmarov, *The Myth*, p. 26.
127. Quoted in Kuzmarov, *The Myth*, p. 27.
128. Quoted in Kuzmarov, *The Myth*, p. 28.
129. Quoted in Shay, *Achilles in Vietnam*, p. 63.
130. Quoted in Kuzmarov, *The Myth*, p. 27.
131. Robins, *The Vietnam Drug User Returns*, p. 57.
132. Quoted in Holmes, *Acts of War*, p. 244.
133. Sedlickas and Stasys, *The War in Chechnya*, p. 152.
134. Seely, *Russo-Chechen Conflict*, p. 272.
135. Tishkov, *Chechnya*, p. 134.
136. Quoted in Tishkov, *Chechnya*, p. 96.
137. Quoted in Tishkov, *Chechnya*, p. 139.
138. Zoroya, "Alcohol Abuse by GIs Soars since 2003," http://www.usatoday.com/news/military/2009-06-18-army-alcohol-problems_N.htm, accessed May 6, 2014.
139. Zoroya, "Alcohol Abuse Weighs on Army," http://www.usatoday.com/news/military/2010-02-09-treatment-army-alcohol_N.htm, accessed May 6, 2014.
140. Bergen-Cico, *War and Drugs*, p. 130.
141. Quoted in Netter, "Army Alcoholics," http://abcnews.go.com/Health/army-alcoholics-soldiers-seek-treatment-alcohol-abuse/story?id=9863321#.T9-rN1K_lqU, accessed May 20, 2014.
142. Quoted in Netter, "Army Alcoholics."
143. Teachman, Anderson, and Tedrow, "Military Service and Alcohol Use," p. 462.
144. *Substance Use Disorders in the U.S. Armed Forces.*
145. Teachman, Anderson, and Tedrow, "Military Service," p. 461.
146. Quoted in Linkner, "Alkohole młodopolskiego cygana," p. 23.
147. Holmes, *Acts of War*, p. 244.

Chapter 1

1. Berridge, *Opium and the People*, p. xxii.
2. Scarborough, "The Opium Poppy," pp. 4–23.
3. Homer, *The Odyssey*, 4.219–27, p. 127.
4. Musto, *The American Disease*, p. 69; Davenort-Hines, *The Pursuit of Oblivion*, pp. 35–6.
5. Quoted in Booth, *Opium*, p. 24.
6. Booth, *Opium*, p. 19.
7. Homer, *The Odyssey*, 9.92–7, p. 192.
8. Shay, *Odysseus in America*, p. 36.
9. Daftary, *The Assassin Legends*, p. 91.
10. *Longman Dictionary of the English Language*, p. 92.
11. Elliot, *Warrior Cults*.

12. Morgan, "The Assassins," p. 40.
13. Daftary, *The Assassin Legends*, pp. 90–3.
14. Rosenthal, *The Herb*, p. 155.
15. Lincoln, "An Early Moment," p. 247.
16. Walton, *Out of It*, p. 67.
17. Polo, *The Description of the World*, p. 139.
18. Polo, *The Description of the World*, p. 131.
19. Lincoln, "An Early Moment," p. 249.
20. Lewis, *The Assassins*, pp. 11–12.
21. Baudelaire, "The Poem of Hashish," p. 37.
22. Eliade, *The Myth of the Eternal Return*, pp. 1–48.
23. Wasson and Wasson, *Mushrooms, Russia and History*, vol. 1, p. 144.
24. Toussaint-Samat, *A History of Food*, p. 53.
25. Rudgley, *The Alchemy of Culture*, pp. 40–1.
26. Wasson and Wasson, *Mushrooms, Russia and History*, vol. 2, p. 318.
27. Rudgley, *The Alchemy of Culture*, p. 40.
28. Quoted in Mann, *Turn on*, p. 120.
29. Mann, *Turn on*, p. 221.
30. Gabriel, *No More Heroes*, p. 138.
31. Fabing, "On Going Berserk," p. 232.
32. Quoted in Fabing, "On Going Berserk," p. 232.
33. Fabing, "On Going Berserk," p. 235.
34. Mann, *Murder, Magic, and Medicine*, p. 79.
35. Hesse, *Narcotics and Drug Addiction*, pp. 103–4.
36. Holmes, *Acts of War*, p. 247.
37. Quoted in Fabing, "On Going Berserk," p. 234.
38. Shay, *Odysseus in America*, p. 2.
39. Quoted in Shay, *Achilles in Vietnam*, pp. 82–3.
40. Tritle, *From Melos to My Lai*, p. 65.
41. Shay, *Achilles*, p. 91.
42. Mann, *Murder, Magic, and Medicine*, p. 79.
43. Carroll, *Alice's Adventures in Wonderland*, p. 38.
44. Sroka, *Teologia narkotyku*, p. 67.
45. Wasson and Wasson, *Mushrooms, Russia and History*, vol. 1, p. 192.
46. Sroka, *Teologia narkotyku*, p. 68.
47. Vespucci, *Letters*, p. 25.
48. Quoted in Streatfeild, *Cocaine*, p. 7.
49. Quoted in Mortimer, *Peru*, pp. 159–60.
50. Madge, *White Mischief*, p. 25.
51. Quoted in Davenport-Hines, *The Pursuit of Oblivion*, p. 28.
52. Ryn, *Medycyna indiańska*, p. 248.
53. Dillehay et al., "Early Holocene Coca Chewing in Northern Peru."
54. Madge, *White Mischief*, p. 42.
55. Mortimer, *Peru*, p. 157.
56. Feiling, *The Candy Machine*, p. 13.
57. Quoted in Hobhouse, *Seeds of Change*, p. 308.
58. Davenport-Hines, *The Pursuit of Oblivion*, p. 200.
59. Quoted in Courtwright, *Dark Paradise*, p. 97.
60. Mortimer, *Peru*, p. 168.
61. Streatfeild, *Cocaine*, p. 65; Davenport-Hines, *The Pursuit of Oblivion*, p. 28.

Chapter 2

1. Crowdy and Hook, *French Soldier*, p. 11.
2. Rosenthal, *The Herb*, pp. 2, 64, 160.

3. Quoted in Rosenthal, *The Herb*, p. 106.
4. Baudelaire, "The Poem of Hashish," p. 37.
5. Courtwright, *Forces of Habit*, pp. 39–40.
6. Robinson, *The Great Book of Hemp*, p. 118.
7. Baudelaire, "On Wine and Hashish," pp. 24–5.
8. Rosenthal, *The Herb*, p. 87.
9. Crowdy and Hook, *French Soldier*, p. 21.
10. Baudelaire, "The Poem of Hashish," p. 80.
11. Quoted in Crowdy and Hook, *French Soldier*, p. 21.
12. Robinson, *The Great Book of Hemp*, p. 118.
13. Quoted in Piomelli, "The Molecular Logic of Endocannabinoid Signaling," p. 873.
14. Mann, *Turn on*, p. 80.
15. Quoted in Robinson, *The Great Book of Hemp*, p. 119.
16. Robinson, *The Great Book of Hemp*, p. 81; Davenport-Hines, *The Pursuit of Oblivion*, pp. 94–8.
17. Baudelaire, "The Poem of Hashish," pp. 33, 45.
18. Davenport-Hines, *The Pursuit of Oblivion*, p. 92.
19. Fage with Tordoff, *A History of Africa*, p. 378.
20. Abun-Nasr, *A History of the Maghrib*, pp. 249–50.
21. Davenport-Hines, *The Pursuit of Oblivion*, pp. 92, 93.
22. Baudelaire, "The Poem of Hashish," p. 66.

Chapter 3

1. Brook and Wakabayashi, "Introduction: Opium's History in China," p. 19.
2. Hanes and Sanello, *The Opium Wars*, p. 20; Brook and Wakabayashi, "Introduction," p. 7.
3. Harding, *Opiate Addiction, Morality and Medicine*, p. 18.
4. See Wong, *Deadly Dreams*.
5. Marx, "Free Trade and Monopoly," http://www.marxists.org/archive/marx/works/1858/09/25.htm, accessed June, 15, 2015.
6. Zheng, "The Social Life of Opium in China 1483–1999."
7. McMahon, *The Fall of the God of Money*, pp. 33–44.
8. Gelber, *Opium, Soldiers and Evangelicals*, p. 34.
9. Baulmer, *The Chinese and Opium under the Republic*, p. 16.
10. Mann, *Murder*, p. 193.
11. Courtwright, *Forces of Habit*, p. 34.
12. Davenport-Hines, *The Pursuit of Oblivion*, p. 46.
13. Brook and Wakabayashi, "Introduction," p. 6.
14. Harding, *Opiate Addiction*, p. 6.
15. Booth, *Opium*, p. 120.
16. Hanes and Sanello, *The Opium Wars*, p. 21; Mann, *Murder*, p. 193.
17. Brook and Wakabayashi, "Introduction," p. 2.
18. Zheng, *The Social Life of Opium in China*, p. 154.
19. Holman, *Travels in China*, p. 254.
20. Holman, *Travels in China*, p. 256.
21. Booth, *Opium*, p. 128.
22. Quoted in Tien, *Chinese Military Theory*, p. 75.
23. Hanes and Sanello, *The Opium Wars*, p. 171.
24. Quoted in Booth, *Opium*, p. 25.
25. Davenport-Hines, *The Pursuit of Oblivion*, p. 187.
26. Courtwright, *Forces of Habit*, p. 140; Bergen-Cico, *War and Drugs*, p. xii.
27. Quoted in *First Report of the Royal Commission on Opium*, p. 113, http://www.archive.org/details/cu31924073053864, accessed March 12, 2015.
28. Quoted in *First Report*, p. 420.
29. Gelber, *Opium*, p. 46.

30. Quoted in Zheng, *The Social Life*, p. 91.
31. Berridge, *Opium and the People*, p. 66.
32. Dikötter, Laamann, and Xun, *Narcotic Culture*, p. 86.
33. Zheng, *The Social Life of China*, p. 92.
34. Quoted in Zheng, *The Social Life of China*, p. 88.
35. Quoted in Zheng, *The Social Life of China*, p. 96.
36. Sun Pin, *Military Methods*, p. 247.
37. Murray, *Doings in China*, p. 109.
38. McMahon, *The Fall*, p. 95.
39. Tien, *Chinese Military Theory*, p. 72.
40. Sun Tzu, *The Art of War*, p. 89.
41. Laozi, *Daodejing*, p. 19.
42. Sun Pin, *Military Methods*, p. 195.
43. Quoted in Gelber, *Opium*, p. 57.
44. Paris, *Pharmacologia*, pp. 109–10.

Chapter 4

1. Courtwright, *Dark Paradise*, p. 43.
2. De Quincey, *Confessions of an English Opium-Eater*.
3. Davenport-Hines, *The Pursuit of Oblivion*, p. 105; Schroeder-Lein, *Encyclopedia*, p. 240.
4. Courtwright, *Dark Paradise*, p. 45.
5. Quoted in Courtwright, *Dark Paradise*, p. 43.
6. Quoted in Courtwright, *Dark Paradise*, p. 50.
7. Davenport-Hines, *The Pursuit of Oblivion*, p. 115.
8. De Quincey, *Confessions of an English Opium-Eater*, p. 50.
9. Quoted in Davenport-Hines, *The Pursuit of Oblivion*, p. 106.
10. Collins, *Armadale*, p. 444.
11. Quoted in Courtwright, *Dark Paradise*, p. 60.
12. Quoted in M. McPherson, *Battle Cry of Freedom*, p. 486.
13. Flannery, *Civil War Pharmacy*, p. 15.
14. "Medical Care, Battle Wounds, and Disease," http://www.civilwarhome.com/civilwarmedicine. htm, accessed February 17, 2014.
15. Flannery, *Civil War Pharmacy*, p. 6.
16. Courtwright, *Dark Paradise*, p. 54.
17. Di Maio, *Gunshot Wounds*, p. 168; Schroeder-Lein, *Encyclopedia*, pp. 213–4.
18. Schroeder-Lein, *The Encyclopedia*, pp. 16–7.
19. Courtwright, "Opiate Addiction," p. 105.
20. Waldorf, Orlick, and Reinarman, *Morphine Maintenance*, p. 35.
21. Schroeder-Lein, *Encyclopedia*, p. 120.
22. Adams, "Caring for the Men," http://www.civilwarhome.com/medicinehistory.htm, accessed March 4, 2014.
23. Adams, "Caring for the Men"; Schroeder-Lein, *Encyclopedia*, pp. 21–3.
24. Metcalfe, "The Influence of the Military," p. 595.
25. Quoted in Metcalfe, "The Influence of the Military," p. 597.
26. Schroeder-Lein, *Encyclopedia*, pp. 155, 160.
27. Smallman-Raynor and Cliff, *War Epidemics*, p. 184.
28. Smallman-Raynor and Cliff, *War Epidemics*, pp. 218–20; "Medical Care."
29. Flannery, *Civil War Pharmacy*, p. 22.
30. "Medical Care"; Griffiths, "Medicine and Surgery," p. 206.
31. Smallman-Raynor and Cliff, *War Epidemics*, p. 189.
32. Marshall, "Medicine in the Confederacy," p. 291.
33. McCallum, *Military Medicine*, p. 772.
34. Grossman, *On Killing*, p. 73.
35. Coker, "War and Disease."

36. Courtwright, *Dark Paradise*, p. 56; Schroeder-Lein, *Encyclopedia*, pp. 85–7.
37. Schroeder-Lein, *Encyclopedia*, p. 219.
38. Booth, *Opium*, p. 73.
39. Booth, *Opium*, p. 72.
40. Mitchell, *Characteristics*, p. 14.
41. Mitchell, *Characteristics*, p. 14.
42. Whitman, "Specimen Days," p. 498.
43. Gabriel, *No More Heroes*, p. 58.
44. Day, *The Opium Habit*, p. 7.
45. Quinones, "Drug Abuse," p. 1012.
46. Quoted in Weld, "A Connecticut Surgeon," pp. 278–9.
47. Quinones, "Drug Abuse," pp. 1018–9.
48. Quinones, "Drug Abuse," pp. 1018–9.
49. Mandel, "The Mythical Roots of U.S. Drug Policy," http://www.druglibrary.org/schaffer/History/soldis.htm, accessed March 20, 2014.
50. Marks, "The Curse of Narcotism," p. 315.
51. Mandel, "The Mythical Roots."
52. Quoted in Courtwright, "Opiate Addiction," p. 103.
53. Trebach, *Fatal Distraction*, p. 168.
54. Starkey, "Use and Abuse," pp. 482–4.
55. Courtwright, *Dark Paradise*, pp. 36, 54–64.
56. Crothers, *Morphinism and Narcomanias*, pp. 75–6.
57. Quoted in Davenport-Hines, *The Pursuit of Oblivion*, p. 9.
58. Courtwright, "Opiate Addiction," pp. 102, 111; Courtwright, *Forces of Habit*, p. 54.
59. Courtwright, "The Hidden Epidemic," p. 66.
60. Courtwright, *Forces of Habit*, p. 101; Quinones, "Drug Abuse," p. 1010.
61. Courtwright, *Dark Paradise*, p. 9.
62. Davenport-Hines, *The Pursuit of Oblivion*, p. 121.
63. Gelber, *Opium*, p. 206.
64. Booth, *Opium*, p. 74.
65. Terry and Pellens, *The Opium Problem*, p. 484.

Chapter 5

1. Holmes, *Acts of War*, p. 247.
2. Krige, *The Social System of the Zulus*, p. 261.
3. Unterhalter, "Confronting Imperialism," p. 103; Yorke, "Isandlwana," p. 172.
4. Krige, *The Social System*, p. 269.
5. Krige, *The Social System*, p. 289.
6. Krige, *The Social System*, p. 274; *Intelezi*, Ulwazi, http://wiki.ulwazi.org/index.php5?title=Intelezi, accessed August 4, 2014.
7. Reader, *Zulu Tribe in Transition*, p. 284.
8. Bryant, *The Zulu People*, vol. 1, p. 222.
9. Kan, *Drugs and Contemporary Warfare*, p. 47.
10. *Day of the Zulu*, PBS, http://www.pbs.org/wnet/secrets/previous_seasons/case_zulu/clues.html, accessed August 10, 2014.
11. Yorke, "Isandlwana," p. 176.
12. Unterhalter, "Confronting Imperialism," pp. 103–4.
13. Quoted in Laband, " 'Bloodstained Grandeur,' " p. 171.
14. Knight, "What Do You Red-Jackets Want," p. 187; Laband, " 'Bloodstained Grandeur,' " p. 169.
15. Livingstone, *Missionary Travels and Research in South Africa*, p. 579.
16. Lehmann and Mihalyi, "Aggression, Bravery, Endurance, and Drugs."
17. Rudgley, *The Alchemy of Culture*, pp. 116–8.
18. Ylikangas, *Unileipää, kuolonvettä, spiidiä*, p. 143.

19. "World Armies Still Use Psychotropic Drugs," http://english.pravda.ru/world/europe/18-11-2008/106714-psychotropic-0, accessed August 21, 2014.
20. Davenport-Hines, *The Pursuit of Oblivion*, p. 153.
21. Fulton, *Moroland*.
22. Fulton, *Moroland*, p. 29.
23. Wolff, *Little Brown Brother*, p. 317.
24. Jones, *From Here to Eternity*, p. 16.
25. Gowing, "Kris and Crescent," p. 8.
26. Quoted in Fulton, *The Legend of the Colt .45*, http://www.morolandhistory.com/Related%20Articles/Legend%20of%20.45.htm, accessed August 23, 2014.
27. Fulton, *The Legend*.
28. Musto, *The American Disease*, p. 7.
29. Kolb, "'Like a Mad Tiger,'" p. 30.
30. Fulton, *The Legend*.

Chapter 6

1. Miller, *Memories of General Miller*, vol. 2, p. 197.
2. Dimeo, *A History of Drug Use*, p. 19.
3. Dimeo, *A History of Drug Use*, p. 20.
4. Erickson et al., *The Steel Drug*, p. 8.
5. Madge, *White Mischief*, p. 52.
6. Quoted in Streatfeild, *Cocaine*, p. 66.
7. Quoted in Plant, *Writing on Drugs*, p. 62.
8. Streatfeild, *Cocaine*, p. 67.
9. Quoted in Davenport-Hines, *The Pursuit of Oblivion*, p. 154.
10. Madge, *White Mischief*, pp. 55–6.
11. Robson, *Forbidden Drugs*, pp. 86–7.
12. Alexander, "Freud's Pharmacy"; Gootenberg, *Andean Cocaine*, pp. 23–4.
13. Quoted in Davenport-Hines, *The Pursuit of Oblivion*, p. 157.
14. See Markel, *An Anatomy of Addiction*.
15. Davenport-Hines, *The Pursuit of Oblivion*, p. 133.
16. Van Creveld, *The Changing Face of War*, p. 24.
17. Streatfeild, *Cocaine*, p. 85.
18. Friman, "Germany and the Transformation of Cocaine," p. 95.
19. Braam, *The Cocaine Salesman*, p. 441.
20. Courtwright, *Forces of Habit*, p. 50.
21. Peters, "Dutch Cocaine," http://www.rnw.nl/english/article/dutch-cocaine-ultimate-weapon, accessed September 3, 2014.
22. Courtwright, *Forces of Habit*, p. 50.
23. De Kort, "Doctors, Diplomats, and Businessmen," p. 132.
24. Braam, *The Cocaine Salesman*, p. 22.
25. Courtwright, *Forces of Habit*, p. 50.
26. Quoted in Woods, *Dangerous Drugs*, p. 42.
27. Streatfeild, *Cocaine*, p. 158.
28. "Forced March," http://www.cocaine.org/forcedmarch.htm, accessed September 16, 2014.
29. Ylikangas, *Unileipää*, p. 144.
30. Quoted in Peters, "Dutch Cocaine."
31. Braam, *The Cocaine Salesman*, pp. 379–80.
32. Braam, *The Cocaine Salesman*, p. 423.
33. Quoted in Kohn, "Cocaine Girls," p. 113.
34. Berridge, *Opium and the People*, p. 256.
35. Erickson et al., *The Steel Drug*, p. 5.
36. Davenport-Hines, *The Pursuit of Oblivion*, p. 196.
37. Davenport-Hines, *The Pursuit of Oblivion*, p. 164.

38. Dalaby, "Sherlock Holmes's Cocaine Habit," pp. 73–4.
39. Doyle, *The Sign of the Four*, p. 8.
40. Berridge, "Drugs and Social Policy," p. 20; Streatfeild, *Cocaine*, p. 159; Robson, *Forbidden Drugs*, p. 175.
41. Quoted in Streatfeild, *Cocaine*, p. 159.
42. Berridge, *Opium and the People*, p. 252.
43. Quoted in Davenport-Hines, *The Pursuit of Oblivion*, p. 220.
44. Quoted in Berridge, *Opium and the People*, p. 249.
45. Berridge, "Drugs and Social Policy," p. 20.
46. Berridge, "War Conditions and Narcotic Control," pp. 285–304.
47. Quoted in Berridge, "War Conditions and Narcotic Control," p. 303.
48. Kohn, "Cocaine Girls," pp. 134–9.

Chapter 7

1. Rasmussen, *On Speed*, p. 6.
2. Abadinsky, *Drug Use and Abuse*, p. 151; Courtwright, *Forces of Habit*, p. 78; Davenport-Hines, *The Pursuit of Oblivion*, p. 375.
3. Hobhouse, *Seeds of Change*, p. 338.
4. Grunberger, *Social History of The Third Reich*, p. 528.
5. Metzner, "Nazis on Speed," p. 289.
6. "Hochdosiert," pp. 276–8.
7. Bullock, *Hitler*, p. 388.
8. Bullock, *Hitler*, p. 717.
9. "Hochdosiert," pp. 265–76.
10. Eberle and Uhl, *The Hitler Book*, p. 57.
11. Quoted in Bullock, *Hitler*, pp. 373–4.
12. Bullock, *Hitler*, p. 374.
13. Doyle, "Adolf Hitler's Medical Care," p. 77; Whitaker, *Global Connection*, p. 85.
14. Ohler, *Der totale Rausch*, pp. 124 ff.
15. Metzner, "Nazis on Speed," p. 290; Ohler, *Der totale Rausch*, pp. 185 ff.
16. Quoted in Trevor-Roper, *The Last Days of Hitler*, p. 108.
17. Wade, "The Treatment of a Dictator," p. 121.
18. Bullock, *Hitler*, p. 742; Streatfeild, *Cocaine*, p. 184.
19. Doyle, "Adolf Hitler's," p. 77.
20. "A Fresh Light," http://www.dw.com/en/a-fresh-light-on-the-nazis-wartime-drug-addiction/a-18703678, accessed October 5, 2015.
21. "A Fresh Light," http://www.dw.com/en/a-fresh-light-on-the-nazis-wartime-drug-addiction/a-18703678, accessed October 5, 2015.
22. Braswell, *Crazy Town*, p. 14.
23. Trevor-Roper, *The Last Days of Hitler*, p. 116.
24. Rasmussen, *On Speed*, p. 54.
25. Dimeo, *A History of Drug Use*, p. 5.
26. Iversen, *Speed, Ecstasy, Ritalin*, p. 71; Robson, *Forbidden Drugs*, p. 99.
27. Kemper, "Pervitin," p. 126.
28. Steinkamp, "Pervitin (Methamphetamine) Tests," pp. 63–4.
29. Kemper, "Pervitin," p. 128.
30. Rasmussen, *On Speed*, p. 54.
31. Quoted in Grinspoon and Hedblom, *The Speed Culture*, p. 18.
32. Quoted in Ulrich, "The Nazi Death Machine."
33. Nöldecke, "Einsatz von leistungssteigernden," p. 135.
34. Rasmussen, *On Speed*, p. 55.
35. Quoted in Steinkamp, "Pervitin," p. 67.
36. Quoted in Steinkamp, "Pervitin," p. 68.
37. Quoted in Keating, "Flying on Amphetamines," pp. 18–9.
38. Quoted in Ulrich, "The Nazi Death Machine."

39. Quoted in Cross, *The Battle of Kursk*, p. 180.
40. Ohler, *Der totale Rausch*, p. 154.
41. Grunberger, *A Social History*, p. 296.
42. Houlihan, *Dying to Win*, p. 45.
43. Quoted in Ulrich, "The Nazi Death Machine."
44. Kemper, "Pervitin," p. 131.
45. Vasagar, "Nazis Tested Cocaine on Camp Inmates," http://www.guardian.co.uk/world/2002/nov/19/research.germany, accessed September 2, 2014; Tsur, "Nazis Attempted to Make Robots of Their Soldiers," http://english.pravda.ru/science/tech/14-02-2003/1872-nazi- accessed September 2, 2014; Ulrich, "The Nazi Death Machine"; Ohler, *Der totale Rausch*, pp. 268 ff.
46. Rasmussen, *On Speed*, p. 59; Dimeo, *A History of Drug Use*, p. 48.
47. Rasmussen, *On Speed*, pp. 60–1.
48. Quoted in Brodie, *Strategy in the Missile Age*, p. 116.
49. Quoted in Rasmussen, *On Speed*, p. 62.
50. Rasmussen, *On Speed*, p. 64.
51. Rasmussen, *On Speed*, p. 65.
52. Rasmussen, *On Speed*, p. 65.
53. Davenport-Hines, *The Pursuit of Oblivion*, p. 307.
54. Ellis, *The Sharp End of War*, p. 293.
55. Quoted in Ellis, *The Sharp End of War*, p. 293.
56. Atkinson, *An Army at Dawn*, p. 419.
57. Rasmussen, *On Speed*, p. 71.
58. Quoted in Dimeo, *A History of Drug Use*, p. 46.
59. Quoted in Dimeo, *A History of Drug Use*, p. 47.
60. Quoted in Dimeo, *A History of Drug Use*, p. 47.
61. Rasmussen, *On Speed*, p. 78.
62. Rasmussen, *On Speed*, p. 84.
63. Bayer, "The Abuse of Psychotropic Drugs," http://www.unodc.org/unodc/en/data-and-analysis/bulletin/bulletin_1973-01-01_3_page003.html, accessed October 18, 2014.
64. Rasmussen, "America's First Amphetamine Epidemic," p. 975.
65. Rasmussen, *On Speed*, p. 71.
66. Clodfelter, *Warfare and Armed Conflicts*, p. 541.
67. Hynes, *The Soldiers' Tale*, p. 163.
68. Stephenson, *Cryptonomicon*.
69. Rasmussen, *On Speed*, p. 76.
70. Lind, "With a B–29 over Japan—A Pilot's Story," p. SM3.
71. Wakabayashi, "From Peril to Profit," p. 66.
72. Vaughn, Huang, and Ramirez, "Drug Abuse and Anti-Drug Policy in Japan," pp. 493–4.
73. Hill, *The Japanese Mafia*, p. 98.
74. Russell, *Egyptian Service*, p. 253.
75. Kobayashi, "Drug Operations by Resident Japanese in Tianjin," p. 152.
76. *International Military Tribunal for the Far East, Judgment of 4 November 1948*, http://werle.rewi.hu-berlin.de/tokio.pdf, accessed October 22, 2014.
77. Brook and Wakabayashi, "Introduction," pp. 18–9.
78. Brook and Wakabayashi, "Introduction," p. 15.
79. Brook and Wakabayashi, "Introduction," pp. 17–8.
80. Brook and Wakabayashi, "Introduction," p. 17.
81. Kobayashi, "Drug Operations," p. 157.
82. Quoted in Kobayashi, "An Opium Tug-of-War," p. 351.
83. Booth, *Opium*, p. 168.
84. Brook and Wakabayashi, "Introduction," p. 18.
85. Brook and Wakabayashi, "Introduction," p. 17.
86. Booth, *Opium*, p. 163.
87. Quoted in Davenport-Hines, *The Pursuit of Oblivion*, p. 274.
88. Kobayashi, "An Opium Tug-of-War," p. 356.

89. Satō, "Methamphetamine Use in Japan," p. 718.
90. Satō, "Japan's Long Association with Amphetamines," p. 151.
91. Kato, "An Epidemiological Analysis"; Schoenberger, "Japan Faces Widespread Drug Problems," p. 34; Yokoyama, "Japan: Changing Drugs Laws."
92. Quoted in Durst, *Weimar Modernism*, p. 175.
93. Kato, "An Epidemiological Analysis," p. 592.
94. Vaughn, Huang, and Ramirez, "Drug Abuse," p. 497.
95. Kan, *Drugs*, p. 156.
96. Satō, "Methamphetamine Use," p. 720.
97. Daizen, *Zen at War*, p. 105.
98. Ohnuki-Tierney, *Kamikaze, Cherry Blossoms*, p. 183.
99. Confucius, *The Analects*, p. 8.
100. Nitobe, *Bushido*, p. 21.
101. Quoted in Ohnuki-Tierney, *Kamikaze Diaries*, p. 172.
102. Benedict, *The Chrysanthemum and the Sword*, p. 167.
103. Kaplan and Dubro, *Yakuza*, p. 61; Hill, *The Japanese Mafia*, p. 100.
104. Courtwright, *Forces of Habit*, p. 83.
105. Satō, "Methamphetamine Use," p. 720; Satō, "Japan's Long Association," p. 151.
106. Hill, *The Japanese Mafia*, p. 99; Brill and Hirose, "The Rise and Fall of a Methamphetamine Epidemic"; Grinspoon and Hedblom, *The Speed Culture*, p. 189.
107. Bayer, "The Abuse."
108. Satō, "Methamphetamine Use," p. 723.
109. Vaughn, Huang, and Ramirez, "Drug Abuse," p. 498.
110. Ylikangas, *Unileipää*, p. 129.
111. Ylikangas, *Unileipää*, p. 77. All translations are kindly provided by Mikko Ylikangas.
112. Ylikangas, author's correspondence, January 2015.
113. Ylikangas, *Unileipää*, p. 128.
114. Ylikangas, *Unileipää*, p. 183.
115. Nieminen, "Finland—a Leading Consumer of Heroin," http://www.hs.fi/english/article/Finland+-+a+leading+consumer+of+heroin+from+the+1930s+to+the+1950s/1135245022270, accessed November 4, 2014; Rantanen, "History: Amphetamine Overdose," http://www2.hs.fi/english/archive/news.asp?id=20020528IE9, accessed November 4, 2014.
116. Ylikangas, *Unileipää*, p. 127.
117. Trotter, *A Frozen Hell*, p. 35.
118. Trotter, *A Frozen Hell*, p. 42.
119. Ylikangas, *Unileipää*, p. 147.
120. Ylikangas, *Unileipää*, p. 148.
121. Quoted in Nieminen, "Finland."
122. Ylikangas, *Unileipää*, p. 149.
123. Quoted in Ylikangas, *Unileipää*, p. 150.
124. Quoted in Ylikangas, *Unileipää*, p. 149.
125. Quoted in Ylikangas, *Unileipää*, p. 155.
126. Trotter, *A Frozen Hell*, p. 62.
127. Quoted in Langdon-Davies, *Invasion in the Snow*, pp. 120–1.
128. Ylikangas, *Unileipää*, p. 154.
129. Ylikangas, *Unileipää*, p. 153.
130. Ylikangas, *Unileipää*, p. 153.
131. Quoted in Ylikangas, *Unileipää*, p. 156.
132. Ylikangas, *Unileipää*, p. 162.
133. Quoted in Ylikangas, *Unileipää*, p. 166.
134. Quoted in Ylikangas, *Unileipää*, p. 163.
135. Quoted in Ylikangas, *Unileipää*, p. 165.
136. Quoted in Ylikangas, *Unileipää*, p. 165.
137. Ylikangas, *Unileipää*, p. 166.
138. Quoted in Ylikangas, *Unileipää*, p. 173.
139. Quoted in Ylikangas, *Unileipää*, p. 174.

140. Rantanen, "History."
141. Ylikangas, author's correspondence, January 2015.
142. Rantanen, "History."
143. Ylikangas, *Unileipää*, p. 202.
144. Smith, *The Most Dangerous Animal*, p. 153.
145. "World Armies Still Use."
146. Quoted in Trotter, *A Frozen Hell*, p. 83.
147. Trotter, *A Frozen Hell*, p. 83.
148. Quoted in Trotter, *A Frozen Hell*, p. 84.
149. Lucas, *Amphetamines*, pp. 16–7.
150. Dimeo, *A History of Drug Use*, p. 134.

Chapter 8

1. Rasmussen, *On Speed*, p. 192.
2. Menhard, *The Facts About Amphetamines*, p. 30.
3. Iversen, *Speed, Ecstasy, Ritalin*, p. 72.
4. Grinspoon and Hedblom, *The Speed Culture*, p. 20.
5. Quoted in Davenport-Hines, *The Pursuit of Oblivion*, p. 306.
6. Courtwright, *Forces of Habit*, p. 80.
7. "Before Prohibition," http://wings.buffalo.edu/aru/preprohibition.htm, accessed December 3, 2014.
8. Walton, *Out of It*, p. 102.
9. Plant, *Writing on Drugs*, p. 116.
10. Walton, *Out of It*, p. 101.
11. Rasmussen, *On Speed*, pp. 168–9.
12. Courtwright, "The Rise and Fall and Rise of Cocaine," p. 224.
13. McCallum, *Military Medicine*, p. 108; Abadinsky, *Drug Use and Abuse*, pp. 60, 24.
14. Edwards, *The Korean War*, p. 156.
15. MacDonald, *Korea*, p. 224.
16. Edwards, *The Korean War*, p. 156.
17. Quoted in Blackman, *Chilling Out*, p. 37.
18. Leary, *Perilous Missions*; Booth, *Opium*, p. 258.
19. MacDonald, *Korea*, p. 224.
20. Booth, *Opium*, p. 257.
21. Quoted in Sandler, *The Korean War*, p. 120.
22. See Mott and Kim, *Philosophy of Chinese Military Culture*, pp. 103–29.
23. Edwards, *The Korean War*, p. 138, 144.
24. Quoted in Watson, *Far Eastern Tour*, p. 91.
25. Booth, *Opium*, pp. 168–9.
26. Booth, *Opium*, pp. 168–9.
27. Watson, *Far Eastern Tour*, p. 91.
28. MacDonald, *Korea*, p. 134.
29. Best, *War and Law Since 1945*, pp. 141–2, 352–4.
30. Casey, *Selling the Korean War*, p. 282; MacDonald, *Korea*, p. 145.
31. Hunter, "'Brain-Washing' Tactics."
32. Hunter, *Brainwashing in Red China*.
33. Schein, "Chinese Methods of Handling Prisoners of War," pp. 324–7.
34. Meerloo, *Mental Seduction and Menticide*, p. 49.
35. MacDonald, *Korea*, pp. 146, 150–1.
36. Carruthers, *Cold War Captives*, pp. 193–4.
37. Streatfeild, *Brainwash*, p. 7; Meerloo, *Mental Seduction*, p. 19.
38. Wubben, "American Prisoners of War in Korea," p. 5.
39. Biderman, "The Image of 'Brainwashing,'" p. 548.
40. Carruthers, "Redeeming the Captives," p. 277.
41. Quoted in Streatfeild, *Brainwash*, p. 22.

42. See Seed, *Brainwashing*.
43. Quoted in Wubben, "American Prisoners," p. 18.
44. Wubben, "American Prisoners," p. 18.
45. Carruthers, *Cold War Captives*, p. 186.
46. Meerloo, *Mental Seduction*, p. 34.
47. Sandler, *The Korean War*, p. 265; Biderman, "The Image," p. 550.
48. Streatfeild, *Brainwash*, pp. 11–2.
49. Quoted in Albarelli Jr., *A Terrible Mistake*, pp. 191–2.
50. Bowart, *Operation Mind Control*, p. 56.
51. Powers and Gentry, *Operation Overflight*, pp. 238–9.

Chapter 9

1. Ketchum, *Chemical Warfare Secrets*, pp. 245–6.
2. Albarelli, *A Terrible Mistake*, p. 375.
3. Streatfeild, *Brainwash*, p. 20.
4. *Brainwashing: A Synthesis of the Communist Textbook on Psychopolitics*, http://www.alor. org/Library/BrainWashing.htm, accessed January 12, 2015.
5. Quoted in Streatfeild, *Brainwash*, p. 25.
6. Ketchum, *Chemical Warfare Secrets*, p. 15.
7. Cook, "Chemical Weapons," pp. 291, 289.
8. Van Creveld, *The Changing Face*, p. 53.
9. Duffy, "Weapons of War—Poison Gas," August 22, 2009, http://www.firstworldwar. com/weaponry/gas.htm, accessed January 14, 2015.
10. Brophy, "Origins of the Chemical Corps," p. 218.
11. Quoted in Moreno, *Undue Risk: Secret State Experiments on Humans*, p. 40.
12. Brophy, "Origins," p. 226.
13. Moreno, *Undue Risk*, p. 28.
14. Phillsbury, "Penicilin Therapy of Early Syphilis," pp. 139–50.
15. Quoted in Moreno, *Undue Risk*, pp. 29–30.
16. Pechura and Rall, eds., *Veterans at Risk: The Health Effects of Mustard Gas and Lewisite*, p. 379.
17. Pechura and Rall, *Veterans at Risk*, p. 1.
18. Moreno, *Undue Risk*, p. 33.
19. Hunt, *Secret Agenda*, p. 162; Albarelli, *A Terrible Mistake*, p. 362.
20. Hofmann, *LSD: My Problem Child*, pp. 12–8.
21. *Project MKULTRA*, p. 98.
22. Quoted in Bowart, *Operation Mind Control*, p. 91.
23. Ketchum, *Chemical Warfare Secrets*, p. 8.
24. Ketchum, *Chemical Warfare Secrets*, pp. 25, 32–3, 58.
25. Ketchum, *Chemical Warfare Secrets*, p. 103.
26. Ketchum, *Chemical Warfare Secrets*, p. 29.
27. Moreno, *Undue Risk*, pp. 251–2.
28. Quoted in Bowart, *Operation Mind Control*, pp. 91–2.
29. Ketchum, *Chemical Warfare Secrets*, pp. 51, 253.
30. Quoted in Moreno, *Undue Risk*, p. 251.
31. Hornblum, *Acres of Skin*, p. 131.
32. Hornblum, *Acres of Skin*, p. 147.
33. Moreno, *Undue Risk*, p. 230.
34. Quoted in Hornblum, *Acres of Skin*, p. 123.
35. Quoted in Hornblum, *Acres of Skin*, p. 141.
36. Albarelli, *A Terrible Mistake*, p. 557.
37. "U.S. Chemical Weapons Stockpile Information Declassified," http://www.defense. gov/releases/release.aspx?releaseid=729, accessed January 22, 2015; "Russia, Chemical

Notes

329

Weapons," Federation of American Scientists, http://www.fas.org/nuke/guide/russia/cbw/cw.htm, accessed January 22, 2015.

38. DeLillo, *End Zone*, pp. 81, 83.
39. Toffler and Toffler, *War and Anti-War*, p. 125.
40. Ketchum, *Chemical Warfare Secrets*, p. 36.
41. Ketchum, *Chemical Warfare Secrets*, pp. 12–3.
42. Ketchum, *Chemical Warfare Secrets*, p. 14.
43. Mann, *Murder*, p. 25.
44. Ketchum, *Chemical Warfare Secrets*, p. 14–5.
45. Ketchum, *Chemical Warfare Secrets*, p. 36.
46. Albarelli, *A Terrible Mistake*, p. 62.
47. Albarelli, *A Terrible Mistake*, p. 370.
48. Hunt, *Secret Agenda*, p. 162.
49. Cook, "Chemical Weapons," p. 292.
50. Quoted in Baar, "Army Seeks Poison Gas Missiles," p. 10.
51. Sherwin, *A World Destroyed*, pp. 307–8.
52. *Summary of Major Events and Problems*. https://www.osti.gov/opennet/servlets/purl/16006842-VXqarW/16006842.pdf, accessed January 25, 2015.
53. Quoted in Lee and Shlain, *Acid Dreams. The Complete Social History of LSD*, p. 37.
54. Creasy, "Can We Have War Without Death?," p. 74.
55. Ketchum, *Chemical Warfare Secrets*, p. 5.
56. Lee and Shlain, *Acid Dreams*, p. 40.
57. Quoted in Bowart, *Operation Mind Control*, p. 85.
58. Coates, *Nonlethal and Nondestructive Combat in Cities Overseas*.
59. Coates, *Nonlethal*, p. 20.
60. Coates, *Nonlethal*, p. 90.
61. Sun Tzu, *The Art of War*, p. 77.
62. Bowart, *Operation Mind Control*, p. 85.
63. Coker, *Humane Warfare*, p. 14.
64. Ketchum, *Chemical Warfare Secrets*, p. 37.
65. Albarelli, *A Terrible Mistake*, pp. 366–73.
66. Albarelli, *A Terrible Mistake*, p. 210.
67. Cleick, "Humane Warfare for International Peacekeeping," http://www.au.af.mil/au/afri/aspj/airchronicles/aureview/1968/sep-oct/celick.html, accessed January 27, 2015.
68. Stafford, *Psychodelic Encyclopedia*, p. 48.
69. *Field Testing of Hallucinogenic Agents*, http://mcm.dhhq.health.mil/cb_exposures/cold_war/cwfieldtesting.aspx, accessed January 26, 2015.
70. Lee and Shlain, *Acid Dreams*, p. 39.
71. Bowart, *Operation Mind Control*, p. 86.
72. Ketchum, *Chemical Warfare Secrets*, pp. 155–6; *British Soldiers in LSD Trial*, http://www.youtube.com/watch?v=SX7m4fqTLKU&feature=player_embedded, accessed February 10, 2015.
73. *Czechoslovak Military LSD Experiment*, http://www.youtube.com/watch?v=5HXMHdhQL_8&NR=1, accessed February 10, 2015.
74. Lee and Shlain, *Acid Dreams*, p. 41.
75. Ketchum, *Chemical Warfare Secrets*, p. 129.
76. Ketchum, *Chemical Warfare Secrets*, pp. 24, 43–7, 52.
77. Quoted in Bowart, *Operation Mind Control*, p. 83.
78. Ketchum, *Chemical Warfare Secrets*, p. 244, 327.
79. Quoted in Lee and Shlain, *Acid Dreams*, p. 41.
80. Lee and Shlain, *Acid Dreams*, p. 41.
81. Ketchum, *Chemical Warfare Secrets*, pp. 141–52.
82. Lee and Shlain, *Acid Dreams*, p. 43.
83. Ketchum, *Chemical Warfare Secrets*, p. 110.
84. Ketchum, *Chemical Warfare Secrets*, pp. 109–16.

85. Jason R. Odeshoo, "Truth or Dare?: Terrorism and 'Truth Serum' in the Post–9/11 World," pp. 216–7; *Project MKULTRA*, p. 27.
86. Meerloo, *Mental Seduction*, p. 65.
87. Odeshoo, "Truth or Dare," p. 217.
88. Marks, *The Search for the "Manchurian Candidate,"* p. 6.
89. Moreno, *Undue Risk*, p. 191.
90. Marks, *The Search*, p. 38.
91. Streatfeild, *Brainwash*, pp. 36–7.
92. Moreno, *Undue Risk*, p. 190; Cockburn and St. Clair, *Whiteout: the CIA, Drugs, and the Press*, p. 151.
93. *Project MKULTRA*, p. 67.
94. Quoted in Marks, *The Search*, p. 40.
95. Marks, *The Search*, pp. 40–2.
96. Lee and Shlain, *Acid Dreams*, p. 14.
97. Pechura and Rall, *Veterans at Risk*, p. 46.
98. *Project MKULTRA*, p. 92.
99. Quoted in Albarelli, *A Terrible Mistake*, p. 583.
100. Stafford, *Psychodelic Encyclopedia*, pp. 48–9; *Project MKULTRA*, pp. 94–5.
101. Lee and Shlain, *Acid Dreams*, p. 40.
102. Ketchum, *Chemical Warfare Secrets*, p. 222.
103. Moreno, *Undue Risk*, pp. 194–8.
104. Hunt, *Secret Agenda*, p. 170.
105. Moreno, *Undue Risk*, p. 196; Bowart, *Operation Mind Control*, p. 90.
106. Albarelli, *A Terrible Mistake*, p. 163.
107. Quoted in Moreno, *Undue Risk*, p. 198.

Chapter 10

1. Caputo, *A Rumor of War*, p. 354.
2. Quoted in Plant, *Writing on Drugs*, p. 116.
3. Brush, "Higher and Higher," http://www.library.vanderbilt.edu/central/Brush/American-drug-use-vietnam.htm, accessed March 9, 2015.
4. Courtwright, *Dark Paradise*, p. 98.
5. Lewy, *America in Vietnam*, p. 154.
6. Dubberly, "Drugs and Drug Use," pp. 179–80.
7. Krogh Jr., "Heroin Politics," p. 40.
8. Herr, *Dispatches*, p. 5.
9. Iversen, *Speed, Ecstasy, Ritalin*, p. 72.
10. Rasmussen, *On Speed*, p. 190.
11. Gray, *Postmodern War*, p. 209.
12. Keating, "Flying on Amphetamines," pp. 18–9.
13. Rasmussen, *On Speed*, p. 191.
14. Kuzmarov, *The Myth*, p. 17.
15. Dubberly, "Drugs and Drug Use," p. 180.
16. Rasmussen, *On Speed*, p. 191.
17. Grossman, *On Killing*, p. 270.
18. Clayton and Nash, "Medication Management," p. 235.
19. Bourne, *Men, Stress, and Vietnam*, p. 74; McCallum, "Medicine, Military," p. 425.
20. Grossman, *On Killing*, p. 271.
21. Quoted in Coleman, *Flashback*, pp. 113–4.
22. Caputo, *Indian Country*, p. 382.
23. Tritle, *From Melos to My Lai*, p. 63.
24. Grossman, *On Killing*, p. 247.
25. Taylor, "Post-Traumatic Stress Disorder," p. 582.
26. O'Brien, *The Things They Carried*, p. 230.

27. Herr, *Dispatches*, p. 5.
28. Rasmussen, *On Speed*, p. 190.
29. Buzzanco, *Vietnam*, p. 114.
30. Quoted in Kuzmarov, *The Myth*, p. 17.
31. Quoted in Dubberly, "Drugs and Drug Use," p. 180.
32. Quoted in Mauer, *Strange Ground*, p. 219.
33. Courtwright, *Forces of Habit*, p. 42.
34. Grinspoon and Hedblom, *The Speed Culture*, pp. 183–4.
35. Quoted in Szasz, *Ceremonial Chemistry*, p. 201.
36. Hoff Jr., "Drug Abuse," p. 171.
37. Hoff Jr., "Drug Abuse," p. 180.
38. Parks, "Statistics Versus Actuality in Vietnam," http://www.airpower.maxwell.af.mil/airchronicles/aureview/1981/may-jun/parks.htm, accessed March 15, 2015.
39. Brush, "Higher and Higher."
40. Holmes, *Acts of War*, p. 252.
41. Brush, "Higher and Higher."
42. Dubberly, "Drugs and Drug Use," p. 181.
43. Lewy, *America in Vietnam*, p. 154.
44. Robins, Davis, and Nurco, "How Permanent Was Vietnam Drug Addiction?," p. 39.
45. Quoted in Brush, "Higher and Higher."
46. Booth, *Opium*, pp. 270–1.
47. Baker, "U.S. Army Heroin Abuse Identification Program," p. 423; Kuzmarov, *The Myth*, p. 18.
48. Robins and Slobodyan, "Post-Vietnam Heroin Use," 8, p. 1054.
49. Kuzmarov, *The Myth*, p. 19; Baker Jr., "U.S. Army Heroin Abuse," p. 544.
50. Quoted in Booth, *Opium*, p. 272.
51. Booth, *Opium*, p. 272.
52. Buzzanco, *Vietnam*, p. 114.
53. Quoted in Mauer, *Strange Ground*, p. 518.
54. Buzzanco, *Vietnam*, p. 114.
55. Helmer, quoted in Kuzmarov, *The Myth*, p. 22.
56. O'Brien, *The Things*, pp. 14–5.
57. Caputo, *A Rumor of War*, pp. 59, 60.
58. Webb, *Fields of Fire*, p. 75.
59. O'Brien, *The Things*, p. 40.
60. Quoted in DeGroot, *A Noble Cause?*, p. 144.
61. Heinl Jr., "The Collapse of the Armed Forces," http://chss.montclair.edu/english/furr/Vietnam/heinl.pdf, accessed March 18, 2015.
62. Hynes, *The Soldiers' Tale*, p. 183.
63. Caputo, *A Rumor of War*, p. xix.
64. Caputo, *A Rumor of War*, p. 311.
65. Caputo, *A Rumor of War*, p. 355.
66. Kovic, *Born on the Fourth of July*, p. 214.
67. O'Brien, *The Things They Carry*, p. 44.
68. Vonnegut, *Fates Worse Than Death*, p. 209.
69. Herring, *America's Longest War*, p. 268.
70. Buzzanco, *Vietnam*, p. 241.
71. Bergen-Cico, *War and Drugs*, p. 81.
72. Davenport-Hines, *The Pursuit of Oblivion*, pp. 431, 529.
73. Coleman, *Flashback*, p. 114.
74. Musto and Korsmeyer, *Quest for Drug Control*, p. 48.
75. Mauer, *Strange Ground*, p. 161.
76. Rotter, "*Musisz kierować się instynktem przetrwania*," p. 73. Translated by Michelle Atallah.
77. Shay, *Achilles in Vietnam*, p. 203.

78. Robins, "Vietnam: Drug Use," http://www.encyclopedia.com/doc/1G2-3403100469. html, accessed March 22, 2015.
79. Dubberly, "Drugs and Drug Use," p. 180.
80. Brush, "Higher and Higher;" Bey, *Wizard 6*, p. 120.
81. Krogh Jr., "Heroin Politics," pp. 39–40.
82. Holmes, *Acts of War*, p. 251.
83. Booth, *Opium*, p. 271.
84. Quoted in Lewy, *America in Vietnam*, p. 160.
85. Jünger, "Wojna i technika," p. 13. Translated by Michelle Atallah.
86. Caputo, *A Rumor of War*, p. 43.
87. Quoted in Mauer, *Strange Ground*, p. 220.
88. O'Brien, *The Things*, p. 34.
89. Robins, *The Vietnam Drug User Returns*, p. 25.
90. Caputo, *A Rumor of War*, pp. 68–9.
91. Lewy, *America in Vietnam*, p. 160.
92. Grossman, *On Killing*, pp. 266–7.
93. Kuzmarov, *The Myth*, p. 22.
94. Shay, *Achilles in Vietnam*, p. 34; Bunker, "Booby Traps," p. 76.
95. O'Brien, *The Things They Carry*, pp. 82–3.
96. Freud, *Civilisation and Its Discontents*, p. 16.
97. Caputo, *A Rumor of War*, p. xv.
98. Herr, *Dispatches*, p. 71.
99. Quoted in Kuzmarov, *The Myth*, pp. 21–2.
100. Mauer, *Strange Ground*, p. 361.
101. Quoted in Mauer, *Strange Ground*, p. 361.
102. O'Brien, *The Things*, p. 21.
103. Caputo, *A Rumor of War*, p. 276.
104. Quoted in Kuzmarov, *The Myth*, p. 23.
105. Robins, *The Vietnam Drug User*, p. ix.
106. Robins, "Vietnam: Drug Use."
107. Freud, *Civilisation and Its Discontents*, p. 13.
108. Quoted Musto and Korsmeyer, *Quest for Drug Control*, p. 51.
109. Nixon, "Remarks," http://www.presidency.ucsb.edu/ws/?pid=3047; Nixon, "Special Message," http://www.presidency.ucsb.edu/ws/?pid=3048, both accessed March 21, 2015.
110. Nixon, "Special Message."
111. Nixon, "Special Message."
112. Musto and Korsmeyer, *Quest for Drug Control*, pp. 98–9.
113. Helzer, "Significance," p. 220.
114. Brush, "Higher and Higher."
115. Kuzmarov, *The Myth*, pp. 4–5.
116. Weimer, "Drugs-as-a-Disease," p. 269.
117. Alsop, "Worse than My Lai," p. 108.
118. Kuzmarov, *The Myth*, p. 44.
119. Kuzmarov, *The Myth*, p. 44.
120. Dove, "The Holocaust," http://xroads.virginia.edu/~cap/holo/image.html, accessed October 1, 2015.
121. Quoted in Pach Jr., "TV News," p. 460.
122. Kuzmarov, *The Myth*, p. 189.
123. Quoted in Kuzmarov, *The Myth*, p. 71.
124. Epstein, *Agency of Fear*, p. 181.
125. Herr, *Dispatches*, p. 181.
126. Ingraham, "Sense and Nonsense," p. 61.
127. Campbell, *Writing Security*.
128. Weimer, "Drugs-as-a-Disease," p. 266.
129. Weimer, "Drugs-as-a-Disease," p. 267.

130. Finlator, *The Drugged Nation*, p. 8.
131. Mauer, *Strange Ground*, p. 364.
132. MacPherson, *Long Time Passing*, p. 53.
133. Robins, Davis, and Nurco, "How Permanent," p. 40.
134. Davenport-Hines, *The Pursuit of Oblivion*, p. 423.
135. Shay, *Odysseus in America*, p. 36.
136. Shay, *Odysseus in America*, p. 95.

Chapter 11

1. Sarin and Dvoretsky, *The Afghan Syndrome*, pp. 95–6, 100.
2. Sarin and Dvoretsky, *The Afghan Syndrome*, p. 187.
3. Hauner, *The Soviet War in Afghanistan*, p. 100; Bradsher, *Afghan Communism and Soviet Intervention*, p. 251.
4. Alexievich, *Zinky Boys*, p. 77.
5. Merridale, "The Collective Mind," p. 53.
6. Mahoney, "The Wounds of Two Wars," p. A61.
7. Quoted in Heinämaa, Leppänen, and Yurchenko, *The Soldiers' Story*, p. 33.
8. Cooley, *Unholy Wars*, p. 131.
9. Bradsher, *Afghan Communism*, pp. 251, 248.
10. Urban, *War in Afghanistan*, p. 128.
11. Alexiev, *Inside the Soviet Army*, pp. 41–4.
12. Sarin and Dvoretsky, *The Afghan Syndrome*, pp. 89–90.
13. Alexiev, *Inside the Soviet Army*, p. 50.
14. Heinämaa, Leppänen, and Yurchenko, *The Soldiers' Story*, p. 100.
15. Urban, *War in Afghanistan*, p. 127; Alexiev, *Inside the Soviet Army*, pp. 35–40.
16. Quoted in Galeotti, *Afghanistan*, p. 51.
17. O'Ballance, *Afghan Wars*, p. 136.
18. Quoted in Heinämaa, Leppänen, and Yurchenko, *The Soldiers' Story*, p. 12.
19. Galeotti, *Afghanistan*, p. 52; Alexiev, *Inside the Soviet Army*, p. 50.
20. Quoted in Heinämaa, Leppänen, and Yurchenko, *The Soldiers' Story*, p. 46.
21. Quoted in Galeotti, *Afghanistan*, p. 52.
22. Cooley, *Unholy Wars*, p. 164.
23. Cordovez and Harrison, *Out of Afghanistan*, p. 247.
24. Borovik, *The Hidden War*, p. 13.
25. Borovik, *The Hidden War*, p. 14.
26. Reese, *Red Commanders*, pp. 231–2.
27. Alexievich, *Zinky Boys*, p. 80.
28. Alexiev, *Inside the Soviet Army*, p. 52.
29. Quoted in Alexiev, *Inside the Soviet Army*, p. 50.
30. Reese, *Soviet Military Experience*, p. 173.
31. Cooley, *Unholy Wars*, pp. 130–1; Alexiev, *Inside the Soviet Army*, p. 50.
32. Carew, *Jihad!*, p. 217.
33. "Afghan Soldiers Report Getting Hashish Rations."
34. Quoted in Borovik, *The Hidden War*, p. 186.
35. Quoted in Alexiev, *Inside the Soviet Army*, p. 51.
36. Quoted in Heinämaa, Leppänen, and Yurchenko, *The Soldiers' Story*, p. 111.
37. Alexiev, *Inside the Soviet Army*, p. 51.
38. Quoted in Alexievich, *Zinky Boys*, p. 80.
39. Alexievich, *Zinky Boys*, p. 94.
40. Quoted in Urban, *War in Afghanistan*, p. 128.
41. Braithwaite, *Afgantsy*, p. 179.
42. Quoted in Heinämaa, Leppänen, and Yurchenko, *The Soldiers' Story*, p. 12.
43. Quoted in Heinämaa, Leppänen, and Yurchenko, *The Soldiers' Story*, p. 18.
44. Urban, *War in Afghanistan*, p. 128.

45. Alexiev, *Inside the Soviet Army*, p. 53.
46. Alexiev, *Inside the Soviet Army*, p. 54; Reese, *Soviet Military Experience*, p. 173.
47. Cooley, *Unholy Wars*, p. 130.
48. Bradsher, *Afghan Communism*, p. 249.
49. Galeotti, *Afghanistan*, p. 47.
50. Bradsher, *Afghan Communism*, p. 249.
51. Bradsher, *Afghan Communism*, p. 249.
52. Quoted in Alexievich, *Zinky Boys*, p. 19.
53. Reese, *Soviet Military Experience*, p. 157.
54. Cooley, *Unholy Wars*, p. 170.
55. Braithwaite, *Afgantsy*, p. 191.
56. Galeotti, *Afghanistan*, p. 53.
57. Quoted in Heinämaa, Leppänen, and Yurchenko, *The Soldiers' Story*, p. 46.
58. Cooley, *Unholy Wars*, p. 128.
59. Cooley, *Unholy Wars*, p. 129.
60. Feifer, *The Great Gamble*, pp. 182, 183.
61. Scott, *The Road to 9/11*, pp. 124–5.
62. Misdaq, *Afghanistan*, p. 160.
63. Asad and Harris, *Drug Production on the Pakistan-Afghanistan Border*, pp. 53–4.
64. Misdaq, *Afghanistan*, p. 155.
65. Hauner, *The Soviet War*, p. 144; Misdaq, *Afghanistan*, p. 159.
66. Cordovez and Harrison, *Out of Afghanistan*, p. 161.
67. Michael, *The Taliban Movement in Afghanistan*, p. 146.
68. Michael, *The Taliban Movement in Afghanistan*, p. 149.
69. Urban, *War in Afghanistan*, p. 78.
70. Cordovez and Harrison, *Out of Afghanistan*, p. 161.
71. MacDonald, *Drugs in Afghanistan*, pp. 60–1, 90.
72. Borovik, *The Hidden War*, p. 46.
73. Saikal, *Modern Afghanistan*, p. 199.
74. Klass, *Afghanistan*, pp. 20–1.
75. Lohbeck, *Holy War, Unholy Victory*, p. 244.
76. Borovik, *The Hidden War*, pp. 185–6.
77. O'Ballance, *Afghan Wars*, p. 247.
78. Carlisle, *America At War*, p. xi.
79. Bradsher, *Afghan Communism*, p. 400.
80. Inkster and Comolli, *Drugs, Insecurity and Failed States*, p. 68.
81. *Addiction, Crime and Insurgency*, http://www.unodc.org/documents/data-and-analysis/Afghanistan/Afghan_Opium_Trade_2009_web.pdf, accessed April 2, 2015.

Chapter 12

1. Perry, "Fallouja Insurgents Fought Under Influence of Drugs," http://articles.latimes.com/2005/jan/13/world/fg-iraqdrugs13, accessed April 9, 2015.
2. Kan, *Drugs*, p. 53.
3. Kronstadt, *Terrorist Attacks in Mumbai*, http://www.fas.org/sgp/crs/terror/R40087.pdf, accessed April 12, 2015; Rabasa et al., *The Lessons of Mumbai*.
4. "Mumbai Terrorists," http://news.ebru.tv/en/central_asia/8763.html, accessed April 9, 2015; McElroy, "Mumbai Attacks," http://www.telegraph.co.uk/news/worldnews/asia/india/3540964/Mumbai-attacks-Terrorists-took-cocaine-to-stay-awake-during-assault.html, accessed April 9, 2015.
5. Kan, *Drugs*, p. 50.
6. "The Drug of ISIS," http://anfenglish.com/news/the-drug-of-isis-and-al-nusra-captagon, accessed October 3, 2015.
7. Perlmutter, "ISIS Meth Heads," http://www.frontpagemag.com/fpm/252783/isis-meth-heads-tweeking-name-islam-dawn-perlmutter, accessed October 3, 2015.

8. Perlmutter, "ISIS Meth Heads," http://www.frontpagemag.com/fpm/252783/isis-meth-heads-tweeking-name-islam-dawn-perlmutter, accessed October 3, 2015; Baker, "Syria's Breaking Bad," http://world.time.com/2013/10/28/syrias-breaking-bad-are-amphetamines-funding-the-war, accessed October 3, 2015.

9. "Two Tons of IS Drugs," http://bignews2day.com/en/news/raskryt-sekret-zhivotnoj-svireposti-islamistov----eto-tabletka-uzhasa, accessed October 2, 2015.

10. Quoted in Perlmutter, "ISIS Meth Heads," http://www.frontpagemag.com/fpm/252783/isis-meth-heads-tweeking-name-islam-dawn-perlmutter, accessed October 3, 2015.

11. Perlmutter, "ISIS Meth Heads," http://www.frontpagemag.com/fpm/252783/isis-meth-heads-tweeking-name-islam-dawn-perlmutter, accessed October 3, 2015.

12. "Red Bull," http://www.thelocal.at/20141110/red-bull-fuelling-syrian-islamists, accessed October 3, 2015.

13. Holley, "The Tiny Pill," https://www.washingtonpost.com/news/worldviews/wp/2015/11/19/the-tiny-pill-fueling-syrias-war-and-turning-fighters-into-super-human-soldiers/?tid=sm_tw, accessed November 23, 2015.

14. "Captagon—Saudi Mind Control," https://therearenosunglasses.wordpress.com/2014/03/08/captagon-saudi-mind-control-drug-of-choice, accessed October 2, 2015.

15. Watson, "'They Would Torture You,'" http://edition.cnn.com/2014/10/28/world/meast/syria-isis-prisoners-watson, accessed October 4, 2015.

16. Fuchs, "Spain Says Bombers Drank Water from Mecca and Sold Drugs," http://www.nytimes.com/2004/04/15/world/spain-says-bombers-drank-water-from-mecca-and-sold-drugs.html, accessed April 10, 2015.

17. Maxwell, "Operation Enduring Freedom."

18. Quoted in Kan, *Drugs*, p. 64.

19. Bergen-Cico, *War and Drugs*, p. 9.

20. Meyer, "Japan and the World Narcotics Traffic," p. 194; *Department of Justice Examples of Terrorism Convictions*, http://www.justice.gov/opa/pr/2006/June/06_crm_389.html, accessed April 10, 2015.

21. Quoted in "Afghan Opium Market Plummets," http://www.unodc.org/unodc/en/press/releases/2009/September/afghan-opium-market-plummets-says-unodc.html, accessed April 10, 2015.

22. Quoted in Kan, *Drugs*, p. 2.

23. "Colombia: The Status of the FARC," http://www.stratfor.com/memberships/118140/analysis/colombia_status_farc, accessed April 11, 2015.

24. Echevarria, *Preparing for One War*, p. 17.

25. Quoted in Madge, *White Mischief*, p. 149.

26. Castells, *The Rise of The Network Society*.

27. Friedman, *The World is Flat*.

28. Kan, *Drugs*, p. 53.

29. Kan, *Drugs*, pp. 54–5.

30. Kan, *Drugs*, p. 38.

31. *Coca Mama*.

32. Streatfeild, "My Deal with Old King Coke," http://www.theguardian.com/film/2001/may/20/features, accessed September 30, 2015.

33. Booth, *Opium*, p. 338.

34. Ehrenfeld, *Funding Evil*, pp. 166–70.

35. Quoted in Ehrenfeld, *Funding Evil*, p. 166.

36. Carter, "Hezbollah Uses Mexican Drug Routes into U.S.," http://www.washingtontimes.com/news/2009/mar/27/hezbollah-uses-mexican-drug-routes-into-us/?page=all#pagebreak, accessed April 15, 2015; Stewart, "Hezbollah Radical, but Rational," http://www.stratfor.com/weekly/20100811_hezbollah_radical_rational, accessed April 15, 2015.

37. "Drug Addiction Among the Beslan Terrorists," http://english.pravda.ru/news/russia/18-10-2004/59836-0, accessed April 17, 2015.

Chapter 13

1. "Special Air Service (SAS)," http://www.eliteukforces.info/special-air-service/sas-operations/operation-barras, accessed May 14, 2015.
2. Singer, "Caution: Children at War," http://www.carlisle.army.mil/usawc/Parameters/Articles/01winter/singer.htm, accessed May 14, 2015.
3. *Convention on the Rights of the Child*, http://www.ohchr.org/en/professionalinterest/pages/crc.aspx, accessed May 14, 2015.
4. *Cape Town Principles*, p. 12, http://www.unicef.org/emerg/files/Cape_Town_Principles%281%29.pdf, accessed May 14, 2015.
5. *Global Report on Child Soldiers*, p. 96.
6. *Child Soldiers: Global Report 2008*, p. 9.
7. *Child Soldiers: Global Report 2008*, p. 9.
8. Singer, *Children at War*, p. 15.
9. Pearn, "Children and War," p. 169.
10. Kaldor, *New and Old Wars*; Münkler, *The New Wars*.
11. Holsti, *The State, War, and the State of War*.
12. Van Creveld, *The Transformation of War*.
13. Lind et al., "The Changing Face of War."
14. Newman, "The 'New Wars' Debate."
15. Coker, *Ethics and War*, pp. 17–20.
16. Van Creveld, *The Transformation of War*, p. 104.
17. Singer, "The Enablers of War," p. 100.
18. Kapuściński, *The Shadow of the Sun*, p. 149.
19. Burrows, *Kalashnikov AK 47*, p. 7; *Small Arms Survey 2005*, p. 261.
20. "World Population Prospects," http://www.un.org/esa/population/publications/wpp2006/wpp2006.htm, accessed May 18, 2015.
21. *Child Soldiers*, p. 15, http://www.dtic.mil/cgi-bin/GetTRDoc?Location=U2&doc=GetTRDoc.pdf&AD=ADA433182, accessed May 18, 2015.
22. Singer, "Caution: Children at War."
23. Münkler, *The New Wars*, p. 80.
24. Quoted in Brest and McCallin, *Children*, p. 97.
25. See Brett and Specht, *Young Soldiers*.
26. Quoted in Cortes and Buchanan, "The Experience of Columbian Child Soldiers," p. 48.
27. Vautravers, "Why Child Soldiers," p. 104.
28. Nordstrom, "Backyard Front," p. 271.
29. Otis, "Rebel Held: Child Warriors," http://www.chron.com/default/article/Child-warriors-2021604.php, accessed May 20, 2015.
30. Ellis, "Young Soldiers," http://www.ascleiden.nl/pdf/conference24042003-ellis.pdf, accessed May 19, 2015.
31. Dallaire with Humphreys, *They Fight Like Soldiers*, pp. 88–9.
32. Meerloo, *Mental Seduction*, p. 59.
33. Murphy, "Military Patrimonialism," p. 65.
34. Murphy, "Military Patrimonialism," p. 77.
35. See Pham, *Child Soldiers, Adult Interests*, pp. 88, 104; Abdullah and Muana, "Revolutionary United Front of Sierra Leone," p. 190; Denov, "Girl Soldiers and Human Rights," p. 181.
36. Beah, *A Long Way Gone*, pp. 121, 122.
37. Wessells, *Child Soldiers*, p. 76.
38. Wessells, *Child Soldiers*, p. 76.
39. Masland, "Voices of the Children," p. 24.
40. Quoted in Wessells, *Child Soldiers*, p. 76.
41. *Global Report on Child Soldiers*, p. 378.
42. Ashby, "Child Combatants," p. 12.
43. *Easy Prey*, p. 14.
44. *Easy Prey*, p. 37.
45. Quoted in Ellis, "Young Soldiers," p. 169.

46. "How to Fight," p. 29.
47. *Children in Combat*, p. 13.
48. Quoted in "How to Fight," p. 28.
49. *Victims, Perpetrators or Heroes?*, p. 21.
50. Quoted in "How to Fight," p. 28.
51. Singer, *Children at War*, p. 81.
52. Singer, *Children at War*, p. 80.
53. Machel, *Impact of Armed Conflict on Children*, http://www.unicef.org/emerg/files/report_machel.pdf, accessed May 23, 2015.
54. Coulter, *Bush Wives and Girl Soldiers*, p. 102.
55. Coulter, *Bush Wives and Girl Soldiers*, pp. 54–5.
56. Singer, *Children at War*, p. 82.
57. "Mai Mai Child Soldier Recruitment and Use," p. 4.
58. Quoted in Wessells, *Child Soldiers*, p. 77.
59. Denov and Maclure, "Turnings and Epiphanies," p. 256.
60. Singer, *Children at War*, p. 107.
61. Wessells, "Child Soldiers," p. 36.
62. *"My Gun Was as Tall as Me,"* p. 86.
63. Quoted in *No Childhood At All*, p. 50.
64. Quoted in Brest and McCallin, *Children*, p. 98.
65. Gates, "Recruitment and Allegiance"; Andvig and Gates, "Recruiting Children for Armed Conflict."
66. Gates, "Recruitment and Allegiance," p. 114.
67. Utas and Jörgel, "The West Side Boys," p. 499.
68. *Child Soldiers: Implications*, p. 27.
69. Quoted in Bindu, "Congo (DRC): Drug Addiction," http://iwpr.net/report-news/drug-addiction-hinders-child-soldier-reintegration, accessed May 24, 2015.
70. Beah, *A Long Way Gone*, p. 139.
71. Denov and Maclure, "Turnings and Epiphanies," p. 251.
72. Quoted in Denov, "Girl Soldiers," p. 829.
73. Dukuly, "Liberia," http://www.afrika.no/Detailed/4782.html, accessed May 24, 2015.
74. Bindu, "Congo (DRC)."
75. Singer, *Children at War*, p. 82.
76. McNeil, "Drugs Banned," http://www.nytimep.com/2007/09/10/health/10pain.html?pagewanted=all, accessed May 24, 2015.
77. Quoted in Ashby, "Child Combatants," p. 12.
78. Quoted in Dukuly, "Liberia."
79. Shepler, "The Rites of the Child," p. 199.
80. Daly, "First American to Die in Afghanistan," http://articles.nydailynews.com/2010-01-05/news/17945156_1_forward-operating-base-chapman-special-forces-tora-bora, accessed May 24, 2015.
81. Dallaire with Humphreys, *They Fight Like Soldiers*, pp. 117–8.
82. "Officials: Taliban Recruiting Children as Bombers," http://www.usatoday.com/news/world/2009-07-28-taliban-children_N.htm, accessed May 24, 2015; Boone, "Groomed for Suicide," http://www.guardian.co.uk/world/2011/may/17/groomed-suicide-taliban-recruits-afghan-children-murder, accessed May 24, 2015.
83. "2,000 Former Afghan Child Soldiers," http://www.unicef.org/media/media_19165.html, accessed May 25, 2015.
84. Singer, "The Enables of War," 94.
85. Sullivan, "Child Soldiers," http://www.airpower.maxwell.af.mil/apjinternational/apj-s/2008/1tri08/sullivaneng.htm, accessed May 25, 2015.
86. Pincus, "U.S. Has Detained 2,500 Juveniles as Enemy Combatants," http://www.washingtonpost.com/wp-dyn/content/article/2008/05/14/AR2008051403365.html, accessed May 25, 2015.
87. Cocks, "Iraqi Girl Tells of Ordeal as Suicide Bomber," http://www.reuters.com/article/2008/08/29/us-iraq-girl-idUSLP60382820080829, accessed May 25, 2015; Haynes,

"Young Iraqi Girls Turned into Perfect Weapon," http://www.timesonline.co.uk/tol/news/world/iraq/article4849336.ece, accessed May 25, 2015.

88. "Alarm Over Somalia's Child Soldiers," http://news.bbc.co.uk/2/hi/8173079.stm, accessed May 25, 2015.

89. "Child Soldiers Sent by Gaddafi," http://www.channel4.com/news/child-soldiers-sent-by-gaddafi-to-fight-libyan-rebels, accessed May 27, 2015.

90. Dowdney, *Children of the Drug Trade*, p. 51.

91. Graham, "Mexican Teenage Girls," http://www.reuters.com/article/2011/06/17/us-mexico-drugs-teenagers-idUSTRE75G5F820110617, accessed May 26, 2015.

92. Williams and Felbab-Brown, *Drug Trafficking*, p. 17; Inkster and Comolli, *Drugs, Insecurity and Failed States*, p. 92.

93. "U.S. Boy, 14, Sentenced in Mexico for Cartel Killings," http://www.msnbc.msn.com/id/43900421/ns/world_news-americas/t/us-boy-sentenced-mexico-cartel-killings, accessed May 26, 2015.

94. Grayson, *La Familia Drug Cartel*, p. 37.

95. Brands, *Mexico's Narco-Insurgency*, p. 4.

96. Ignatieff, *The Warrior's Honor*, p. 12.

97. McMahan, "An Ethical Perspective on Child Soldiers," p. 28.

98. Grossman, *On Killing*, pp. 266–7.

99. Singer, *Children at War*, p. 170.

100. Münkler, *The New Wars*, p. 80.

101. Singer, "Caution: Children at War."

102. Sullivan, "Child Soldiers."

103. See Coker, *Humane Warfare*.

Chapter 14

1. Virilio, *Speed and Politics*, p. 43.

2. Miller, Panagiotis, and Shattuck, "Fatigue and Its Effect," p. 231.

3. Helmer, "Chief of Staff Shares Views on Global Strike Task Force," http://www.combat-sim.com/memb123/cnews/arch/cnews-arc146.htm#chstff, accessed October 5, 2015.

4. Kenagy et al., "Dextroamphetamine Use," pp. 381–2.

5. Virilio, *Speed and Politics*, pp. 153, 167.

6. Quoted in Fontenot, Degen, and Tohn, *On Point*, p. 117.

7. Quoted in Miller, Panagiotis, and Shattuck, "Fatigue and Its Effect," p. 231.

8. See Arnedt et al., "Simulated Driving Performance"; Williamson et al., "Developing Measures of Fatigue"; Dawson and Reid, "Fatigue, Alcohol and Performance Impairment," p. 235.

9. Roehrs et al., "Ethanol and Sleep Loss," p. 984.

10. Caldwell and Caldwell, "Fatigue in Military Aviation," p. C39.

11. Westcott, "Modafinil," p. 333; Buguet, Moroz, and Radomski, "Modafinil," p. 659; Lagarde and Batejat, "Disrupted Sleep-Wake Rhythm," p. 166.

12. Dinges, "An Overview of Sleepiness and Accidents."

13. Martin, *Counting Sheep*, p. 33.

14. See Wojtczak-Jaroszowa and Jarosz, "Time-Related Distribution of Occupational Accidents"; Lauridsen and Tønnesen, "Injuries Related to Shift Working"; Laundry and Lees, "Industrial Accident Experience."

15. Quoted in Kasindorf, "Accidental Deaths Exceed Those in Combat," http://usatoday30.usatoday.com/news/world/iraq/2003-03-26-count_usat_x.htm, accessed October 7, 2015.

16. Lagarde and Batejat, "Disrupted Sleep-Wake Rhythm," p. 166.

17. Sample, "Wired Awake," http://www.guardian.co.uk/education/2004/jul/29/research.highereducation, accessed October 9, 2015.

18. Caldwell et al., "Fatigue Countermeasures in Aviation," p. 37.

19. Buguet, Moroz, and Radomski, "Modafinil," p. 659.

20. Martin, *Counting Sheep*, p. 108.

21. Caldwell and Caldwell, "Fatigue in Military Aviation," p. C43; Batéjat et al., "Prior Sleep with Zolpidem," p. 515.
22. Cornum, Cornum, and Storm, "Use of Stimulants," pp. 37–42.
23. Caldwell, Caldwell, and Schmidt, "Alertness Management Strategies," p. 267; Caldwell, "Dextroamphetamine and Modafinil," pp. 31–4, http://ftp.rta.nato.int/public//PubFullText/RTO/MP/RTO-MP-HFM-124///MP-miscMatter-10-31.pdf, accessed October 16, 2014.
24. Flora, *Taking America Off Drugs*, p. 79; Lovell and Kluger, *Apollo 13*, p. 314.
25. Braswell, *American Meth*, p. 44.
26. Keating, "Flying on Amphetamines," pp. 18–9.
27. Jones and Marsh, *Flight Surgeon*, p. 128.
28. Jones and Marsh, *Flight Surgeon*, p. 128.
29. Cornum, Cornum, and Storm, "Use of Stimulants," p. 37–41.
30. Atkinson, *Crusade*, p. 525.
31. *Performance Maintenance*, p. 10, http://www.med.navy.mil/directives/Pub/6410.pdf, accessed October 14, 2014; Emonson and Vanderbeek, "The Use of Amphetamines."
32. Quoted in Cornum, Cornum, and Storm, "Use of Stimulants," p. 37–43.
33. Cornum, Cornum, and Storm, "Use of Stimulants," p. 37–41.
34. Mehlman, *The Price of Perfection*, p. 21.
35. Bonné, "'Go Pills,'" http://www.msnbc.msn.com/id/3071789/ns/us_news-only/t/go-pills-war-drugs/#.UMsrUazTlzw, accessed October 15, 2014.
36. Cornum, Caldwell, and Cornum, "Stimulant Use," p. 57.
37. Caldwell, "Dextroamphetamine and Modafinil," p. 100.
38. Bonné, "Go Pills."
39. *Performance Maintenance*, p. 21.
40. Dowty, *Christian Fighter Pilot*, p. 5.
41. "51st Fighter Wing Instruction," pp. 2–5, http://static.e-publishing.af.mil/production/1/51fw/publication/51fwi44-102/51fwi44-102.pdf, accessed October 17, 2015.
42. Interviewed by the author on April 19, 2012.
43. *Performance Maintenance*, p. 10.
44. Jones and Marsh, *Flight Surgeon*, p. 137.
45. Caldwell, Caldwell, and Schmidt, "Alertness Management," p. C40–2.
46. *Performance Maintenance*, p. 11.
47. Quoted in Jones and Marsh, *Flight Surgeon*, p. 144.
48. See Coker, *Humane Warfare*.
49. Schultz and Miller, *Fatigue and Use of Go/No Go Pills*, pp. v, 3.
50. Schultz and Miller, *Fatigue and Use of Go/No Go Pills*, p. 6.
51. Caldwell and Caldwell, "Fatigue in Military Aviation," p. C48.
52. Kenagy et al., "Dextroamphetamine Use," pp. 383, 384.
53. Quoted in Elliott, "'Go Pills,'" http://www.aetc.randolph.af.mil/se2/torch/back/2003/0304/gopill.htm, accessed October 20, 2014.
54. "Dexedrine Spansule: Prescribing Information," http://dailymed.nlm.nih.gov/dailymed/lookup.cfm?setid=a37b6ef9-78b4-4b18-8797-ecb583502500, accessed August 13, 2015.
55. Miller, "'Go' Pills for F-16 Pilots," http://www.sfgate.com/cgi-bin/article.cgi?f=/c/a/2003/01/04/MN191592.DTL&ao=all, accessed October 21, 2014.
56. Bergen-Cico, *War and Drugs*, p. 129.
57. Caldwell et al., "Fatigue Countermeasures in Aviation," p. 50.
58. Friscolanti, *Friendly Fire*.
59. Bonné, "'Go Pills'"; Braswell, *American Meth*, p. 141.
60. Braswell, *American Meth*, p. 142.
61. Smith, "Harry Schmidt's War," http://www.chicagomag.com/Chicago-Magazine/April-2005/Harry-Schmidts-War, accessed October 25, 2014.
62. Killgore et al., "Restoration of Risk-Propensity," pp. 868, 872.
63. Franzak, *A Nightmare's Prayer*, pp. 124–5.

64. "U.S. Air Force Verdict," http://www.cbc.ca/news2/background/friendlyfire/verdict. html, accessed October 25, 2014.
65. *Brain Waves Module 3*, p. 6.
66. Stivalet et al., "Effects of Modafinil," p. 501.
67. Pigeau et al., "Modafinil."
68. See Lyons and French, "Modafinil"; Krueger, "Sustained Military Performance"; Baranski et al., "Modafinil."
69. Miller, *Encyclopedia of Addictive Drugs*, p. 302; Westcott, "Modafinil, Sleep Deprivation," p. 334.
70. Killgore et al., "Effects of Dextroamphetamine, Caffeine and Modafinil," p. 318.
71. Stivalet et al., "Effects of Modafinil," p. 502; Baranski et al. "Modafinil."
72. Estrada et al., "Modafinil as a Replacement," p. 556.
73. Kim, "Practical Use and Risk of Modafinil," http://dx.doi.org/10.5620/eht.2012.27. e2012007, accessed August 11, 2015.
74. Buguet, Moroz, and Radomski, "Modafinil," p. 659; Lawton, "Get Up and Go."
75. Volkow et al., "Effects of Modafinil."
76. Lawton, "Get Up and Go."
77. Caldwell, Caldwell, and Schmidt, "Alertness Management," p. 267.
78. Armstrong, "Brave Neuro World," p. 58.
79. Flower, "The Osler Lecture 2012," p. 827.
80. See Kamieński, "Cosmetic Pharmacology."
81. Quoted in Westcott, "Modafinil, Sleep Deprivation," p. 334.
82. Didier, Louisy, and Matton, *Gestion de la vigilance*.
83. Lagarde and Batejat, "Disrupted Sleep-Wake Rhythm"; Baranski et al., "Modafinil."
84. Caldwell et al., "A Double-Blind."
85. Pearson, "Sleep It Off," p. 263.
86. Caldwell et al., "Modafinil's Effects on Simulator Performance."
87. *Caffeine for the Sustainment of Mental Task Performance*, p. 74.
88. Estrada et al., "Modafinil," p. 557.
89. Caldwell et al., "Fatigue Countermeasures in Aviation," p. 50.
90. Saul, "Merck Cancels Work," http://www.nytimes.com/2007/03/29/business/29sleep. html?ref=health&_r=0, accessed July 29, 2015.
91. Moore, *The 24/7 Society*.
92. Quoted in Su, "Merck Plans to File Its Novel Sleeping Pill," http://www.pharmatopics. com/2012/02/merck-plans-to-file-its-novel-sleeping-pill-suvorexant-with-fda, accessed July 24, 2015.
93. Kramer, *Listening to Prozac*.
94. Von Zeilbauer, "For U.S. Troops at War," http://www.nytimes.com/2007/03/13/world/ middleeast/13alcohol.html?pagewanted=print, accessed July 25, 2015.
95. Kan, *Drugs*, p. 63.
96. Hoge et al., "Combat Duty in Iraq and Afghanistan," p. 13.
97. Tanielian and Jaycox, *Invisible Wounds of War*, p. xxi, http://www.rand.org/pubs/ monographs/2008/RAND_MG720.pdf, accessed July 27, 2015.
98. *Army Health Promotion*, pp. 56, i, https://army.deps.mil/army/sites/APP/OPMG/ Policy/DocumentsLibrary/ArmyRedBook.pdf, accessed September 27, 2015.
99. Quoted in Allen, "The Iraq War—On Drugs," http://www.inthesetimes.com/article/ 2670, accessed July 28, 2015.
100. Kan, *Drugs*, p. 63.
101. Von Zeilbauer, "For U.S. Troops at War."
102. McKinley, "Despite Army Efforts, Soldier Suicides Continue," http://www.nytimes. com/2010/10/11/us/11suicides.html?pagewanted=all, accessed July 28, 2015.
103. Bergen-Cico, *War and Drugs*, p. 127.
104. Quoted in Allen, "The Iraq War—On Drugs."
105. "U.S. Soldiers Implicated in Italian Steroid Bust," http://www.abc.net.au/news/2005- 07-17/us-soldiers-implicated-in-italian-steroidbust/2060024, accessed July 28, 2015.

106. Jaffe, "Army's Recruiting Push."

107. Bergen-Cico, *War and Drugs*, p. 132.

108. Roug, "Witnesses Tell of Troop Stress," http://articles.latimes.com/2006/aug/09/world/fg-iraq9, accessed July 28, 2015; "Soldier: 'Death Walk' Drives Troops 'Nuts,'" http://edition.cnn.com/2006/WORLD/meast/08/08/iraq.mahmoudiya/index.html, accessed July 28, 2015.

Conclusion

1. Booth, *Opium*, p. 19.

2. Berridge, *Opium and the People*, p. xxiii.

3. Matthee, "Exotic Substances," p. 26.

4. Matthee, "Exotic Substances," p. 26.

5. Matthee, "Exotic Substances," p. 44.

6. Quoted in Porter, *War and the Rise of the State*, p. xix.

7. Knipe, *Culture, Society, and Drugs*, p. 1.

8. Dally, "Anomalies and Mysteries in the 'War on Drugs,'" p. 199.

9. Plato, *Republic*, p. 138.

10. Walzer, *Just and Unjust Wars*, p. 252.

11. Camus, *Caligula*, p. 258.

12. Niebuhr, *Moral Man and Immoral Society*.

13. Courtwright, *Forces of Habit*, p. 14.

14. Szasz, *Ceremonial Chemistry*, p. 75.

15. Foucault, *Discipline and Punish*, p. 137.

16. Plant, *Writing on Drugs*, p. 152.

17. Quoted in Plant, *Writing on Drugs*, p. 152.

18. Plant, *Writing on Drugs*, p. 152.

19. Foucault, *Discipline and Punish*, p. 168.

20. Foucault, *Discipline and Punish*, p. 138.

21. Harner, *The Way of the Shaman*, p. 40.

22. Eliade, *Shamanism*, p. 223.

23. Eliade, *Shamanism*, p. 401.

24. Harner, "Introduction," p. xi.

25. Coker, *Waging War*, p. 6.

26. Coker, *The Warrior Ethos*, p. 94.

27. Foucault, *Discipline and Punish*, p. 136.

28. Taylor, *The Principles of Scientific Management*, p. 7.

29. Tether, "Statement," http://www.darpa.mil/WorkArea/DownloadAsset.aspx?id=1781, accessed August 12, 2015.

Epilogue

1. Aron, *The Opium of the Intellectuals*.

2. Quoted in Walton, *Out of It*, p. 237.

3. Slawney, "Hallucinogenric Literature," p. 42.

4. Ronell, *Crack Wars*, p. 78.

5. Ehrenreich, *Blood Rites*, p. 13.

6. Partridge, *The Psychology of Nations*, p. 23.

7. Hillman, *A Terrible Love of War*.

8. Hynes, *The Soldiers' Tale*, p. 28.

9. Brænder, "Adrenaline Junkies," p. 5.

10. Ronell, *Crack Wars*, pp. 118–9.

11. Hedges, *War Is a Force*, p. 3.

12. Hedges, *War Is a Force*, p. 10.

13. Hedges, *War Is a Force*, p. 3.
14. Hillman, *A Terrible Love of War*, p. 10.
15. Hynes, *The Soldiers' Tale*, p. 23.
16. James, *The Moral Equivalent of War*, http://www.constitution.org/wj/meow.htm, accessed August 13, 2015.
17. Quoted in Alexievich, *Zinky Boys*, p. 59.
18. Ehrenreich, *Blood Rites*, p. 129.
19. Weil, *The Iliad or Poem of Force*, p. 11.
20. Gray, *The Warriors*, p. 55.
21. Quoted in Holmes, *Acts of War*, p. 18.
22. Hedges, *War Is a Force*, p. 25.
23. Hynes, *The Soldiers' Tale*, pp. 201–2.
24. Quoted in Jaśkiewicz, "Witkacego kreatory sztucznych jaźni," p. 130.
25. Hillman, *A Terrible Love of War*, p. 159.
26. Tritle, *From Melos to My Lai*, p. 55.
27. Quoted in Jones, *All-out For Victory!*, p. 54.
28. Caputo, *A Rumor of War*, p. 6.
29. Hynes, *The Soldiers' Tale*, p. 178.
30. Hedges, *War Is a Force*, p. 3.
31. Alexievich, *Zinky Boys*, p. 26.
32. Collin, *Altered State*, p. 25.
33. Collin, *Altered State*, p. 32.
34. Collin, *Altered State*, p. 54.
35. Robson, *Forbidden Drugs*, p. 138.
36. *MDMA/PTSD U.S. Study (Veterans of War)*, http://www.maps.org/research/mdma/mdma_ptsd_u.s._study_veterans_of_war, accessed August 13, 2015.
37. Collin, *Altered State*, p. viii.
38. Anderson, "The Agony and the Ecstasy," http://motherboard.vice.com/2011/8/16/the-agony-and-the-ecstasy-the-quiet-mission-to-fight-ptsd-with-psychedelic-drugs, accessed August 13, 2015.

BIBLIOGRAPHY

"2,000 Former Afghan Child Soldiers to Be Demobilized and Rehabilitated," *News Note*, UNICEFF, 8 February 2004, http://www.unicef.org/media/media_19165.html.

"51st Fighter Wing Instruction 44-102(51FWI44-102), Medication Use with Flying Operations," 16 April 2012, http://static.e-publishing.af.mil/production/1/51fw/publication/51fwi44-102/51fwi44-102.pdf.

Abadinsky, Howard, *Drug Use and Abuse: A Comprehensive Introduction*, Belmont, CA: Thomson Wadsworth, 2008.

Abdullah, Ibrahim and Patrick Muana, "The Revolutionary United Front of Sierra Leone," in Christopher Clapham (ed.), *African Guerillas*, Oxford: James Currey, 1998.

Abun-Nasr, Jamil M., *A History of the Maghrib in the Islamic Period*, Cambridge: Cambridge University Press, 1987.

Adams, George W., "Caring for the Men: The History of Civil War Medicine," in *The Image of War: 1861–1865*, Doubleday: National Historical Society, 1983, vol. 4, http://www.civilwarhome.com/medicinehistory.htm.

Addiction, Crime and Insurgency. The Transnational Threat of Afghan Opium, Vienna: United Nations Office on Drugs and Crime, 2009, http://www.unodc.org/documents/data-and-analysis/Afghanistan/Afghan_Opium_Trade_2009_web.pdf.

"Afghan Opium Market Plummets, Says UNOD," *Press Release*, United Nations Office on Drugs and Crime, 2 September 2009, http://www.unodc.org/unodc/en/press/releases/2009/September/afghan-opium-market-plummets-says-unodc.html.

"Afghan Soldiers Report Getting Hashish Rations," *St. Louis Dispatch*, 25 May 1989: 18A.

"Alarm Over Somalia's Child Soldiers," *BBC News*, 29 July 2009, http://news.bbc.co.uk/2/hi/8173079.stm.

Albarelli, Hank P., Jr., *A Terrible Mistake: The Murder of Frank Olson and the CIA's Secret Cold War Experiments*, Walterville, OR: Trine Day, 2011.

Alexander, Anna, "Freud's Pharmacy: Cocaine and the Corporeal Unconscious," in Anna Alexander and Mark S. Roberts (eds.), *High Culture. Reflections on Addiction and Modernity*, New York: State University of New York Press, 2003: 209–32.

Alexiev, Alexander, *Inside the Soviet Army in Afghanistan*, Santa Monica, CA: RAND Corporation, 1988.

Alexievich, Svetlana, *Zinky Boys. Soviet Voices from the Afghanistan War*, New York: W.W. Norton, 1992.

Allen, Terry J., "The Iraq War—On Drugs," *In These Times*, 31 May 2006, http://www.inthesetimes.com/article/2670.

Alsop, Stewart, "Worse than My Lai," *Newsweek*, May 24, 1971: 104.

Anderson, Brian, "The Agony and the Ecstasy: The Quiet Mission to Fight PTSD with Psychedelic Drugs," Mother Board, 16 August 2011, http://motherboard.vice.com/2011/8/16/the-agony-and-the-ecstasy-the-quiet-mission-to-fight-ptsd-with-psychedelic-drugs.

Andvig, Jens Christopher and Scott Gates, "Recruiting Children for Armed Conflict," in Scott Gates and Simon Reich (eds.), *Child Soldiers in the Age of Fractured States*, Pittsburgh: University of Pittsburgh Press, 2010: 77–92.

Armstrong, Walter, "Brave Neuro World," *Pharmaceutical Executive*, 30:4, 2010: 58–60, 62, 64.

Army Health Promotion, Risk Reduction Suicide Prevention Report 2010, Washington, DC: United States Army/DIANE, 2010, https://army.deps.mil/army/sites/APP/OPMG/Policy/DocumentsLibrary/ArmyRedBook.pdf.

Arnedt, J. Todd, Gerald J. S. Wilde, Peter W. Munt, and Alistair W. MacLean, "Simulated Driving Performance Following Prolonged Wakefulness and Alcohol Consumption: Separate and Combined Contributions to Impairment," *Journal of Sleep Research*, 9:3, 2000: 233–41.

Aron, Raymond, *The Opium of the Intellectuals*, London: Secker & Warburg, 1957.

Asad, Amir Zada and Robert Harris, *The Politics and Economics of Drug Production on the Pakistan-Afghanistan Border*, Burlington, VT: Ashgate, 2003.

Ashby, Phil, "Child Combatants: A Soldier's Perspective," *The Lancet*, Supplement, 360, 2002: 11–2.

Atkinson, Rick, *An Army at Dawn: The War in North Africa 1942–1943*, New York: Henry Holt & Co., 2002.

Atkinson, Rick, *Crusade: The Untold Story of the Persian Gulf War*, Boston: Houghton Mifflin, 1993.

Baar, James, "Army Seeks Poison Gas Missiles," *Missiles and Rockets*, 16 May 1960: 10–1.

Baker, Aryn, "Syria's Breaking Bad: Are Amphetamines Funding the War?" *Time*, October 28, 2013, http://world.time.com/2013/10/28/syrias-breaking-bad-are-amphetamines-funding-the-war.

Baker, Stewart L., Jr., "Drug Abuse in the United States Army," *Bulletin of the New York Academy of Medicine*, 47:6, 1971: 541–9.

Baker, Stewart L., Jr., "U.S. Army Heroin Abuse Identification Program in Vietnam: Implications for a Methadone Program," *American Journal of Public Health*, 62:6, 1972: 857–60.

Baranski, Joseph, Corinne Cian, Dominique Esquivié, Ross Pigeau, and Christian Raphel, "Modafinil during 64 Hours of Sleep Deprivation: Dose-Related Effects on Fatigue, Alertness, and Cognitive Performance," *Military Psychology*, 10:3, 1998: 173–93.

Barthes, Roland, *Mythologies* (trans. Annette Lavers), New York: Hill and Wang, 1972.

Batéjat, Denise, Olivier Coste, Pascal van Peers, Didier Lagarde, and Christophe Piérard, "Prior Sleep with Zolpidem Enhances the Effect of Caffeine or Modafinil during 18 Hours Continuous Work," *Aviation, Space, and Environmental Medicine*, 77:5, 2006: 515–25.

Baudelaire, Charles, "On Wine and Hashish," in Charles Baudelaire, *Artificial Paradises* (trans. Stacy Diamond), Secaucus, NJ: Carol, 1998: 1–26.

Baudelaire, Charles, "The Poem of Hashish," in Charles Baudelaire, *On Wine and Hashish* (trans. Andrew Brown), London: Hesperus 2002.

Baulmer, Adam, *The Chinese and Opium under the Republic: Worse than Floods and Wild Beasts*, Albany: State University of New York Press, 2007.

Bayer, Istvan, "The Abuse of Psychotropic Drugs," *Bulletin on Narcotics*, 3 January 1973, http://www.unodc.org/unodc/en/data-and-analysis/bulletin/bulletin_1973-01-01_3_page003.html.

Beah, Ishmael, *A Long Way Gone: Memoirs of a Boy Soldier*, London: Fourth Estate, 2007.

"Before Prohibition," Addiction Research Unit, Department of Psychology, University at Buffalo, http://wings.buffalo.edu/aru/preprohibition.htm.

Benedict, Ruth, *The Chrysanthemum and the Sword: Patterns of Japanese Culture*, New York: Houghton Mifflin Harcourt, 2005 (original publication 1946).

Bergen-Cico, Dessa K., *War and Drugs: The Role of Military Conflict in the Development of Substance Abuse*, Boulder, CO: Paradigm, 2012.

Berridge, Virginia, "Drugs and Social Policy: The Establishment of Drug Control in Britain 1900–30," *British Journal of Addiction*, 79:1, 1984: 17–29.

Berridge, Virginia, *Opium and the People: Opiate Use and Drug Control Policy in Nineteenth and Early Twentieth Century England*, London: Free Association Books, 1999.

Berridge, Virginia, "War Conditions and Narcotic Control: The Passing of Defence of the Realm Act Regulation 40B," *Journal of Social Policy*, 7:3, 1978: 285–304.

Best, Geoffrey, *War and Law Since 1945*, Oxford: Clarendon Press, 2001.

Bey, Douglas, *Wizard 6: A Combat Psychiatrist in Vietnam*, College Station: Texas A&M University Press, 2006.

Biderman, Albert D., "The Image of 'Brainwashing,'" *Public Opinion Quarterly*, 26:4, 1962: 547–63.

Bindu, Lucie, "Congo (DRC): Drug Addiction Hinders Child Soldier Reintegration," *Report News*, Institute for War and Peace Reporting, January 2010, http://iwpr.net/report-news/drug-addiction-hinders-child-soldier-reintegration.

Blackman, Shane J., *Chilling Out: The Cultural Politics of Substance Consumption, Youth and Drug Policy*, Berkshire: McGraw-Hill Education, 2004.

Bonné, Jon, "'Go Pills': A War on Drugs?," MSNBC.com, 9 January 2003, http://www.msnbc.msn.com/id/3071789/ns/us_news-only/t/go-pills-war-drugs/#.UMsrUazTlzw.

Boone, Jon, "Groomed for Suicide: How Taliban Recruits Children for Mass Murder," *Guardian*, 17 May 2011, http://www.guardian.co.uk/world/2011/may/17/groomed-suicide-taliban-recruits-afghan-children-murder.

Booth, Martin, *Opium. A History*, New York: St. Martin's Press, 1998.

Borovik, Artyom, *The Hidden War: A Russian Journalist's Account of the Soviet War in Afghanistan*, London: Faber and Faber, 1990.

Bourne, Peter G., *Men, Stress, and Vietnam*, Boston: Little Brown, 1970.

Bowart, Walter, *Operation Mind Control*, New York: Dell, 1978.

Braam, Conny, *The Cocaine Salesman* (trans. Jonathan Reeder), London: Haus, 2011.

Bradsher, Henry S., *Afghan Communism and Soviet Intervention*, Oxford: Oxford University Press, 1999.

Brænder, Morten, "Adrenaline Junkies: Why Soldiers Return from War Wanting More," *Armed Forces and Society*, first published online 13 February 2015.

Brain Waves Module 3: Neuroscience, Conflict, and Security, London: The Royal Society, 2012.

Brainwashing: A Synthesis of the Communist Textbook on Psychopolitics, 1956 [?], see http://www.alor.org/Library/BrainWashing.htm.

Braithwaite, Rodric, *Afgantsy: The Russians in Afghanistan, 1979–89*, New York: Oxford University Press, 2011.

Brands, Hal, *Mexico's Narco-Insurgency and U.S. Counterdrug Policy*, Carlisle Barracks, PA: Strategic Studies Institute, U.S. Army War College, 2009.

Braswell, Sterling R., *American Meth: A History of the Methamphetamine Epidemic in America*, New York: iUniverse, 2005.

Braswell, Sterling R., *Crazy Town: Money. Marriage. Meth*, Wilkes-Barre, PA: Kallisti, 2008.

Brest, Rachel and Margaret McCallin, *Children: The Invisible Soldiers*, Stockholm: Rädda Baren, Save the Children Sweden, 1998.

Brett, Rachel and Irma Specht, *Young Soldiers: Why They Choose to Fight*, Boulder, CO: Lynne Rienner, 2004.

Brill, Henry and Tetsuya Hirose, "The Rise and Fall of a Methamphetamine Epidemic: Japan 1945–1955," *Seminars in Psychiatry*, 1:2, 1969: 179–94.

British Soldiers in LSD Trial, You Tube, http://www.youtube.com/watch?v=SX7m4fqTLKU&feature=player_embedded.

Brodie, Bernard, *Strategy in the Missile Age*, Princeton: Princeton University Press, 1959.

Brook, Timothy and Bob Tadashi Wakabayashi, "Introduction: Opium's History in China," in Timothy Brook and Bob Tadashi Wakabayashi (eds.), *Opium Regimes: China, Britain and Japan, 1839–1952*, Berkeley: University of California Press, 2000: 1–27.

Brophy, Leo P., "Origins of the Chemical Corps," *Military Affairs*, 20:4, 1956: 217–26.

Brush, Peter, "Higher and Higher: Drug Use Among U.S. Forces in Vietnam," *Vietnam*, 15:5, 2002, http://www.library.vanderbilt.edu/central/Brush/American-drug-use-vietnam.htm.

Bryant, Alfred T., *The Zulu People as They Were Before the White Man Came*, Pietermaritzburg: Shuter and Shooter, 1949, vol. 1.

Buguet, Alain, Dianne E. Moroz and Manny W. Radomski, "Modafinil—Medical Considerations for Use in Sustained Operations," *Aviation, Space, and Environmental Medicine*, 74:6, 2003: 659–63.

Bullock, Alan, *Hitler: A Study in Tyranny*, New York: Harper & Row, 1964.

Bunker, Robert J., "Booby Traps," in Spencer C. Tucker (ed.), *Encyclopedia of the Vietnam War. A Political, Social and Military History*, Santa Barbara, CA: ABC-CLIO, 1998, vol. 1: 76.

Burns, Eric, *The Spirits of America. A Social History of Alcohol*, Philadelphia: Temple University Press, 2004.

Burrows, Gideon, *Kalashnikov AK 47*, Oxford: New Internationalist, 2006.

Bushnell, John, "The Tsarist Officer Corps, 1881–1914: Customs, Duties, Inefficiency," *The American Historical Review*, 86:4, 1981: 753–80.

Buzzanco, Robert, *Vietnam and the Transformation of American Life*, Oxford: Blackwell, 1999.

Caffeine for the Sustainment of Mental Task Performance: Formulations for Military Operations, Washington, DC: National Academy Press (Committee on Military Nutrition Research, Food and Nutrition Board, Institution of Medicine), 2001.

Caldwell, John, "Dextroamphetamine and Modafinil Are Effective Countermeasures for Fatigue in the Operational Environment," in *Strategies to Maintain Combat Readiness during Extended Deployments—A Human Systems Approach*, Meeting Proceedings RTO-MP-HFM-124, Paper 31, Neuilly-sur-Seine: NATO Research and Technology Organisation, 2005: 31-1–31-16, http://ftp.rta.nato.int/public//PubFullText/RTO/MP/RTO-MP-HFM-124///MP-HFM-124-31.pdf.

Caldwell, John, "Go Pills in Combat: Prejudice, Propriety, and Practicality," *Air and Space Power Journal*, 22:3, 2008: 97–104.

Caldwell, John and Lynn Caldwell, "Fatigue in Military Aviation: An Overview of U.S. Military-Approved Pharmacological Countermeasures," *Aviation, Space, and Environmental Medicine*, 76:7:Section II, 2005: C39–C51.

Caldwell, John, Lynn Caldwell, and Regina Schmidt, "Alertness Management Strategies for Operational Contexts," *Sleep Medicine Reviews*, 12:4, 2008: 257–73.

Caldwell, John, Lynn Caldwell, Jennifer Smith, and David Brown, "Modafinil's Effects on Simulator Performance and Mood in Pilots during 37 Hours without Sleep," *Aviation, Space, and Environmental Medicine*, 75:9, 2004: 777–84.

Caldwell, John, Lynn Caldwell, Nicholas Smythe III, and Kecia Hall, "A Double-blind, Placebo-controlled Investigation of the Efficacy of Modafinil for Sustaining the Alertness and Performance of Aviators: A Helicopter Simulator Study," *Psychopharmacology*, 150:3, 2000: 272–82.

Caldwell, John, Melissa Mallis, Lynn Caldwell, Michel Paul, James Miller, and David Neri (Aerospace Medical Association Aerospace Fatigue Countermeasures Subcommittee of the Human Factors Committee), "Fatigue Countermeasures in Aviation," *Aviation, Space, and Environmental Medicine*, 80:1, 2009: 29–59.

Campbell, David, *Writing Security: United States Foreign Policy and the Politics of Identity*, Minneapolis: The University of Minnesota Press, 1992.

Camus, Albert, *Caligula and Three Other Plays*, London: Vintage Books, 1962.

Cape Town Principles and Best Practices on the Recruitment of Children into the Armed Forces and on Demobilization and Social Reintegration of Child Soldiers in Africa, Cape Town: UNICEF, April 1997, http://www.unicef.org/emerg/files/Cape_Town_Principles%281%29.pdf.

"Captagon—Saudi Mind Control Drug of Choice," *ThereAreNoSunglasses*, https://therearenosunglasses.wordpress.com/2014/03/08/captagon-saudi-mind-control-drug-of-choice.

Caputo, Philip, *A Rumor of War*, New York: Henry Holt and Company, 1996.

Caputo, Philip, *Indian Country*, New York: Vintage, 2004.

Carew, Tom, *Jihad! The Secret War in Afghanistan*, Edinburgh: Mainstream, 2000.

Carlisle, Rodney P., *America At War: Afghanistan War*, New York: Chelsea House, 2010.

Carroll, Lewis, *Alice's Adventures in Wonderland and Through the Looking-Glass*, New York: Bantam Dell, 2006.

Carruthers, Susan L., "Redeeming the Captives: Hollywood and the Brainwashing of America's Prisoners of War in Korea," *Film History*, 10:3, 1998: 275–94.

Carruthers, Susan L., *Cold War Captives: Imprisonment, Escape, and Brainwashing*, Berkeley: University of California Press, 2009.

Carter, Sara A., "Hezbollah Uses Mexican Drug Routes into U.S.," *Washington Times*, 27 March 2009, http://www.washingtontimes.com/news/2009/mar/27/hezbollah-uses-mexican-drug-routes-into-us/?page=all#pagebreak.

Casey, Steven, *Selling the Korean War: Propaganda, Politics, and Public Opinion in the United States, 1950–1953*, Oxford: Oxford University Press, 2008.

Castells, Manuel, *The Rise of The Network Society*, Oxford: Wiley-Blackwell, 1996.

"Child Soldiers Sent by Gaddafi to Fight Libyan Rebels," *Channel 4 News*, 23 April 2011, http://www.channel4.com/news/child-soldiers-sent-by-gaddafi-to-fight-libyan-rebels.

Child Soldiers: Global Report 2008, London: Coalition to Stop the Use of Child Soldiers, 2008.

Child Soldiers: Implications for U.S. Forces, Seminar Report, Quantico: Center for Emerging Threats and Opportunities, Marine Corps Warfighting Laboratory, November 2002, http://www.dtic.mil/cgi-bin/GetTRDoc?Location=U2&doc=GetTRDoc.pdf&AD=ADA433182.

Children in Combat, Human Rights Watch, Children's Rights Project, 8, 1 January 1996.

Clausewitz, Carl von, *On War* (ed. Michael Howard and Peter Paret), Princeton: Princeton University Press, 1989.

Clayton, Nancy M. and William P. Nash, "Medication Management of Combat and Operational Stress Injuries in Active Duty Service Members," in (eds.) Charles R. Figley and William P. Nash, *Combat Stress Injury. Theory, Research and Management*, New York: Routledge, 2007: 219–46.

Cleick, Arnold J., "Humane Warfare for International Peacekeeping," *Air University Review*, September–October 1968, http://www.au.af.mil/au/afri/aspj/airchronicles/aureview/1968/sep-oct/celick.html.

Clodfelter, Michael, *Warfare and Armed Conflicts: A Statistical Encyclopedia of Casualty and Other Figures, 1494–2007*, Jefferson, NC: McFarland, 2008.

Coates, Joseph F., *Nonlethal and Nondestructive Combat in Cities Overseas*, Paper P-569, Arlington, VA: Institute for Defense Analyses, Science and Technology Division, 1970.

Coca Mama: The War on Drugs, a documentary by Jan Thielen, 2001.

Cockburn, Alexander and Jeffrey St. Clair, *Whiteout: The CIA, Drugs, and the Press*, London: Verso, 1998.

Cocks, Tim, "Iraqi Girl Tells of Ordeal as Suicide Bomber," Reuters, 29 August 2008, http://www.reuters.com/article/2008/08/29/us-iraq-girl-idUSLP60382820080829.

Coker, Christopher, *Ethics and War in the 21st Century*, London: Routledge, 2008.

Coker, Christopher, *Humane Warfare*, London: Routledge, 2001.

Coker, Christopher, *Waging War Without Warriors? The Changing Culture of Military Conflict*, London–Bolder: Lynne Rienner, 2002.

Coker, Christopher, "War and Disease," paper presented at the Disease and Security, 21st Century Trust, Villa Monastero, Lake Como, Italy, April–May 2004.

Coker, Christopher, *The Warrior Ethos. Military Culture and the War on Terror*, London: Routledge, 2007.

Coleman, Penny, *Flashback. Posttraumatic Stress Disorder, Suicide, and the Lessons of War*, Boston: Beacon Press, 2006.

Collin, Matthew, *Altered State: The Story of Ecstasy Culture and Acid House*, London: Serpent's Tail, 2009.

Collins, Wilkie, *Armadale*, London: Penguin 1995 (original publication 1866).

"Colombia: The Status of the FARC," *Stratfor*, 12 June 2008, http://www.stratfor.com/memberships/118140/analysis/colombia_status_farc.

Confucius, *The Analects* (trans. Raymond Dawson), Oxford: Oxford University Press, 2008.

Convention on the Rights of the Child, United Nations, Treaty Series, 1989, vol. 1577: 3, see http://www.ohchr.org/en/professionalinterest/pages/crc.aspx.

Cook, Tim, "Chemical Weapons," in Spencer C. Tucker (ed.), *Encyclopedia of World War I, 1914–1918: A Political, Social, and Military History*, Denver: ABC-CLIO, 2005, vol. 1: 289–92.

Cooley, John K., *Unholy Wars: Afghanistan, America and International Terrorism*, London: Pluto Press, 2000.

Cordovez, Diego and Selig S. Harrison, *Out of Afghanistan: The Inside Story of the Soviet Withdrawal*, Oxford: Oxford University Press, 1995.

Cornum, Rhonda, John Caldwell, and Kory Cornum, "Stimulant Use in Extended Flight Operations," *Airpower Journal*, 11:1, 1997: 53–8.

Cornum, Kory, Rhonda Cornum, and William Storm, "Use of Stimulants in Extended Flight Operations: A Desert Shield Experience," paper presented at the Aerospace Medical Panel Symposium on "Neurological Limitations of Aircraft Operations: Human Performance Implications," Köln, Germany, October 1995: 37-1–37-3.

Cortes, Liliana and Marla Jean Buchanan, "The Experience of Columbian Child Soldiers from a Resilience Perspective," *International Journal for the Advancement of Counselling*, 29:1, 2007: 43–55.

Coulter, Chris, *Bush Wives and Girl Soldiers: Women's Lives Through War and Peace in Sierra Leone*, Ithaca: Cornell University Press, 2009.

Courtwright, David T., *Dark Paradise: A History of Opiate Addiction in America*, Cambridge, MA: Harvard University Press, 1982.

Courtwright, David T., *Forces of Habit: Drugs and the Making of the Modern World*, Cambridge, MA: Harvard University Press, 2001.

Courtwright, David T., "The Hidden Epidemic: Opiate Addiction and Cocaine Use in the South, 1860–1920," *Journal of Southern History*, 49:1, 1983: 57–72.

Courtwright, David T., "Opiate Addiction as a Consequence of the Civil War," *Civil War History*, 24:2, 1978: 101–11.

Courtwright, David T., "The Rise and Fall and Rise of Cocaine in the United States," in Jordon Goodman, Paul E. Lovejoy and Andrew Sherratt (eds.), *Consuming Habits. Global and Historical Perspectives on How Cultures Define Drugs*, London: Routledge, 2007: 215–37.

Creasy, William M., "Can We Have War Without Death?," *Reader's Digest*, September 1959: 74 f.

Cross, Robin, *The Battle of Kursk: Operation Citadel 1943*, London: Penguin, 2002.

Crothers, Tomas Davison, *Morphinism and Narcomanias from Other Drugs*, Philadelphia: W.B. Saunders, 1902.

Crowdy, Terry and Christa Hook, *French Soldier in Egypt 1798–1801: The Army of the Orient*, Reading: Osprey, 2003.

Czechoslovak Military LSD Experiment, YouTube, http://www.youtube.com/watch?v= 5HXMHdhQL_8&NR=1.

Czubiński, Antoni, *Historia Powszechna XX wieku*, Poznań: Wydawnictwo Poznańskie, 2009 [20th Century World History].

Daftary, Farhad, *The Assassin Legends: Myths of the Isma'ilis*, London: Tauris, 1994.

Daizen, Victoria, *Zen at War*, Lanham, MD: Rowman & Littlefield, 2006.

Dalaby, J. Thomas, "Sherlock Holmes's Cocaine Habit," *Irish Journal of Psychological Medicine*, 8, 1991: 73–4.

Dallaire, Roméo with Jessica Dee Humphreys, *They Fight Like Soldiers: They Die Like Children. The Global Quest to Eradicate the Use of Child Soldiers*, Toronto: Random House Canada, 2010.

Dally, Ann, "Anomalies and Mysteries in the 'War on Drugs,'" in Roy Porter and Mikuláš Teich (eds.), *Drugs and Narcotics in History*, Cambridge: Cambridge University Press, 1996: 199–215.

Daly, Michael, "First American to Die in Afghanistan, Nathan Chapman, Remembered Eight Years Later," *New York Daily News*, 5 January 2010, http://articles.nydailynews.com/2010-01-05/news/17945156_1_forward-operating-base-chapman-special-forces-tora-bora.

Davenport-Hines, Richard, *The Pursuit of Oblivion. A Global History of Narcotics*, London: W.W. Norton, 2004.

Dawson, Drew and Kathryn Reid, "Fatigue, Alcohol and Performance Impairment," *Nature*, 388:235, 17 July 1997: 235.

Day of the Zulu, Public Broadcasting Service, 2004, http://www.pbs.org/wnet/secrets/previous_seasons/case_zulu/clues.html.

Day, Horace B., *The Opium Habit, with Suggestions as to the Remedy*, New York: Harper & Brothers, 1868.

De Kort, Marcel, "Doctors, Diplomats, and Businessmen: Conflicting Interest in the Netherlands and Dutch East Indies, 1860–1950," in Paul Gootenberg (ed.), *Cocaine: Global Histories*, London: Routledge, 1999: 123–45.

De Quincey, Thomas, *Confessions of an English Opium-Eater and Other Writings*, Oxford: Oxford University Press, 2013 (original publication 1821).

DeGroot, Gerard J., *A Noble Cause? America and the Vietnam War*, Harlow: Longman, 2000.

DeLillo, Don, *End Zone*, London: Penguin, 1986.

Denov, Myriam, "Girl Soldiers and Human Rights: Lessons from Angola, Mozambique, Sierra Leone and Northern Uganda," *International Journal of Human Rights*, 12:5, 2008: 813–36.

Denov, Myriam and Richard Maclure, "Turnings and Epiphanies: Militarization, Life Histories, and the Making and Unmaking of Two Child Soldiers in Sierra Leone," *Journal of Youth Studies*, 10:2, 2007: 243–61.

Department of Justice Examples of Terrorism Convictions Since September 11, 2001, Washington, DC: Department of Justice, 23 June 2006, http://www.justice.gov/opa/pr/2006/June/06_crm_389.html.

Derrida, Jacques, "The Rhetoric of Drugs," in Anna Alexander and Mark S. Roberts (eds.), *High Culture. Reflections on Addiction and Modernity*, New York: State University of New York Press, 2003.

"Dexedrine Spansule: Prescribing Information," DailyMed, http://dailymed.nlm.nih.gov/dailymed/lookup.cfm?setid=a37b6ef9-78b4-4b18-8797-ecb583502500.

Di Maio, Vincent J. M., *Gunshot Wounds: Practical Aspects of Firearms, Ballistics, and Forensic Techniques*, Boca Raton: CRC Press, 1998.

Didier Lagarde and Denise Batejat, "Disrupted Sleep-Wake Rhythm and Performance: Advantages of Modafinil," *Military Psychology*, 7:3, 1995: 165–91.

Didier, Lagarde, F. Louisy, and T. Matton, *Gestion de la vigilance au cours des opérations soutenues: Application au conflit du Golfe Persique (1990–1991)*, Brétigny sur Orge: CERMA, 1991.

Dikötter, Frank, Lars Peter Laamann, and Zhou Xun, *Narcotic Culture: A History of Drugs in China*, Chicago: University of Chicago Press, 2004.

Dillehay, Tom D., Jack Rossen, Donald Ugent, Anathasios Karathanasis, Víctor Vásquez and Patricia J. Netherly, "Early Holocene Coca Chewing in Northern Peru," *Antiquity*, 84:326, 2010: 939–53.

Dimeo, Paul, *A History of Drug Use in Sport 1876–1976: Beyond Good and Evil*, London: Routledge, 2007.

Dinges, David, "An Overview of Sleepiness and Accidents," *Journal of Sleep Research*, 4, Supplement II, 1995: 4–14.

Dove, Laura, "The Holocaust in the American Imagination 1945–1978," in *Memory Made Manifest: The United States Holocaust Memorial Museum*, 1995, http://xroads.virginia.edu/~cap/holo/image.html.

Dowdney, Luke, *Children of the Drug Trade. A Case Study of Children in Organised Armed Violence in Rio de Janeiro*, Rio de Janeiro: 7Letras, 2003.

Dowty, Jonathan C., *Christian Fighter Pilot Is Not an Oxymoron*, J.C. Dowty, 2007.

Doyle, Arthur Conan, *The Sign of the Four*, London: Penguin Books, 1993 (original publication 1890).

Doyle, D., "Adolf Hitler's Medical Care," *Journal of the Royal College of Physicians of Edinburgh*, 35:1, 2005: 75–82.

"Drug Addiction Among the Beslan Terrorists," *Pravda*, 18 October 2004, http://english.pravda.ru/news/russia/18-10-2004/59836-0.

Dubberly, Benjamin C., "Drugs and Drug Use," in Spencer C. Tucker (ed.), *Encyclopedia of the Vietnam War. A Political, Social and Military History*, Santa Barbara, CA: ABC-CLIO, 1998, vol. 1: 179–80.

Duffy, Michael, "Weapons of War—Poison Gas," Firstworldwar.com. A Multimedia History of World War One, 22 August 2009, http://www.firstworldwar.com/weaponry/gas.htm.

Dukuly, Abdullah, "Liberia: Civil War Leaves a Legacy of Drug Addiction," *Inter Press Service*, 29 January 2004, http://www.afrika.no/Detailed/4782.html.

Dunn, Walter Scott, *Frontier Profit and Loss: The British Army and the Fur Traders, 1760–1764*, Westport, CT: Greenwood, 1998.

Durst, David C., *Weimar Modernism: Philosophy, Politics, and Culture in Germany, 1918–1933*, Lanham: Lexington Books, 2004.

Easy Prey: Child Soldiers in Liberia, New York: Human Rights Watch, September 1994.

Eberle, Henrik and Matthias Uhl (eds.), *The Hitler Book: The Secret Dossier Prepared for Stalin from the Interrogations of Hitler's Personal Aides*, New York: Public Affairs, 2005.

Echevarria, Antulio J., II, *Preparing for One War and Getting Another?*, Carlisle, PA: Strategic Studies Institute, U.S. Army War College, 2010.

Edwards, Paul M., *The Korean War*, Westport: Greenwood, 2006.

Ehrenfeld, Rachel, *Funding Evil. How Terrorism Is Financed and How To Stop It*, New Rochelle, NY: Multi Educator, 2011.

Ehrenreich, Barbara, *Blood Rites: Origins and History of the Passions of War*, London: Virago, 1997.

Eliade, Mircea, *The Myth of the Eternal Return, or Cosmos and History* (trans. Willard R. Trask), Princeton, NJ: Princeton University Press, 1991.

Eliade, Mircea, *Shamanism Archaic Techniques of Ecstasy* (trans. Willard R. Trask), London: Routledge & Kegan Paul, 1964.

Elliot, Paul, *Warrior Cults: A History of Magical, Mystical and Murderous Organizations*, London: Blandford, 1995.

Elliott, Scott, "Go Pills: Stimulant Is Pilots' Last Tool," *Air Force Print News*, January 2003, http://www.aetc.randolph.af.mil/se2/torch/back/2003/0304/gopill.htm.

Ellis, John, *The Sharp End of War: The Fighting Man in World War II*, Newton Abbot: David & Charles, 1980.

Ellis, Stephen, "Liberia's Warlord Insurgency," in Christopher Clapham (ed.), *African Guerillas*, Oxford: James Currey, 1998: 155–71.

Ellis, Stephen, "Young Soldiers and the Significance of Initiation: Some Notes from Liberia," Leiden: African Studies Centre, 2003, http://www.ascleiden.nl/pdf/conference24042003-ellis.pdf.

Emonson, David and Rodger Vanderbeek, "The Use of Amphetamines in U.S. Air Force Tactical Operations during Desert Shield and Storm," *Aviation Space, and Environmental Medicine*, 66:3, 1995: 260–63.

Epstein, Edward Jay, *Agency of Fear: Opiates and Political Power in America*, London: Verso, 1990.

Erickson, Patricia G., Edward M. Adlaf, Glenn F. Murray, and Reginald G. Smart, *The Steel Drug. Cocaine in Perspective*, Toronto: Lexington Books, 1987.

Estrada, Arthur, Amanda Kelley, Catherine Webb, Jeremy Athy, and John Crowley, "Modafinil as a Replacement for Dextroamphetamine for Sustaining Alertness in Military Helicopter Pilots," *Aviation, Space, and Environmental Medicine*, 83:6, 2012: 556–64.

Fabing, Howard D., "On Going Berserk: a Neurochemical Inquiry," *Scientific Monthly*, 83:5, 1956: 232–7.

Fage, John Donnelly with William Tordoff, *A History of Africa*, London: Routledge, 2002.

Feifer, Gregory, *The Great Gamble. The Soviet War in Afghanistan*, New York: Harper, 2009.

Feiling, Tom, *The Candy Machine. How Cocaine Took Over the World*, London: Penguin Books, 2009.

Field Testing of Hallucinogenic Agents, Force Health Protection & Readiness Policy & Programs, Falls Church, VA, http://mcm.dhhq.health.mil/cb_exposures/cold_war/cwfieldtesting.aspx.

Figes, Orlando, "The Red Army and Mass Mobilization during the Russian Civil War 1918–1920," *Past & Present*, 129, 1990: 168–211.

Finlator, John, *The Drugged Nation: a "Narc's" Story*, Michigan: Simon and Schuster, 1973.

First Report of the Royal Commission on Opium: with Minutes of Evidence and Appendices, 29th January to 22nd February 1894, London: H.M. Stationery Office, 1894, see http://www.archive.org/details/cu31924073053864.

Flannery, Michael A., *Civil War Pharmacy. A History of Drugs, Drug Supply and Provision, and Therapeutics for the Union and Confederacy*, Binghamton: Haworth Press, 2004.

Flora, Stephen Ray, *Taking America Off Drugs: Why Behavioral Therapy Is More Effective for Treating ADHD, OCD, Depression, and Other Psychological Problems*, Albany: State University of New York Press, 2007.

Flower, Rod, "The Osler Lecture 2012: 'Pharmacology 2.0, Medicines, Drugs and Human Enhancement,'" *QJM: An International Journal of Medicine*, 105:9, 2012: 823–30.

Fontenot, Gregory, E. J. Degen and David Tohn, *On Point: The United States Army in Operation Iraqi Freedom*, Annapolis, MD: Naval Institute Press, 2005.

"Forced March," http://www.cocaine.org/forcedmarch.htm.

Foucault, Michel, *Discipline and Punish: The Birth of the Prison* (trans. Alan Sheridan), New York: Vintage Books, 1995.

Franzak, Michael, *A Nightmare's Prayer: A Marine Corps Harrier Pilot's War in Afghanistan*, New York: Threshold Editions, 2010.

"A Fresh Light on the Nazis' Wartime Drug Addiction," *Deutsche Welle*, September 9, 2015, http://www.dw.com/en/a-fresh-light-on-the-nazis-wartime-drug-addiction/a-18703678.

Freud, Sigmunt, *Civilisation and Its Discontents* (trans. David McLintock), London: Penguin Books, 2002.

Fried, Morton, Marvin Harris, and Robert Murphy (eds.), *War: The Anthropology of Armed Conflict and Aggression*, Garden City, NY: Natural History Press, 1967.

Friedman, Thomas L., *The World Is Flat: A Brief History of the Twenty-First Century*, New York: Farrar, Straus and Giroux, 2005.

Friman, H. Richard, "Germany and the Transformation of Cocaine, 1880–1920," in Paul Gootenberg (ed.), *Cocaine: Global Histories*, London: Routledge, 1999: 83–104.

Friscolanti, Michael, *Friendly Fire: The Untold Story of the U.S. Bombing That Killed Four Canadian Soldiers in Afghanistan*, Mississauga: J. Wiley & Sons Canada, 2005.

Fuchs, Daler, "Spain Says Bombers Drank Water from Mecca and Sold Drugs," *New York Times*, 15 April 2004, http://www.nytimes.com/2004/04/15/world/spain-says-bombers-drank-water-from-mecca-and-sold-drugs.html.

Fulton, Robert A., *The Legend of the Colt .45 Caliber Semi-Automatic Pistol and the Moros*, 2007, http://www.morolandhistory.com/Related%20Articles/Legend%20of%20.45.htm.

Fulton, Robert A., *Moroland: The History of Uncle Sam and the Moros 1899–1920*, Bend: Tumalo Creek Press, 2009.

Fussell, Paul, *The Great War and Modern Memory*, Oxford: Oxford University Press, 2000 (original publication 1975).

Gabriel, Richard, *No More Heroes: Madness and Psychiatry in War*, New York: Hill and Wang, 1987.

Gabriel, Richard, *The New Red Legion: An Attitudinal Portrait of the Soviet Soldier*, Westport, CT: Greenwood Press, 1980.

Galeotti, Mark, *Afghanistan: The Soviet Union's Last War*, London: Frank Cass 1995.

Gately, Iain, *Drink: A Cultural History of Alcohol*, New York: Gotham Books, 2008.

Gates, Scott, "Recruitment and Allegiance: The Microfoundations of Rebellion," *Journal of Conflict Resolution*, 46:1, 2002: 111–30.

Gelber, Harry G., *Opium, Soldiers and Evangelicals. Britain's 1840–1842 War with China, and its Aftermath*, London: Palgrave, 2004.

Global Report on Child Soldiers, London: Coalition to Stop the Use of Child Soldiers, 2001.

Gootenberg, Paul, *Andean Cocaine: The Making of a Global Drug*, Chapel Hill: University of North Carolina Press, 2009.

Gowing, Peter G., "Kris and Crescent," *Saudi Aramco World*, 16:4, 1965: 2–11.

Graham, Dave, "Mexican Teenage Girls Train as Drug Cartel Killers," Reuters, 17 June 2011, http://www.reuters.com/article/2011/06/17/us-mexico-drugs-teenagers-idUSTRE75G5F820110617.

Granier-Doyeux, Marcel, "Native Hallucinogenic Drugs Piptadenias," *Bulletin on Narcotics*, 17:2, 1965: 29–38, http://www.unodc.org/unodc/en/data-and-analysis/bulletin/bulletin_1965-01-01_2_page006.html.

Gray, Chris Hables, *Postmodern War. The New Politics of Conflict*, New York: Gulford Press, 1997.

Gray, John Glenn, *The Warriors: Reflections on Men in Battle*, Lincoln: University of Nebraska Press, 1998.

Grayson, George W., *La Familia Drug Cartel: Implications for U.S.-Mexican Security*, Carlisle Barracks: Strategic Studies Institute, U.S. Army War College, 2010.

Greenaway, John R., *Drink and British Politics since 1830: A Study in Policy-Making*, Basingstoke: Palgrave Macmillan, 2003.

Griffin, Michael, *Reaping the Whirlwind. The Taliban Movement in Afghanistan*, London: Pluto Press, 2001.

Griffith, Samuel B., "Introduction," in Sun Tzu, *The Art of War* (trans. Samuel B. Griffith), Oxford: Oxford University Press, 1971: 1–56.

Griffiths, D.L., "Medicine and Surgery in the American Civil War," *Proceedings of the Royal Society of Medicine*, 59:3, 1966: 204–8.

Grinspoon, Lester and Peter Hedblom, *The Speed Culture. Amphetamine Use and Abuse in America*, Cambridge, MA: Harvard University Press, 1975.

Grossman, David, *On Killing. The Psychological Cost of Learning to Kill in War and Society*, Boston: Little, Brown and Company, 1995.

Grunberger, Richard, *A Social History of the Third Reich*, London: Phoenix, 2005.

Hanes, W. Travis III and Frank Sanello, *The Opium Wars: The Addiction of One Empire and the Corruption of Another*, Naperville: Source Books, 2002.

Hanson, Victor Davis, *The Western Way of War: Infantry Battle in Classical Greece*, Berkeley: University of California Press, 2000.

Harding, Geoffrey, *Opiate Addiction, Morality and Medicine. From Moral Illness to Pathological Disease*, London: Macmillan Press, 1988.

Harner, Michael J., "Introduction," in Michael J. Harner (ed.), *Hallucinogens and Shamanism*, New York: Oxford University Press, 1973: xi–xv.

Harner, Michael J., *The Way of the Shaman*, San Francisco: Harper & Row, 1990.

Hauner, Milan, *The Soviet War in Afghanistan. Patterns of Russian Imperialism*, Philadelphia: University of America, 1991.

Haynes, Deborah, "Young Iraqi Girls Turned into Perfect Weapon," *The Times*, 30 September 2008, http://www.timesonline.co.uk/tol/news/world/iraq/article4849336.ece.

Hedges, Chris, *War Is a Force That Gives Us Meaning*, New York: Anchor Books, 2002.

Heinämaa, Anna, Maija Leppänen, and Yuri Yurchenko, *The Soldiers' Story: Soviet Veterans Remember the Afghan War* (trans. A.D. Haun), Berkeley: University of California at Berkeley, 1994.

Heinl, Robert D., Jr., "The Collapse of the Armed Forces," *Armed Forces Journal*, 108, 1971: 30–8, http://chss.montclair.edu/english/furr/Vietnam/heinl.pdf.

Helmer, Gail, "Chief of Staff Shares Views on Global Strike Task Force," *Air Force News Archive*, 31 October 2001, http://www.combatsim.com/memb123/cnews/arch/cnews-arc146.htm#chstff.

Helzer, John E., "Significance of the Robins et al. Vietnam Veterans Study," *The American Journal of Addictions*, 19:3, 2010: 218–21.

Herlihy, Patricia, *Alcoholic Empire: Vodka and Politics in Late Imperial Russia*, New York: Oxford University Press, 2001.

Herr, Michael, *Dispatches*, London: Picador, 2004.

Herring, George C., *America's Longest War. The United States and Vietnam, 1950–1975*, New York: McGraw–Hill, 1996.

Hesse, Erich, *Narcotics and Drug Addiction*, New York: Philosophical Library, 1946.

Hill, Peter B.E., *The Japanese Mafia: Yakuza, Law, and the State*, Oxford: Oxford University Press, 2003.

Hillman, James, *A Terrible Love of War*, London: Penguin Books, 2004.

Hobhouse, Henry, *Seeds of Change: Six Plants That Transformed Mankind*, London: Papermac 1999.

"Hochdosiert: Adolf Hitler und sein Reichsspritzenmesiter Dr. Morell," in Werner Pieper (ed.), *Nazis on Speed: Drogen im 3. Reich,* Lohrbach: Grüne Kraft, 2002: 263–78.

Hoff, Charles G., Jr., "Drug Abuse," *Military Law Review,* 51, 1971: 147–210.

Hofmann, Albert, *LSD: My Problem Child. Reflection on Sacred Drugs, Mysticism and Science,* New York: McGraw–Hill, 1980.

Hoge, Charles W., Castro Carl A., Messer Stephen C., McGurk Dennis, Cotting Dave I., and Koffman Robert L., "Combat Duty in Iraq and Afghanistan, Mental Health Problems, and Barriers to Care," *The New England Journal of Medicine,* 351:1, 2004: 13–22.

Holden, Wendy, *Shell Shock,* London: Channel 4 Books, 1998.

Holley, Peter, "The Tiny Pill Fueling Syria's War and Turning Fighters Into Superhuman Soldier," *Washington Post,* November 19, 2015, https://www.washingtonpost.com/news/worldviews/wp/2015/11/19/the-tiny-pill-fueling-syrias-war-and-turning-fighters-into-super-human-soldiers/?tid=sm_tw.

Holman, James, *Travels in China, New Zealand, New South Wales, Van Diemen's Land, Cape Horn, Etc., Etc.,* London: G. Routledge, 1840.

Holmes, Richard, *Acts of War: The Behavior of Men in Battle,* New York: Free Press, 1985.

Holmes, Richard, *Tommy: The British Soldier on the Western Front, 1914–1918,* London: Harper Collins, 2004.

Holsti, Kalevi Jaakko, *The State, War, and the State of War,* Cambridge: Cambridge University Press, 1998.

Homer, *The Odyssey* (trans. Rodney Merrill), Ann Arbor: University of Michigan Press, 2002.

Hornblum, Allen M., *Acres of Skin. Human Experiments at Holmesburg Prison,* New York: Routledge, 1998.

Houlihan, Barrie, *Dying to Win. Doping in Sport and the Development of Anti-doping Policy,* Strasbourg: Council of Europe, 1999.

"How to Fight, How to Kill: Child Soldiers in Liberia," *Human Rights Watch,* 16:2, 2004.

Hunt, Linda, *Secret Agenda: the United States Government, Nazi Scientists, and Project Paperclip, 1945 to 1990,* New York: St. Martin's Press, 1991.

Hunter, Edward, *Brainwashing in Red China,* New York: Vanguard, 1951.

Hunter, Edward, "'Brain-Washing' Tactics Force Chinese into Ranks of Communist Party," *Miami News,* September 24, 1950.

Huxley, Aldous, *The Doors of Perception,* New York: Harper & Brothers, 1954.

Hynes, Samuel, *The Soldiers' Tale: Bearing Witness to Modern War,* London: Penguin Books, 1997.

Ignatieff, Michael, *The Warrior's Honor: Ethnic War and the Modern Conscience,* New York: Viking Penguin, 1998.

Ingraham, Larry H., "Sense and Nonsense in the Army's Drug Abuse Prevention Effort," *Parameters,* 11:1, 1981: 60–70.

Inkster, Nigel and Virginia Comolli, *Drugs, Insecurity and Failed States: The Problems of Prohibition,* London: Routledge 2012.

Intelezi, Ulwazi. Sharing Indigenous Knowledge, Durban, http://wiki.ulwazi.org/index.php5?title=Intelezi.

International Military Tribunal for the Far East, Judgment of 4 November 1948, Part A, Chapter III (Obligations Assumed and Rights Acquired by Japan), see http://werle.rewi.hu-berlin.de/tokio.pdf.

Iversen, Leslie, *Speed, Ecstasy, Ritalin: The Science of Amphetamines,* Oxford: Oxford University Press, 2008.

Jaffe, Greg, "Army's Recruiting Push Appears to Have Met Goals," *Wall Street Journal,* 10 July 2006: 3.

James, William, *The Moral Equivalent of War,* 1910, see http://www.constitution.org/wj/meow.htm.

Jandora, John W., "War and Culture. A Neglected Relation," *Armed Forces & Society,* 25:4, 1999: 541–56.

JASON, *Human Performance,* McLean, VA: MITRE Corporation, 2008.

Jaśkiewicz, Ewa, "Witkacego kreatory sztucznych jaźni," in Tadeusz Linker (ed.), *Używki w literaturze. Od Młodej Polski do współczesności*, Gdańsk: Instytut Filologii Polskiej Uniwersytetu Gdańskiego, 2002, vol. 2: 127–36 ["Witkacy's Creations of Artificial Egos," in *Drugs in Literature: From Young Poland Movement to Present Day*].

Jones, David and Royden Marsh, *Flight Surgeon Support to United States Air Force Fliers in Combat*, Brooks City-Base, TX: U.S. Air Force School of Aerospace Medicine, Clinical Science Division, 2003.

Jones, James, *From Here to Eternity*, New York: Delta, 1998.

Jones, John Bush, *All-out For Victory! Magazine Advertising and the World War II Home Front*, Waltham, MA: Brandeis University Press, 2009.

Jünger, Ernst, *Storm of Steel*, London: Penguin Books, 2004.

Jünger, Ernst, *Sturm*, Toruń: Tako, 2006.

Jünger, Ernst, "Wojna i technika," in *Publicystyka polityczna 1919–1936*, Kraków: Arcana, 2007 (original publication 1930): 390–400 ["War and Technology," in *Political Writings 1919–1936*].

Kaldor, Mary, *New and Old Wars: Organized Violence in a Global Era*, Stanford: Stanford University Press, 1999.

Kamieński, Łukasz, "Cosmetic Pharmacology in (Con)Temporary Societies," in Cecile Lawrence and Natalie Churn (eds.), *Movements in Time: Revolution, Social Justice and Times of Change*, Newcastle upon Tyne: Cambridge Scholars, 2012: 227–40.

Kan, Paul Rexton, *Drugs and Contemporary Warfare*, Washington, DC: Potomac Books, 2009.

Kaplan, David E. and Alec Dubro, *Yakuza. Japan's Criminal Underworld*, Berkeley: University of California Press, 2003.

Kapuściński, Ryszard, *The Shadow of the Sun: My African Life*, London: Penguin, 2001.

Kasindorf, Martin, "Accidental Deaths Exceed Those in Combat," *USA Today*, 26 March 2003, http://usatoday30.usatoday.com/news/world/iraq/2003-03-26-count_usat_x.htm.

Kato, Masaaki, "An Epidemiological Analysis of the Fluctuation of Drug Dependence in Japan," *Substance Use and Misuse*, 4:4, 1969: 591–621.

Keating, Susan Katz, "Flying on Amphetamines Is No Departure from Tradition," *Washington Times*, 22 August 1988: 18–9.

Keegan, John, *A History of Warfare*, London: Pimlico, 1994.

Keep, John L.H., *Soldiers of the Tsar: Army and Society in Russia, 1462–1874*, New York: Oxford University Press, 1985.

Kemper, Wolf-R., "Pervitin—die Endsieg-Droge?," in Werner Pieper (ed.), *Nazis on Speed: Drogen im 3. Reich*, Lohrbach: Grüne Kraft, 2002: 122–33.

Kenagy, David, Christopher Bird, Christopher Webber, and Joseph Fischer, "Dextroamphetamine Use during B-2 Combat Missions," *Aviation, Space, and Environmental Medicine*, 75:5, 2004: 381–86.

Ketchum, James S., *Chemical Warfare Secrets Almost Forgotten*, Santa Rosa, CA: ChemBooks, 2006.

Kiernan, Victor Gordon, *European Empires from Conquest to Collapse, 1815–1960*, Leicester: Leicester University Press, 1982.

Killgore, William, Nancy Grugle, Desiree Killgore, Brian Leavitt, George Watlington, Shanelle McNair and Thomas Balin, "Restoration of Risk-Propensity During Sleep Deprivation: Caffeine, Dextroamphetamine, and Modafinil," *Aviation, Space, and Environmental Medicine*, 79:9, 2008a: 867–74.

Killgore, William, Tracy Rupp, Nancy Grugle, Rebecca Reichardt, Erica Lipizzi and Thomas Balkin, "Effects of Dextroamphetamine, Caffeine and Modafinil on Psychomotor Vigilance Test Performance after 44 Hours of Continuous Wakefulness," *Journal of Sleep Research*, 17:3, 2008b: 309–21.

Kim, Dongsoo, "Practical Use and Risk of Modafinil, A Novel Waking Drug," *Environmental Health and Toxicology*, 22 February 2012, http://dx.doi.org/10.5620/eht.2012.27.e2012007.

Kittel, W., "Alkohol und Wehrmacht," in Werner Pieper (ed.), *Nazis on Speed: Drogen im 3. Reich*, Lohrbach: Grüne Kraft, 2002: 543–8.

Klass, Rosanne (ed.), *Afghanistan. The Game Revisited*, London: Freedom House, 1987.

Knight, Ian, "'What Do You Red-Jackets Want in Our Country?' The Zulu Response to the British Invasion of 1879," in Benedict Carlton, John Laband, and Jabulani Sithole (eds.), *Zulu Identities. Being Zulu, Past and Present*, New York: Columbia University Press, 2009: 177–89.

Knipe, Ed, *Culture, Society, and Drugs*, Prospect Heights: Waveland Press, 1995.

Kobayashi, Motohiro, "Drug Operations by Resident Japanese in Tianjin," in Timothy Brook and Bob Tadashi Wakabayashi (eds.), *Opium Regimes: China, Britain and Japan, 1839–1952*, Berkeley: University of California Press, 2000: 152–66.

Kobayashi, Motohiro, "An Opium Tug-of-War. Japan versus the Wang Jingwei Regime," in Timothy Brook and Bob Tadashi Wakabayashi (eds.), *Opium Regimes: China, Britain and Japan, 1839–1952*, Berkeley: University of California Press, 2000: 344–59.

Kohn, Marek, "Cocaine Girls: Sex, Drugs and Modernity in London During and After the First World War," in Paul Gootenberg (ed.), *Cocaine: Global Histories*, London: Routledge, 1999: 105–22.

Kolb, Richard K., "'Like a Mad Tiger': Fighting Islamic Warriors in the Philippines 100 Years Ago," *Veterans of Foreign Wars Magazine*, 89:9, 2002: 26–30.

Kopperman, Paul E., "'The Cheapest Pay': Alcohol Abuse in the Eighteenth-Century British Army," *Journal of Military History*, 60:3, 1996: 445–70.

Kovic, Ron, *Born on the Fourth of July*, New York: Akashic Books, 2005.

Kramer, Peter, *Listening to Prozac*, New York: Viking, 1993.

Krige, Eileen Jensen, *The Social System of the Zulus*, London: Longmans, Green, 1936.

Krogh, Egil, Jr., "Heroin Politics and Policy Under President Nixon," in David F. Musto (ed.), *One Hundred Years of Heroin*, Westport, CT: Auburn House, 2002: 39–53.

Kronstadt, Alan K., *Terrorist Attacks in Mumbai, India, and Implications for U.S. Interests*, Washington, DC: Congressional Research Service, 2008, http://www.fas.org/sgp/crs/terror/R40087.pdf.

Krueger, Gerald P., "Sustained Military Performance in Continuous Operations: Combat Fatigue, Rest and Sleep Needs," in Gal Reuven and A. David Mangelsdorf (eds.), *Handbook of Military Psychology*, Chichester: Wiley, 1991: 255–77.

Kuzmarov, Jeremy, *The Myth of the Addicted Army. Vietnam and the Modern War on Drugs*, Amherst, MA: University of Massachusetts Press, 2009.

Laband, John, "'Bloodstained Grandeur': Colonial and Imperial Stereotypes of Zulu Warriors and Zulu Warfare," in Benedict Carlton, John Laband, and Jabulani Sithole (eds.), *Zulu Identities. Being Zulu, Past and Present*, New York: Columbia University Press, 2009: 168–76.

Lagarde, Didier and Denise Batejat, "Disrupted Sleep-Wake Rhythm and Performance: Advantages of Modafinil," *Military Psychology*, 7:3, 1995: 165–91.

Langdon-Davies, John, *Invasion in the Snow: A Study of Mechanized War*, Boston: Houghton Mifflin, 1941.

Laozi, *Daodejing* (trans. Edmund Ryden), Oxford: Oxford University Press, 2008.

Laundry, Brian R. and Ronald E.M. Lees, "Industrial Accident Experience of One Company on 8- and 12-hour Shifts Systems," *Journal of Occupational Medicine*, 33:8, 1991: 903–6.

Lauridsen, Øyvind and Tor Tønnesen, "Injuries Related to the Aspects of Shift Working: A Comparison of Different Offshore Shift Arrangements," *Journal of Occupational Accidents*, 12:1–3, 1990: 167–76.

Lawton, Graham, "Get Up and Go," *New Scientist*, 189:2539, 19 February 2006: 34–8.

Lazarus, Richard S., *Psychological Stress and the Coping Process*, New York: McGraw–Hill, 1966.

Leary, William M., *Perilous Missions: Civil Air Transport and the CIA Covert Operations in Asia*, Washington, DC: Smithsonian Institution Press, 2002.

Lee, Martin A. and Bruce Shlain, *Acid Dreams. The Complete Social History of LSD: The CIA, The Sixties, and Beyond*, New York: Grove Weidenfeld, 1992.

Lehmann, Arthur C. and Louis J. Mihalyi, "Aggression, Bravery, Endurance, and Drugs: A Radical Re-evaluation and Analysis of the Masai Warrior Complex," *Ethnology*, 21:4, 1982: 335–47.

Lewin, Louis, *Phantastica: A Classic Survey on the Use and Abuse of Mind-Altering Plants* (trans. P.H.A. Wirth), Rochester: Park Street Press, 1998 (original publication 1931).

Lewis, Bernard, *The Assassins. A Radical Sect in Islam*, New York: Octagon Books, 1980.

Lewis, Sinclair, *Babbitt*, Mineola, NY: Courier Dover, 2003.

Lewy, Gunter, *America in Vietnam*, Oxford: Oxford University Press, 1980.

Lifton, Robert Jay, *Thought Reform and the Psychology of Totalism: A Study of "Brainwashing" in China*, New York: W.W. Norton, 1961.

Lincoln, Bruce, "An Early Moment in the Discourse of 'Terrorism': Reflections on a Tale from Marco Polo," *Society for Comparative Study of Society and History*, 48:2, 2006: 242–59.

Lind, Welfred N., "With a B–29 over Japan—A Pilot's Story," *New York Times Magazine*, 25 March 1945: SM3.

Lind, William P., Keith Nightengale, John F. Schmitt, Joseph W. Sutton, and Gary I. Wilson, "The Changing Face of War: into the Fourth Generation," *Marine Corps Gazette*, 1989: 22–27.

Lingis, Alphonso, "The Will to Power," in David B. Allison (ed.), *The New Nietzsche: Contemporary Styles of Interpretation*, New York: Dell, 1977: 37–63.

Linkner, Tadeusz, "Alkohole młodopolskiego cygana," in Tadeusz Linker (ed.) *Używki w literaturze. Od Młodej Polski do współczesności*, Gdańsk: Instytut Filologii Polskiej Uniwersytetu Gdańskiego, 2002, vol. 2: 13–31 ["Alcoholic Drinks of a Young Poland Bohemian,"] in *Drugs in Literature: From Young Poland Movement to Present Day*].

Livingstone, David, *Missionary Travels and Research in South Africa*, New York: Harper & Brothers, 1870 (original publication 1857).

Logan, John Frederick, "The Age of Intoxication," *Yale French Studies*, 50, 1974: 81–94.

Lohbeck, Kurt, *Holy War, Unholy Victory. Eyewitness to the CIA's Secret War in Afghanistan*, Washington, DC: Regnery Gateway, 1993.

Longman Dictionary of the English Language, Harlow: Longman, 1993.

Lovell, Jim and Jeffrey Kluger, *Apollo 13*, Boston: Houghton Mifflin, 2006.

Loyd, Anthony, *My War Gone By, I Miss It So*, New York: Atlantic Monthly Press, 1999.

Lucas, Scott, *Amphetamines: Danger in the Fast Lane*, London: Burke, 1985.

Lyons, T.J. and J. French, "Modafinil: the Unique Properties of a New Stimulant," *Aviation Space Environmental Medicine*, 62:5, 1991: 432–35.

MacArthur, Douglas, "Address to Congress," 19 April 1951, Harry S. Truman Library and Museum, http://www.trumanlibrary.org/whistlestop/study_collections/koreanwar/documents/index.php?documentdate=1951-04-19&documentid=ma-2-18&pagenumber=1.

MacDonald, Callum A., *Korea: The War Before Vietnam*, New York: Free Press, 1986.

MacDonald, David, *Drugs in Afghanistan: Opium, Outlaws and Scorpion Tales*, London: Pluto Press, 2007.

Machel, Graca, *Impact of Armed Conflict on Children*, Report of the Expert of the Secretary-General, Ms. Graca Machel, Submitted Pursuant to General Assembly Resolution 48/157, United Nations, 1996, http://www.unicef.org/emerg/files/report_machel.pdf.

Machiavelli, Niccolo, *The Art of War* (trans. Henry Neville), Mineola, NY: Dover Publications Inc., 2006.

MacPherson, Myra, *Long Time Passing, New Edition: Vietnam and the Haunted Generation*, Bloomington: Indiana University Press, 2001 (original publication 1984).

Madge, Tim, *White Mischief. A Cultural History of Cocaine*, Edinburg–London: Mainstream, 2001.

Mahoney, Peter P. "The Wounds of Two Wars," *New York Times*, 11 June 1989: A61.

"Mai Mai Child Soldier Recruitment and Use: Entrenched and Unending," *Briefing Paper. Democratic Republic of Congo*, London: Coalition to Stop the Use of Child Soldiers, 2010.

Mandel, Jerry, "The Mythical Roots of U.S. Drug Policy: Soldier's Disease and Addiction in the Civil War," in Arnold S. Trebach and Kevin B. Zeese (eds.), *Drug Policy 1989–1990: A Reformer's Catalogue*, Washington, DC: Drug Policy Foundation, 1989, http://www.druglibrary.org/schaffer/History/soldis.htm.

Mann, John, *Murder, Magic, and Medicine*, Oxford: Oxford University Press, 2000.

Mann, John, *Turn on and Tune in: Psychedelics, Narcotics, and Euphoriants*, Cambridge: Royal Society of Chemistry, 2009.

Markel, Howard, *An Anatomy of Addiction: Sigmund Freud, William Halsted, and the Miracle Drug, Cocaine*, New York: Pantheon Books, 2011.

Marks, Jeannette, "The Curse of Narcotism in America—A Reveille," *American Journal of Public Health*, 5:4, 1915: 314–22.

Marks, John, *The Search for the "Manchurian Candidate,"* New York: W.W. Norton, 1991.

Marshall, Mary Louise, "Medicine in the Confederacy," *Bulletin of Medical Library Association*, 30:4, 1942: 278–99.

Martin, Paul, *Counting Sheep: The Science and Pleasure of Sleep and Dreams*, London: Flamingo, 2003.

Marx, Karl, "Free Trade and Monopoly," *New York Daily Tribune*, 25 September 1858, http://www.marxists.org/archive/marx/works/1858/09/25.htm.

Masland, Tom, "Voices of the Children: We Beat and Killed People . . . ," *Newsweek*, 139:19, 13 May 2002: 24–9.

Matthee, Rudi, "Exotic Substances: the Introduction and Global Spread of Tobacco, Coffee, Cocoa, Tea, and Distilled Liquor, Sixteenth to Eighteenth Centuries," in Roy Porter and Mikuláš Teich (eds.), *Drugs and Narcotics in History*, Cambridge: Cambridge University Press, 1996: 24–51.

Mauer, Harry, *Strange Ground. An Oral History of Americans In Vietnam, 1945–1975*, New York: Da Capo Press, 1998.

Maxwell, David S., "Operation Enduring Freedom—Philippines. What Would Sun Tzu Say?," *Military Review*, 84:3, 2004: 20–3.

McCallum, Jack Edward, *Military Medicine: from Ancient Times to the 21st Century*, Santa Barbara, CA: ABC-CLIO, 2008.

McCallum, Jack, "Medicine in War," in Spencer C. Tucker (ed.), *Encyclopedia of World War I, 1914–1918: A Political, Social, and Military History*, Denver: ABC-CLIO, 2005, vol. 3: 770–73.

McCallum, Jack, "Medicine, Military," in Spencer C. Tucker (ed.), *Encyclopedia of the Vietnam War: A Political, Social and Military History*, Santa Barbara, CA: ABC-CLIO, 1998, vol. 1: 425.

McElroy, Damien, "Mumbai Attacks: Terrorists Took Cocaine To Stay Awake During Assault," *Telegraph*, 2 December 2008, http://www.telegraph.co.uk/news/worldnews/asia/india/3540964/Mumbai-attacks-Terrorists-took-cocaine-to-stay-awake-during-assault.html.

McGowan, James P., "Alcohol," in Spencer C. Tucker (ed.), *Encyclopedia of World War I, 1914–1918: A Political, Social, and Military History*, Denver: ABC-CLIO, 2005, vol. 1: 82–3.

McKinley, James C., Jr., "Despite Army Efforts, Soldier Suicides Continue," *New York Times*, 11 October 2010: A11, http://www.nytimes.com/2010/10/11/us/11suicides.html?pagewanted=all

McMahan, Jeff, "An Ethical Perspective on Child Soldiers," in Scott Gates and Simon Reich (eds.), *Child Soldiers in the Age of Fractured States*, Pittsburgh: University of Pittsburgh Press, 2010: 27–36.

McMahon, Keith, *The Fall of the God of Money: Opium Smoking in Nineteenth-Century China*, Lanham: Rowman & Littlefield, 2002.

McNeil, Donald G., Jr., "Drugs Banned, Many of World's Poor Suffer in Pain," *New York Times*, 10 September 2007, http://www.nytimep.com/2007/09/10/health/10pain.html?pagewanted=all.

McPherson, James M., *Battle Cry of Freedom. The Civil War Era*, New York: Oxford University Press, 1988.

MDMA/PTSD U.S. Study (Veterans of War), Multidisciplinary Association for Psychodelic Studies, http://www.maps.org/research/mdma/mdma_ptsd_u.s._study_veterans_of_war.

Mead, Margaret, "Warfare Is Only an Invention—Not a Biological Necessity," *Asia*, 40:8, 1940: 402–5.

"Medical Care, Battle Wounds, and Disease," in *The American Civil War: A Multicultural Encyclopedia*, Danbury, CT: Grolier Educational Corp, 1994, vol. 5, see http://www.civil-warhome.com/civilwarmedicine.htm.

Meerloo, Joost A.M., *Mental Seduction and Menticide: The Psychology of Thought Control and Brainwashing*, London: Jonathan Cape, 1957.

Mehlman, Maxwell J., *The Price of Perfection: Individualism and Society in the Era of Biomedical Enhancement*, Baltimore: Johns Hopkins University Press, 2009.

Menhard, Francha Roffé, *The Facts About Amphetamines*, New York: Marshall Cavendish Benchmark, 2006.

Merridale, Catherine, "The Collective Mind: Trauma and Shell-Shock in Twentieth-Century Russia," *Journal of Contemporary History*, 35:1, 2000: 39–55.

Merridale, Catherine, *Ivan's War: Life and Death in the Red Army, 1939–1945*, New York: Picador, 2006.

Metcalfe, N.H., "The Influence of the Military on Civilian Uncertainty about Modern Anaesthesia Between Its Origins in 1846 and the End of the Crimean War In 1856," *Anaesthesia*, 60:6, 2005: 594–601.

Metzner, Ralph, "Nazis on Speed: Drogen im 3. Reich," *Journal of Psychoactive Drugs*, 36:2, 2004: 289–90.

Miller, Greg, "'Go' Pills for F-16 Pilots Get Close Look: Amphetamines Prescribed in Mission That Killed Canadians," *Los Angeles Times*, 4 January 2003: A1, http://www.sfgate.com/cgi-bin/article.cgi?f=/c/a/2003/01/04/MN191592.DTL&ao=all.

Miller, John, *Memories of General Miller in the Service of the Republic of Peru*, London: Longman, Rees, Orme, Brown, and Green, 1828, vol. 2.

Miller, Nita Lewis, Matsangas Panagiotis, and Lawrence Shattuck, "Fatigue and Its Effect on Performance in Military Environments," in *Performance under Stress*, Peter A. Hancock and James L. Szalma (eds.), Aldershot: Ashgate, 2007: 231–49.

Miller, Richard Lawrence, *The Encyclopedia of Addictive Drugs*, Westport, CT: Greenwood Press, 2002.

Misdaq, Nabi, *Afghanistan. Political Frailty and External Interference*, London: Routledge, 2006.

Mitchell, Silas Weir, *Characteristics*, New York: Century, 1892.

Moore, Ede, *The 24/7 Society: The Risks, Costs and Consequences of a World That Never Stops*, London: Piatkus, 1993.

Moreno, Jonathan D., *Undue Risk: Secret State Experiments on Humans*, London: Routledge, 2001.

Morgan, David, "The Assassins: A Terror Cult," in Martha Crenshaw and John Pimlott (eds.), *The International Encyclopedia of Terrorism*, Chicago: Fitzroy Dearborn, 1997: 40–1.

Mortimer, W. Golden, *Peru: History of Coca: "The Divine Plant" of the Incas*, Honolulu: University Press of the Pacific, 2000 (original publication 1901).

Mott, William H. and Jae Chang Kim, *Philosophy of Chinese Military Culture: Shih vs. Li*, New York: Palgrave Macmillan, 2006.

Mulholland, Kim, "'Mon docteur le vin,' Wine and Health in France, 1900–1950," in Mack P. Holt (ed.), *Alcohol: A Social and Cultural History*, New York: Berg, 2006: 77–93.

"Mumbai Terrorists on Drugs During Attacks," *Ebru News*, 2 December 2008, http://news.ebru.tv/en/central_asia/8763.html.

Münkler, Herfried, *The New Wars*, London: Polity, 2005.

Murphy, William P., "Military Patrimonialism and Child Soldier Clientalism in the Liberian and Sierra Leonean Civil Wars," *African Studies Review*, 46:2, 2003: 61–87.

Murray, Alexander, *Doings in China: Being the Personal Narrative of an Officer Engaged in the Late Chinese Expedition, from the Recapture of Chusan in 1841, to the Peace of Nankin in 1842*, London: R. Bentley, 1843.

Musto, David F., *The American Disease. Origins of Narcotic Control*, New Haven, CT: Yale University Press, 1973.

Musto, David F., and Pamela Korsmeyer, *Quest for Drug Control: Politics and Federal Policy in a Period of Increasing Substance Abuse, 1963–1981*, New Haven: Yale University Press, 2002.

"My Gun Was as Tall as Me": Child Soldiers in Burma, New York: Human Rights Watch, 2002.

Myerly, Scott Hughes, *British Military Spectacle: From the Napoleonic Wars through the Crimea*, Cambridge, MA: Harvard University Press, 1996.

Netter, Sarah, "Army Alcoholics: More Soldiers Hitting the Bottle," *ABC News*, 22 February 2010, http://abcnews.go.com/Health/army-alcoholics-soldiers-seek-treatment-alcohol-abuse/story?id=9863321#.T9-rN1K_lqU.

Newman, Edward, "The 'New Wars' Debate: A Historical Perspective Is Needed," *Security Dialogue*, 35:2, 2004: 239–51.

Nicolai, Georg Friedrich, *The Biology of War*, New York: Century, 1918.

Niebuhr, Reinhold, *Moral Man and Immoral Society: A Study of Ethics and Politics*, Louisville: Westminster John Knox Press, 1960 (original publication 1932).

Nieminen, Tommi, "Finland—a Leading Consumer of Heroin from the 1930s to the 1950s," *Helsingin Sanomat. International Edition*, 5 April 2009, http://www.hs.fi/english/article/Finland+-+a+leading+consumer+of+heroin+from+the+1930s+to+the+1950s/1135245022270.

Nietzsche, Friedrich, *The Birth of Tragedy and Other Writings* (eds. Raymond Geuss and Ronald Speirs, trans. Ronald Speirs), Cambridge: Cambridge University Press, 1999.

Nietzsche, Friedrich, *The Gay Science with the Prelude in Rhymes and an Appendix of Songs* (trans. Walter Kaufmann), New York: Vintage Books, 1974.

Nitobe, Inazō, *Bushido: Samurai Ethics and the Soul of Japan*, Mineola: Courier Dover, 2004.

Nixon, Richard, "Remarks About an Intensified Program for Drug Abuse Prevention and Control," 17 June 1971, online by Gerhard Peters and John T. Woolley, *The American Presidency Project*, 1971, http://www.presidency.ucsb.edu/ws/?pid=3047.

Nixon, Richard, "Special Message to the Congress on Drug Abuse Prevention and Control," 17 June 1971, online by Gerhard Peters and John T. Woolley, *The American Presidency Project*, 1971b, http://www.presidency.ucsb.edu/ws/?pid=3048.

No Childhood At All. Child Soldiers in Burma, Chiangmai: Images Asia, 1997.

Nöldecke, Hartmut, "Einsatz von leistungssteigernden Medikamenten bei Heer un Kriegsmarine," in Werner Pieper (ed.), *Nazis on Speed: Drogen im 3. Reich*, Lohrbach: Grüne Kraft, 2002: 134–42.

Nordstrom, Carolyn, "Backyard Front," in Carolyn Nordstrom and JoAnn Martin (eds.), *The Paths to Domination, Resistance, and Terror*, Berkeley: University of California Press, 1992.

O'Ballance, Egar, *Afghan Wars. Battles in a Hostile Land 1839 to the Present*, London: Brassey's, 2002.

O'Brien, Tim, *The Things They Carried*, New York: Broadway, 1998.

Odeshoo, Jason R., "Truth or Dare?: Terrorism and 'Truth Serum' in the Post–9/11 World," *Stanford Law Review*, 57:1, 2004: 209–55.

"Officials: Taliban Recruiting Children as Bombers," *USA Today*, 28 July 2009, http://www.usatoday.com/news/world/2009-07-28-taliban-children_N.htm.

Ohler, Norman, *Der totale Raush: Drogen im Dritten Reich*, Köln: Kiepenheuer & Witsch, 2015.

Ohnuki-Tierney, Emiko, *Kamikaze Diaries: Reflections on Japanese Student Soldiers*, Chicago: University of Chicago Press, 2006.

Ohnuki-Tierney, Emiko, *Kamikaze, Cherry Blossoms, and Nationalism: The Militarization of Aesthetics in Japanese History*, Chicago: University of Chicago Press, 2002.

Otis, John, "Rebel Held: Child Warriors," *Huston Chronicle*, 5 August 2001, http://www.chron.com/default/article/Child-warriors-2021604.php.

Pach, Chester J., Jr., "TV News, the Johnson Administration, and Vietnam," in Marilyn B. Young and Robert Buzzanco (eds.), *A Companion to the Vietnam War*, Oxford: Blackwell, 2006: 450–69.

Paris, John Ayrton, *Pharmacologia Being an Extended Inquiry into the Operations of Medicinal Bodies. . . : the Theory and Art of Prescribing*, New York: Harper & Bros, 1846.

Parks, W. Hays, "Statistics Versus Actuality in Vietnam," *Air University Review*, 32:4, 1981, http://www.airpower.maxwell.af.mil/airchronicles/aureview/1981/may-jun/parks.htm.

Partridge, George Everett, *The Psychology of Nations: A Contribution To the Philosophy of History*, New York: Macmillan, 1919.

Pearn, John, "Children and War," *Journal of Paediatrics and Child Health*, 39:3, 2003: 166–72.

Pearson, Helen, "Sleep It Off," *Nature*, 443:21, 2006: 261–3.

Pechura, Constance M. and David P. Rall (eds.), *Veterans at Risk: The Health Effects of Mustard Gas and Lewisite*, Washington, DC: National Academy Press, 1993.

Performance Maintenance during Continuous Flight Operations: A Guide for Flight Surgeons, NAVMED P-6410, Fallon, NV: Naval Strike and Air Warfare Center, 2000, http://www.med.navy.mil/directives/Pub/6410.pdf.

Perlmutter, Dawn, "ISIS Meth Heads: Tweeking in the Name of Islam," *FrontPage Magazine*, 9 March 2015, http://www.frontpagemag.com/fpm/252783/isis-meth-heads-tweeking-name-islam-dawn-perlmutter.

Perry, Tony, "Fallouja Insurgents Fought Under Influence of Drugs, Marines Say," *Los Angeles Times*, 13 January 2005, http://articles.latimes.com/2005/jan/13/world/fg-iraqdrugs13.

Peters, Marijke, "Dutch Cocaine—the Ultimate Weapon, Radio Netherlands Worldwide," 17 October 2009, http://www.rnw.nl/english/article/dutch-cocaine-ultimate-weapon.

Pham, J. Peter, *Child Soldiers, Adult Interests: the Global Dimensions of the Sierra Leone Tragedy*, New York: Nova Science, 2005.

Phillsbury, Donald M., "Penicilin Therapy of Early Syphilis. Follow-up Examination of 792 Patients Six or More Months After Treatment," *British Journal of Venereal Disease*, 21:4, 1945: 139–50.

Pigeau, Ross, Paul Naitoh, Alain Buguet, Carol McCann, Joseph Baranski, Matthew Taylor, Megan Thompson, and I. Mack, "Modafinil, D-amphetamine and Placebo during 64 Hours of Sustained Mental Work: I. Effects on Mood, Fatigue, Cognitive Performance and Body Temperature," *Journal of Sleep Research*, 4:4, 1995: 212–28.

Pincus, Walter, "U.S. Has Detained 2,500 Juveniles as Enemy Combatants," *Washington Post*, 15 May 2008, A11, http://www.washingtonpost.com/wp-dyn/content/article/2008/05/14/AR2008051403365.html.

Piomelli, Danielle, "The Molecular Logic of Endocannabinoid Signaling," *Nature Reviews Neuroscience*, 4:11, 2003: 873–84.

Plant, Sadie, *Writing on Drugs*, London: Faber and Faber, 1999.

Plato, *The Republic of Plato* (trans. Allan Bloom), New York: Basic Books, 1991.

Polo, Marco, *The Description of the World* (trans. A.C. Moule and Paul Pelliot), London: G. Routledge, 1938.

Porter, Bruce D., *War and the Rise of the State. The Military Foundations of Modern Politics*, New York: Free Press, 1994.

Porter, Patrick, *Military Orientalism. Eastern War Through Western Eyes*, London: Hurst, 2009.

Powers, Francis Gary and Curt Gentry, *Operation Overflight: A Memoir of the U–2 Incident*, Washington, DC: Brassey's, 2004 (original publication 1970).

Prestwich, Particia E., *Drink and the Politics of Social Reform: Antialcoholism in France Since 1870*, Palo Alto, CA: Society for the Promotion of Science and Scholarship, 1988.

Project MKULTRA, the CIA's Program of Research in Behavioral Modification, Joint Hearing Before the Select Committee on Intelligence and the Subcommittee on Health and Scientific Research of the Committee on Human Resources, United States Senate, 95th Congress, 1st Session, 3 August 1977, Washington, DC: U.S. Government Printing Office, 1977.

Quinones, Mark A., "Drug Abuse During the Civil War (1861–1865)," *International Journal of the Addiction*, 10:6, 1975: 1007–20.

Rabasa, Angel, Robert D. Blackwill, Peter Chalk, Kim Cragin, C. Christine Fair, Brian A. Jackson, Brian Michael Jenkins, Seth G. Jones, Nathaniel Shestak, and Ashley J. Tellis, *The Lessons of Mumbai*, Santa Monica, CA: RAND Corporation, 2009.

Rantanen, Miska, "History: Amphetamine Overdose in Heat of Combat," *Helsingin Sanomat, International Edition*, 26 May 2002, http://www2.hs.fi/english/archive/news.asp?id=20020528IE9.

Rasmussen, Nicolas, "America's First Amphetamine Epidemic 1929–1971," *American Journal of Public Health*, 98:6, June 2008: 974–85.

Rasmussen, Nicolas, *On Speed: The Many Lives of Amphetamine*, New York: New York University Press, 2008.

Reader, D. H., *Zulu Tribe in Transition: The Makhanya of Soutern Natal*, Manchester: Manchester University Press, 1966.

"Red Bull Drinks 'Fueling Syrian Islamists,'" *The Local*, 10 November 2014, http://www.thelocal.at/20141110/red-bull-fuelling-syrian-islamists.

Reese, Roger R., *Red Commanders. A Social History of the Soviet Army Officer Corps, 1918–1991*, Kansas: University Press of Kansas, 2005.

Reese, Roger R., *Soviet Military Experience: A History of the Soviet Army, 1917–1991*, London: Routledge, 2000.

Reese, Roger R., *Stalin's Reluctant Soldiers. A Social History of the Red Army, 1925–1941*, Kansas: University Press of Kansas, 1996.

Robins, Lee N. and Sergey Slobodyan, "Post-Vietnam Heroin Use and Injection by Returning U.S. Veterans: Clues to Preventing Injection Today," *Addiction*, 98:8, 2003: 1053–60.

Robins, Lee N., "Vietnam: Drug Use," in *Encyclopedia of Drugs, Alcohol, and Addictive Behavior*, September 16, 2001, http://www.encyclopedia.com/doc/1G2-3403100469.html.

Robins, Lee N., *The Vietnam Drug User Returns. Final Report*, Washington, DC: Special Action Office for Drug Abuse Prevention, 1974.

Robins, Lee, N., Darlene H. Davis, and David N. Nurco, "How Permanent Was Vietnam Drug Addiction?" *American Journal of Public Health*, 64, Supplement, 1974: 38–43.

Robinson, Rowan, *The Great Book of Hemp: the Complete Guide to the Environmental, Commercial, and Medicinal Uses of the World's Most Extraordinary Plant*, Rochester: Park Street Press, 1996.

Robson, Philip, *Forbidden Drugs*, Oxford: Oxford University Press, 1999.

Roehrs, Timothy, Eleni Burduvali, Alicia Bonahoom, Christopher Drake and Thomas Roth, "Ethanol and Sleep Loss: A 'Dose' Comparison of Impairing Effects," *Sleep*, 26:8, 2003: 981–85.

Ronell, Avital, *Crack Wars: Literature Addiction Mania*, Lincoln: University of Nebraska, 1992.

Roosevelt, Franklin Delano, "First Inaugural Address," 4 March 1933, Joint Congressional Committee on Inaugural Ceremonies, http://www.inaugural.senate.gov/swearing-in/address/address-by-franklin-d-roosevelt-1933.

Rosenthal, Franz, *The Herb: Hashish versus Medieval Muslim Society*, Leiden: E.J. Brill, 1971.

Rotter, Małgorzata, *"Musisz kierować się instynktem przetrwania," Analiza tożsamości weteranów wojny w Wietnamie*, unpublished MA thesis, Institute of American Studies and Polish Diaspora, Jagiellonian University, Krakow 2009 [*You Must Follow the Instinct of Self-preservation: Analyzing Identities of Vietnam War Veterans*].

Roug, Louise, "Witnesses Tell of Troop Stress before Attack," *Los Angeles Times*, 9 August 2006, http://articles.latimes.com/2006/aug/09/world/fg-iraq9.

Rudgley, Richard, *The Alchemy of Culture: Intoxicants in Society*, London: British Museum Press, 1993.

Russell, Thomas Wentworth, *Egyptian Service: 1902–1946*, London: J. Murray, 1949.

"Russia, Chemical Weapons," Federation of American Scientists, http://www.fas.org/nuke/guide/russia/cbw/cw.htm.

Ryn, Zdzisław Jan, *Medycyna indiańska*, [*Indian Medicine*], Kraków: Wydawnictwo Literackie, 2007.

Saikal, Amin, *Modern Afghanistan. A History of Struggle and Survival*, London: I.B. Tauris, 2004.

Sajer, Guy, *The Forgotten Soldier*, London: Cassell, 1999 (original publication 1971).

Sample, Ian, "Wired Awake," *The Guardian*, July 29, 2004, http://www.guardian.co.uk/education/2004/jul/29/research.highereducation.

Sandler, Stanley, *The Korean War: No Victors, No Vanquished*, London: Routledge, 1999.

Sarin, Oleg and Lev Dvoretsky, *The Afghan Syndrome: The Soviet Union's Vietnam*, Novato, CA: Presidio, 1993.

Satō, Akihiko, "Japan's Long Association with Amphetamines: What Can We Learn from Their Experiences?," in Richard Pates and Diane Riley (eds.), *Interventions for Amphetamine Misuse*, Oxford: Wiley–Blackwell, 2010: 147–58.

Satō, Akihiko, "Methamphetamine Use in Japan After the Second World War: Transformation of Narratives," *Contemporary Drug Problems*, 35:4, 2008: 717–46.

Saul, Stephanie, "Merck Cancels Work on a New Insomnia Medication," *New York Times*, 29 March 2007, http://www.nytimes.com/2007/03/29/business/29sleep.html?ref=health&_r=0.

Scarborough, John, "The Opium Poppy in Hellenistic and Roman Medicine," in Roy Porter and Mikuláš Teich (eds.), *Drugs and Narcotics in History*, Cambridge: Cambridge University Press, 1996: 4–23.

Schein, Edgar H., "Some Observations on Chinese Methods of Handling Prisoners of War," *The Public Opinion Quarterly*, 20:1, 1956: 321–7.

Schoenberger, Karl, "Japan Faces Widespread Drug Problems, Takes Harsh Measures Against Abusers," *The Wall Street Journal*, 9 December 1987: 34.

Schroeder-Lein, Glenna R., *The Encyclopedia of Civil War Medicine*, New York: M.E. Sharpe, 2008.

Schultz, Darlene and James Miller, *Fatigue and Use of Go/No Go Pills in F-16 Pilots Subjected to Extraordinary Long Combat Sorties*, Brooks City-Base, TX: U.S. Air Force Research Laboratory, Human Effectiveness Directorate, 2004.

Scott, Peter Dale, *The Road to 9/11: Wealth, Empire, and the Future of America*, Berkeley: University of California Press, 2008.

Sedlickas, Romanas and Knezys Stasys, *The War in Chechnya*, College Station, TX: Texas A&M University Press, 1999.

Seed, David, *Brainwashing: The Fictions of Mind Control: A Study of Novels and Films Since World War II*, Kent, OH: Kent State University Press, 2004.

Seely, Robert, *Russo-Chechen Conflict, 1800–2000: A Deadly Embrace*, London: Routledge, 2001.

Segal, Boris Moiseevich, *Russian Drinking: Use and Abuse of Alcohol in Pre-revolutionary Russia*, New Brunswick, NJ: Rutgers Center of Alcohol Studies, 1987.

Shay, Jonathan, *Achilles in Vietnam: Combat Trauma and the Undoing of Character*, New York: Scribner, 2003.

Shay, Jonathan, *Odysseus in America: Combat Trauma and the Trials of Homecoming*, New York: Scribner, 2002.

Shephard, Ben, *A War of Nerves: Soldiers and Psychiatrists in the Twentieth Century*, Cambridge, MA: Harvard University Press, 2003.

Shepler, Susan, "The Rites of the Child: Global Discourses of Youth and Reintegrating Child Soldiers in Sierra Leone," *Journal of Human Rights*, 4:2, 2005: 197–211.

Sherwin, Martin J., *A World Destroyed. The Atomic Bomb and the Grand Alliance*, New York: Vintage Books, 1977.

Sinclair, Andrew, *The Prohibition: The Era of Excess*, Boston: Little, Brown, 1962.

Singer, Peter Warren, "Caution: Children at War," *Parameters*, Winter 2001–02, http://www.carlisle.army.mil/usawc/Parameters/Articles/01winter/singer.htm.

Singer, Peter Warren, *Children at War*, Berkeley: University of California Press, 2006.

Singer, Peter Warren, "The Enablers of War: Casual Factors behind the Child Soldier Phenomenon," in Scott Gates and Simon Reich (eds.), *Child Soldiers in the Age of Fractured States*, Pittsburgh: University of Pittsburgh Press, 2010: 93–107.

Slawney, James, "Hallucinogenric Literature: Avital Ronell's Narcoanalysis," *Diacritics*, 24:4, 1994: 41–9.

Small Arms Survey 2005: Weapons and War, Small Arms Survey, Geneva: Graduate Institute of International Studies, 2007.

Smallman-Raynor, M.R. and A.D. Cliff, *War Epidemics. An Historical Geography of Infectious Diseases in Military Conflict and Civil Strife, 1850–2000*, Oxford: Oxford University Press, 2008.

Smith, Bryan, "Harry Schmidt's War," *Chicago Magazine*, April 2005, http://www.chicago-mag.com/Chicago-Magazine/April-2005/Harry-Schmidts-War.

Smith, David Livingston, *The Most Dangerous Animal: Human Nature and the Origins of War*, New York: St. Martin's Press, 2007.

"Soldier: 'Death Walk' Drives Troops 'Nuts,'" *CNN International*, 9 August 2006, http://edition.cnn.com/2006/WORLD/meast/08/08/iraq.mahmoudiya/index.html.

"Special Air Service (SAS)—Operation Barras—Sierra Leone," Elite UK Forces, http://www.eliteukforces.info/special-air-service/sas-operations/operation-barras.

Sroka, Artur, *Teologia narkotyku. O psychodelikach, szaleństwie, mistycznej paranoi i powrocie do Edenu*, Warszawa: Eneteia, 2008 [*Theology of Drugs. On Psychedelics, Madness, Mystical Insanity and Return to Eden*].

Stafford, Peter, *Psychodelic Encyclopedia*, Berkeley, CA: Ronin, 1992.

Stanley, Peter, "Army Temperance Association," in Jack S. Blocker, David M. Fahey, and Ian R. Tyrrell (eds.), *Alcohol and Temperance in Modern History: An International Encyclopedia*, Santa Barbara, CA: ABC-CLIO, 2003, vol. 1: 55–6.

Starkey, Gerald, "The Use and Abuse of Opiates and Amphetamines," in Patrick Healy and James Manak (eds.), *Drug Dependence and Abuse Resource Book*, Chicago: National District Attorney's Association, 1971: 482–4.

Steinkamp, Peter, "Pervitin (Methamphetamine) Tests, Use and Misuse in the German Wehrmacht," in Wolfgang Uwe Eckart (ed.), *Man, Medicine, and the State: The Human Body as an Object of Government Sponsored Medical Research in the 20th Century*, Stuttgart: Franz Steiner Verlag, 2006: 61–72.

Stephenson, Neal, *Cryptonomicon*, New York: Avon Press, 1999.

Stewart, Scott, "Hezbollah Radical, but Rational," *Stratfor Global Intelligence Security Weekly Report*, 12 August 2010, http://www.stratfor.com/weekly/20100811_hezbollah_radical_rational.

Stivalet, Philippe, Dominique Esquivié, Pierre-Alain Barraud, Daniel Leifflen, and Christian Raphel, "Effects of Modafinil on Attentional Process during 60 Hours of Sleep Deprivation," *Human Psychopharmacology*, 13:7, 1998: 501–7.

Streatfeild, Dominic, "My Deal with Old King Coke," *The Observer*, 20 May 2001, http://www.theguardian.com/film/2001/may/20/features.

Streatfeild, Dominic, *Brainwash: The Secret History of Mind Control*, New York: Thomas Dunne Books, 2007.

Streatfeild, Dominic, *Cocaine*, London: Virgin, 2002.

Su, Edward, "Merck Plans to File Its Novel Sleeping Pill Suvorexant with FDA," *Pharmatropics*, 8 February 2012, http://www.pharmatopics.com/2012/02/merck-plans-to-file-its-novel-sleeping-pill-suvorexant-with-fda.

Substance Use Disorders in the U.S. Armed Forces, Washington, DC: Institute of Medicine, National Academies Press, 2012.

Sullivan, John P., "Child Soldiers: Despair, Barbarization, and Conflict," *Air & Space Power Journal* (Spanish Edition), March 2008, http://www.airpower.maxwell.af.mil/apjinternational/apj-s/2008/1tri08/sullivaneng.htm.

Summary of Major Events and Problems. United States Army Chemical Corps. Fiscal Year 1956, Chemical Corps Historical Office, November 1956, https://www.osti.gov/opennet/servlets/purl/16006842-VXqarW/16006842.pdf.

Sun Pin, *Military Methods* in Sun Tzu and Sun Pin, *The Complete Art of War* (trans. Ralph D. Sawyer), Boulder, CO: Westview Press, 1996.

Sun Tzu, *The Art of War* (trans. Samuel B. Griffith), Oxford: Oxford University Press, 1971.

Szasz, Thomas, *Ceremonial Chemistry: The Ritual Persecution of Drugs, Addicts, and Pushers*, London: Routledge & Kegan Paul, 1974.

Szasz, Thomas, *The Myth of Mental Illness: Foundations of a Theory of Personal Conduct*, New York: Hoeber–Harper, 1961.

Tanielian, Terri and Lisa H. Jaycox (eds.), *Invisible Wounds of War: Psychological and Cognitive Injuries, Their Consequences, and Services to Assist Recovery*, Santa Monica: RAND Corporation, 2008, http://www.rand.org/pubs/monographs/2008/RAND_MG720.pdf.

Taylor, Bernard J., "Post-Traumatic Stress Disorder (PTSD)," in Spencer C. Tucker (ed.), *Encyclopedia of the Vietnam War. A Political, Social and Military History*, Santa Barbara, CA: ABC-CLIO, 1998, vol. 2: 582.

Taylor, Frederick Winslow, *The Principles of Scientific Management*, New York: Harper & Brothers, 1911.

Teachman, Jay, Carter Anderson and Lucky M. Tedrow, "Military Service and Alcohol Use in the United States," *Armed Forces and Society*, vol. 41, no. 3, 2014.

Terry, Charles Edward and Mildred Pellens, *The Opium Problem*, Montclair, NJ: Patterson Smith, 1970 (original publication 1928).

Tether, Anthony, "Statement Submitted to the Subcommittee on Military Research and Development Committee on Armed Services," U.S. House of Representatives,

Washington, DC, 26 June 2001, http://www.darpa.mil/WorkArea/DownloadAsset. aspx?id=1781.

"The Drug of ISIS and Al-Nusra: Captagon," *ANF News*, 24 May 2015, http://anfenglish.com/news/the-drug-of-isis-and-al-nusra-captagon.

The Works of Tacitus: In Four Volumes. To Which are Prefixed, Political Discourses upon That Author by Thomas Gordon, London: T. Woodward and J. Peele, 1737, vol. 4, *A Treatise of the Situation, Customs and People of Germany*, http://oll.libertyfund.org/simple. php?id=787.

Tien, Chen-Ya, *Chinese Military Theory. Ancient and Modern*, Oakville: Mosaic Press 1992.

Tishkov, Valerii Aleksandrovich, *Chechnya: Life in a War-Torn Society*, Berkeley: University of California Press, 2004.

Toffler, Alvin and Heidi Toffler, *War and Anti-War*, New York: Little, Brown, 1993.

Tolstoy, Leo, *War and Peace* (trans. Andrew Bromfield), London: Harper Perennial, 2007.

Toussaint-Samat, Maguelonne, *A History of Food* (trans. Anthea Bell), Chichester: Wiley-Blackwell, 2009.

Trebach, Arnold S., *Fatal Distraction: The War on Drugs in the Age of Islamic Terror*, Bloomington, IN: Unlimited, 2006.

Trevor-Roper, Hugh, *The Last Days of Hitler*, Chicago: University of Chicago Press, 1992.

Tritle, Lawrence, *From Melos to My Lai. War and Survival*, London: Routledge, 2000.

Trotter, William R., *A Frozen Hell: The Russo-Finish Winter War of 1939–1940*, Chapel Hill: Algonquin Books of Chapel Hill, 1991.

Tsur, Semyon, "Nazis Attempted to Make Robots of Their Soldiers," *Pravda*, 14 February 2003, http://english.pravda.ru/science/tech/14-02-2003/1872-nazi-0.

"Two Tons of IS Drugs, Including Captagon, Seized in Western Syria, NATO Connection," Focus Information Agency, 25 May 2015, http://bignews2day.com/en/news/raskryt-sekret-zhivotnoj-svireposti-islamistov----eto-tabletka-uzhasa.

"U.S. Air Force Verdict," *CBC News Online*, 6 July 2004, http://www.cbc.ca/news2/background/friendlyfire/verdict.html.

U.S. Army "Prohibition," 1890–1953, Schaffer Library of Drug Policy, http://druglibrary.org/schaffer/alcohol/prohibit.htm.

"U.S. Boy, 14, Sentenced in Mexico for Cartel Killings," MSNBC, 26 July 2011, http://www.msnbc.msn.com/id/43900421/ns/world_news-americas/t/us-boy-sentenced-mexico-cartel-killings.

"U.S. Chemical Weapons Stockpile Information Declassified," *News Release*, U.S. Department of Defense, Office of the Assistant Secretary of Defense (Public Affairs), 24 January 1996, http://www.defense.gov/releases/release.aspx?releaseid=729.

"U.S. Soldiers Implicated in Italian Steroid Bust," *Australian Broadcasting Corporation News*, 17 July 2005, http://www.abc.net.au/news/2005-07-17/us-soldiers-implicated-in-italian-steroidbust/2060024.

Ulrich, Andreas, "The Nazi Death Machine. Hitler's Drugged Soldier," *Spiegel Online International*, 6 May 2005, http://www.spiegel.de/international/the-nazi-death-machine-hitler-s-drugged-soldiers-a-354606.html.

Unterhalter, Elaine, "Confronting Imperialism: The People of Nquthu and the Invasion of Zululand," in Andrew Duminy and Charles Ballard (eds.), *The Anglo-Zulu War. New Perspectives*, Pietermaritzburg: University of Natal Press, 1981: 98–119.

Urban, Mark, *War in Afghanistan*, London: Macmillan Press, 1988.

Utas, Mats and Magnus Jörgel, "The West Side Boys: Military Navigation in the Sierra Leone Civil War," *Journal of Modern African Studies*, 46:3, 2008: 487–511.

Van Creveld, Martin, *The Changing Face of War: Combat from the Marne to Iraq*, New York: Ballantine Books, 2008.

Van Creveld, Martin, *The Transformation of War*, London: Free Press, 1991.

Vasagar, Jeevan, "Nazis Tested Cocaine on Camp Inmates," *The Guardian*, 19 September 2002, http://www.guardian.co.uk/world/2002/nov/19/research.germany.

Vaughn, Michael S., Frank F.Y. Huang and Christine Rose Ramirez, "Drug Abuse and Anti-Drug Policy in Japan. Past History and Future Directions," *British Journal of Criminology*, 35:4, 1995: 491–524.

Vautravers, Alexandre J., "Why Child Soldiers Are Such a Complex Issue," *Refugee Survey Quarterly*, 27:4, 2009: 96–107.

Vespucci, Amerigo, *Letters of Amerigo Vespucci and Other Documents Illustrative of His Career*, London: Hakluyt Society, 1894.

Victims, Perpetrators or Heroes? Child Soldiers Before the International Criminal Court, London: Redress Trust, 2006.

Virilio, Paul, *Speed and Politics* (trans. Mark Polizzotti), Los Angeles: Semiotext(e), 2006 (original publication 1977).

Volkow, Nora D., Joanna S. Fowler, Jean Logan, David Alexoff, Wei Zhu, Frank Telang, Gene-Jack Wang, Millard Jayne, Jacob M. Hooker, Christopher Wong, Barbara Hubbard, Pauline Carter, Donald Warner, Payton King, Colleen Shea, Youwen Xu, Lisa Muench, and Karen Apelskog-Torres, "Effects of Modafinil on Dopamine and Dopamine Transporters in the Male Human Brain," *JAMA. Journal of the American Medical Association*, 301:11, 2009: 1148–54.

Von Zeilbauer, Paul, "For U.S. Troops at War, Liquor Is Spur to Crime, *New York Times*, March 13, 2007, http://www.nytimes.com/2007/03/13/world/middleeast/13alcohol.html?pagewanted=print.

Vonnegut, Kurt, *Fates Worse Than Death*, New York: Berkley Books, 1992.

Wade, Owen, "The Treatment of a Dictator," *Journal of Medical Biography*, 11:2, 2003: 118–22.

Wakabayashi, Bob Tadashi, "From Peril to Profit: Opium in Late-Edo to Meiji Eyes," in Timothy Brook and Bob Tadashi Wakabayashi (eds.), *Opium Regimes: China, Britain and Japan, 1839–1952*, Berkeley: University of California Press, 2000: 55–75.

Waldorf, Dan, Martin Orlick, and Craig Reinarman, *Morphine Maintenance: The Shreveport Clinic 1919–1923*, Washington, DC: Drug Abuse Council, 1974.

Walton, Stuart, *Out of It. A Cultural History of Intoxication*, London: Hamish Hamilton, 2001.

Walzer, Michael, *Just and Unjust Wars. A Moral Argument with Historical Illustrations*, New York: Basic Books, 2000 (original publication 1977).

Wasson, Valentina Pavlovna and R. Gordon Wasson, *Mushrooms, Russia and History*, 2 vols. Pantheon Books: New York, 1957.

Watson, Brent Byron, *Far Eastern Tour: The Canadian Infantry in Korea, 1950–1953*, Montreal: McGill–Queen's University Press, 2002.

Watson, Ivan, "'They Would Torture You': ISIS Prisoners Reveal Life Inside Terror Group," CNN, 28 October 2014, http://edition.cnn.com/2014/10/28/world/meast/syria-isis-prisoners-watson.

Webb, James, *Fields of Fire*, New York: Bantam Books, 2001 (original publication 1978).

Weil, Andrew, *The Natural Mind. A New Way of Looking at Drugs and the Higher Consciousness*, Boston: Houghton Mifflin, 1972.

Weil, Simone, *The Iliad or Poem of Force*, Wallingford, PA: Pendle Hill, 1956.

Weimer, Daniel, "Drugs-as-a-Disease: Heroin, Metaphors, and Identity in Nixon's Drug War," *Janus Head*, 6:2, 2003: 260–81.

Weld, Stanley B., "A Connecticut Surgeon in the Civil War: The Reminiscences of Dr. Nathan Mayer," *Journal of the History of Medicine and Allied Sciences*, 18:3, 1964: 272–86.

Wessells, Michael, "Child Soldiers," *Bulletin of the Atomic Scientists*, 53:6, 1997: 32–9.

Wessells, Michael, *Child Soldiers: From Violence to Protection*, Cambridge, MA: Harvard University Press, 2006.

Wessells, Michael, "Child Soldiers, Peace Education, and Postconflict Reconstruction for Peace," *Theory Into Practice*, 44:4, 2005: 363–9.

Westcott, Kelli, "Modafinil, Sleep Deprivation, and Cognitive Function in Military and Medical Settings," *Military Medicine*, 170:4, 2005: 333–5.

Whitaker, Ben, *Global Connection: The Crisis of Drug Addiction*, London: Jonathan Cape, 1987.

White, Stephen, *Russia Goes Dry. Alcohol, State and Society*, Cambridge: Cambridge University Press, 1996.

Whitman, Walt, "Specimen Days" (1882), in Michael Warner (ed.), *The Portable Walt Whitman*, London: Penguin Books, 2004.

Williams, Ian, *Rum: A Social and Sociable History of the Real Spirit of 1776*, New York: Nation Books, 2005.

Williams, Phil and Vanda Felbab-Brown, *Drug Trafficking, Violence, and Instability*, Carlisle Barracks: Strategic Studies Institute, U.S. Army War College, 2012.

Williamson, Ann, Anne-Marie Feyer, Richard Mattick, Rena Friswell, and Samantha Finalay-Brown, "Developing Measures of Fatigue Using an Alcohol Comparison to Validate the Effects of Fatigue on Performance," *Accident Analysis and Prevention*, 33:3, 2001: 313–26.

Wilson, George B., *Alcohol and the Nation. A Contribution to the Study of the Liquor Problem in the United Kingdom from 1800 to 1935*, London: Nicholson and Watson Limited, 1940.

Wojtczak-Jaroszowa, Jadwiga and Dorota Jarosz, "Time-Related Distribution of Occupational Accidents," *Journal of Safety Research*, 18:1, 1987: 33–41.

Wolff, Leon, *Little Brown Brother. How the United States Purchased and Pacified the Philippine Islands at the Century's Turn*, Garden City, NY: Doubleday, 1961.

Wong, J.Y., *Deadly Dreams. Opium, Imperialism, and the Arrow War (1856–1860) in China*, Cambridge: Cambridge University Press, 1998.

Woods, Arthur, *Dangerous Drugs: The World Fight Against Illicit Traffic in Narcotics*, New Haven: Yale University Press, 1931.

"World Armies Still Use Psychotropic Drugs to Make Fearless Machines of Their Soldiers," *Pravda*, 18 November 2008, http://english.pravda.ru/world/europe/18-11-2008/106714-psychotropic-0.

"World Population Prospects: The 2006 Revision," UN Department of Economic and Social Affairs, Population Division, 2006, http://www.un.org/esa/population/publications/wpp2006/wpp2006.htm.

Wubben, Harold H., "American Prisoners of War in Korea: A Second Look at the 'Something New in History,'" *American Quarterly*, 22:1, 1970: 3–19.

Ylikangas, Mikko, *Unileipää, kuolonvettä, spiidiä. Huumeet Suomessa 1800–1950* [*Opium, Death's Tincture, Speed. Drugs in Finland 1800–1950*], Jyväskylä: Atena, 2009

Yokoyama, Minoru, "Japan: Changing Drugs Laws: Keeping Pace with the Problem," *Criminal Justice International*, 8:5, 1992: 11–8.

Yorke, Edmund, "Isandlwana 1879: Dividing Your Forces," in John Pimlott (ed.), *The Hutchinson Atlas of Battle Plans: Before and After*, London: Taylor & Francis, 1999: 165–76.

Zheng, Yangwen, "The Social Life of Opium in China, 1483–1999," *Modern Asian Studies*, 37:1, 2003: 1–39.

Zheng, Yangwen, *The Social Life of Opium in China*, Cambridge: Cambridge University Press, 2005.

Znaniecki, Florian, "The Object-Matter of Sociology," *American Journal of Sociology*, 32:4, 1927: 529–84.

Zoroya, Gregg, "Alcohol Abuse by GIs Soars since 2003," *USA Today*, 19 May 2009, 1a, http://www.usatoday.com/news/military/2009-06-18-army-alcohol-problems_N.htm.

Zoroya, Gregg, "Alcohol Abuse Weighs on Army," *USA Today*, 10 February 2010, 1a, http://www.usatoday.com/news/military/2010-02-09-treatment-army-alcohol_N.htm.

INDEX

Abel, Rudolf, 156
Abu Sayyaf Group, 238
Achilles, 42–43
Acosta, José de, 47
addiction, definition of, xix–xxi
adrafinil, 277
Afghanistan
  child soldiers in, 251
  opium production and consumption in,
    223–24, 230, 238
  See also Operation Enduring Freedom—
    Afghanistan (OEF-A); Soviet–Afghan
    War (1979–1989)
Afghantsi, 226–27
Afridi, Muhammad Abid, 238
"Agent Buzz" (BZ), 165, 178–180, 183
Agincourt, battle of (1415), 8
Aguinaldo, Emilio, 188
Ahhayev, Imran, 26
Alam-ad-din Ibn Shukr, 52
Albert the Great (Albertus Magnus), 38
alcohol
  addiction and, xix
  American Civil War and, 10, 72, 77
  American military and, 27–28, 284
  British military and, 8–11, 18–19,
    22, 26
  in Finland, 132
  First World War and, 14–21
  Islam and, 51–52
  Napoleonic wars and, 8, 12, 51, 52–53
  Nazis and, 105
  opium and, 32–33
  popularization of, 292
  posttraumatic stress disorder and, 77
  prohibition and, 14–18
  from religious purposes to hedonistic
    use, 297–98

roles in war of, 5–8
Russian military and, 11–16, 23, 26–27,
  140–41, 223
Second World War and, 21–24
Vietnam War and, 25–26, 191–92
Aleksei Aleksandrovich, Grand Duke of
  Russia, 14
Algeria, 56–57, 292
Ali, Ilyas, 238
Alice's Adventures in Wonderland
  (Carroll), 44–45
Allen, H. Warner, 11
Alles, Gordon, 104
Allyn, Daniel B., 265
Al Qaeda, 238, 259–260
Alsop, Stewart, 211
Amanita muscaria (fly agaric), 38–41,
  44–45, 86
Amanita pantherina, 41, 45
Ambien (zolpidem), 272, 281
American aloe (*maguey*), 8
American Civil War (1861–1865)
  alcohol and, 10, 72, 77
  anesthesia in, 72–74
  child soldiers in, 244
  infectious diseases and epidemics
    in, 74–75
  opium and morphine in, 71–73, 75,
    77–82, 292
  posttraumatic stress disorder
    and, 4, 76–77
  soldiers' disease and, 78–82, 294
American Pharmaceutical Association
  (APhA), 188
American Psychiatric Association (APA), 4
American War of Independence (1775–1783),
  9–10, 68
amobarbital, 202

367

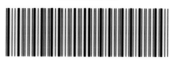